THE
HERBAL DOG

"Rita Hogan readily acknowledges the advances that veterinary medicine has made in diagnostics, surgery, and emergency medicine, but she applies the principles of holistic herbalism with the caveat that the one-size-fits-all approach of modern medicine sometimes overlooks things like environment, stressors, diet, and other factors. . . . The author's calm narrative tone is both inviting and strategic. Her approach will likely help to calm the suspicions of readers who feel that only a fanatic would recommend aloe vera and burdock root instead of an ultrasound scan for a dog's painful abdomen. Even if skeptical readers don't come away completely convinced, they'll be enormously educated—Hogan imparts a huge amount of biological information about dogs, and does it all with an easy readability that will make quite a bit of it stick. *The Herbal Dog* is an informative and sometimes eye-opening examination of natural remedies for helping your dog."

KIRKUS REVIEWS

"*The Herbal Dog* takes the reader far into the realm of true holistic healing, where the underlying causes of what ails millions of companion dogs must be addressed from a perspective that recognizes true wellness as something that cannot occur unless we accept each and every dog as a unique being with a unique set of needs and nuances. Rita expertly and eloquently explains the effective uses of dozens of herbal medicines, and she does so from a deep understanding of the natural system they represent. She accurately conveys that the greatest healing powers of plants do not come from exploitation of a few phytochemicals that science deems useful, but from understanding the natural system of wellness that nature has instilled in all living beings."

GREGORY TILFORD, HERBALIST AND COAUTHOR OF
HERBS FOR PETS: THE NATURAL WAY TO ENHANCE YOUR PET'S LIFE

"Rita Hogan has an incredible understanding of herbal medicine, and I have heard many accolades from clients who have consulted with her on difficult cases. She has an excellent ability to break down the science of herbal therapy into easy-to-understand information."

JUDY MORGAN, DVM, CVA, CVCP, CVFT, HOLISTIC VETERINARIAN,
AND AUTHOR OF *RAISING NATURALLY HEALTHY PETS*

"What a useful and comprehensive guide to herbal remedies for dogs. An insightful naturalist, Rita Hogan has a profound understanding of our connection to the natural world. *The Herbal Dog* is a carefully crafted manual filled with a new perspective on using herbs that pet parents and herbal practitioners alike will find applicable. I'm grateful for Rita's dedication and attention to detail. I know this book will soon be a well-worn treasure on and off my bookshelf!"

BARBARA ROYAL, INTEGRATIVE VETERINARIAN,
AUTHOR, PET FOOD FORMULATOR, AND EDUCATOR

"*The Herbal Dog* by renowned herbalist Rita Hogan brings the power of plants to life, highlighting their remarkable benefits for canine health. This book has become a staple resource in my home and office, helping me provide elevated support for both my patients and my own dogs. Rita's herbal wisdom shines through on every page, reminding us that everything is interconnected, that every dog (and human) is unique, and that holistic herbalism can be used to heal the root causes of ailments for lasting wellness. This book will revolutionize the standards of care for dogs, and I'm a better veterinarian for having read it."

LYNDA LOUDON, INTEGRATIVE EMERGENCY VETERINARIAN,
FOUNDER AND PRESIDENT OF HEALING HAVEN ANIMAL FOUNDATION

"*The Herbal Dog* is a treasure trove of holistic insights to help you deepen your connection to the wisdom and medicine of the plant kingdom. Packed with practical information and guidance, it empowers you to take charge of your dog's well-being. A must-read for anyone committed to natural pet care!"

ODETTE SUTER, DVM, HOLISTIC VETERINARIAN, LECTURER,
AND AUTHOR OF *WHAT YOUR VET NEVER TOLD YOU*

"The entire dog wellness community will be elated with this comprehensive resource that provides extensive plant monographs, herbal applications, and practical protocols for dozens of conditions, including the most common ailments affecting our canine companions. *The Herbal Dog* is a welcome, wonderful resource for guardians who want to use plants as wise medicine."

KAREN SHAW BECKER, DVM, AND RODNEY HABIB,
AUTHORS OF *THE FOREVER DOG* AND *THE FOREVER DOG LIFE*

THE
HERBAL DOG

Holistic Canine Herbalism
Applications and Practice

A Sacred Planet Book

RITA HOGAN, C.H.

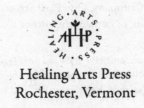

Healing Arts Press
Rochester, Vermont

Healing Arts Press
One Park Street
Rochester, Vermont 05767
www.HealingArtsPress.com

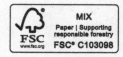

Healing Arts Press is a division of Inner Traditions International

Sacred Planet Books are curated by Richard Grossinger, Inner Traditions editorial board member and cofounder and former publisher of North Atlantic Books. The Sacred Planet collection, published under the umbrella of the Inner Traditions family of imprints, includes works on the themes of consciousness, cosmology, alternative medicine, dreams, climate, permaculture, alchemy, shamanic studies, oracles, astrology, crystals, hyperobjects, locutions, and subtle bodies.

Note to the reader: This book is intended to be an informational guide. The remedies, approaches, and techniques described herein are meant to supplement, and not to be a substitute for, professional veterinary care or treatment. They should not be used to treat a serious ailment without prior consultation with a qualified veterinarian.

Cataloging-in-Publication Data for this title is available from the Library of Congress

ISBN 978-1-64411-959-4 (print)
ISBN 978-1-64411-960-0 (ebook)

Printed and bound in the United States by Lake Book Manufacturing, LLC

10   9   8   7   6   5   4   3

Text design and layout by Kenleigh Manseau
This book was typeset in Garamond Premier Pro with Elmhurst, Frutiger LT Std, Gill Sans MT Pro, and Rig Sans used as display typefaces
Anatomical illustrations on pages 56, 69, 72, 81, and 207 by Catherine Fraisse
Graphic on Contents page is designed by rawpixel.com / Freepik

To send correspondence to the author of this book, mail a first-class letter to the author c/o Inner Traditions • Bear & Company, One Park Street, Rochester, VT 05767, and we will forward the communication, or contact the author directly at **TheHerbalDog.com**.

To my pug Francis,
one of the best friends I've ever had

Contents

PART ONE
· · · · · · · · · · · · ·

Dogs and Plants Are Individuals

1 ⚕ Holistic Canine Herbalism   4

2 ⚕ Food as Medicine   20

PART TWO
. . . .
Herbal Practicum

8 ⚹ Plant and Fungi Monographs   235

Herbs 235

Agrimony, Alfalfa, Aloe, Angelica, Artichoke, Ashwagandha, Astragalus, Bee Balm, Blackberry, Burdock, Calendula, Cayenne, Chamomile, Chickweed, Cleavers, Couch Grass, Dandelion, Echinacea, Elecampane, Fennel, Ginger, Goldenrod, Goldenseal, Gotu Kola, Gravel Root, Hawthorn, Juniper Berry, Lemon Balm, Licorice, Marshmallow, Meadowsweet, Milk Thistle, Milky Oats, Mullein, Nettle, Olive, Oregon Grape Root, Parsley, Passionflower, Pau d'Arco, Plantain, Red Clover, Rose, Rosemary, Skullcap, Slippery Elm, Solomon's Seal, St. John's Wort, Turmeric, Usnea, Uva-Ursi, Violet, Wood Betony, Yarrow, Yellow Dock

Medicinal Mushrooms 329

Chaga, Cordyceps, Lion's Mane, Maitake, Poria, Reishi, Tremella, Turkey Tail

Phytoembryonics 342

Beech, Black Currant, Bramble, Cowberry, Fig, Heather, Horsetail, Mountain Pine, Olive, Walnut, Willow

Flower Essences 354

Agrimony, Aspen, Beech, Bleeding Heart, Boneset, Borage, Bougainvillea, Centaury, Comfrey, Crab Apple, Easter Lily, Fireweed, Gorse, Impatiens, Mimulus, Nasturtium, Oak, Olive, Pine, Red Chestnut, Rescue Remedy, Rock Rose, Star of Bethlehem, Tomato, Vervain, Vine, Walnut, White Chestnut

Appendices

1 ⚹ Herbal Actions   357

2 ⚹ Herbal Constituents   367

3 ⚹ Vitamins and Minerals   370

Foreword

Isla Fishburn, Ph.D.

Nature serves as a reflection of what is happening within. We are in an ecosystem crisis; our planet, ourselves, and our animal friends. Nature is speaking, and we must hear her call and, once again, move toward our ancient roots of connection through our plant allies. As a zoologist and conservation biologist, I'm familiar with Mother Earth and all of the animals that share this planet with us. Through my work with canine wellness and shamanism, I'm able to connect these two worlds and bridge the gap between humans and nature.

Through explorations of the ways of connection, integrated ecosystems, and animal health, openings are beginning to surface on how we can experience and support the interconnectedness of all life. One pathway through which we can all experience our symbiotic dependence is our internal terrain. How healthy are we inside? How resilient is our inner ecosystem to negative outside forces? When we take care of the internal workings of our own ecosystem, the external reflects that work and we thrive.

Rita's knowledge of how to support resiliency continues to evolve and allow for the understanding that our animal friends are individuals, just like all of us. Her constant statement that "dogs are individuals" helps us all remember that dogs, like people, should be treated as such.

In my own work, I was able to study both wolves and domesticated dogs. Looking at study after study in my research, I found that they were all based on the foundation that a dog is a dog. There was little consideration of individuality or of the differing levels of internal health and emotional complexity of each animal, let alone the quality of their diet and environmental stressors. Acceptance of the idea that animals are "one size fits all" is limited, unhelpful, and entirely unstable, especially when decisions are being made based on this limited-scope research methodology.

We have almost forgotten that animals are each themselves a complex ecosystem of interconnected living systems and energy flow. *The Herbal Dog* reintroduces us to the concept of individual medicine, ecosystem health, and terrain resilience. Rita considers not only your dog's ecosystem but the reflection of your own individuality and health.

I met Rita when she interviewed me about how I connect and practice intuitive plant medicine through my work with essential oils and hydrosols. Rita's connection, knowledge, friendship, expertise, dedication, and love for our plant friends is infectious to witness and inspiring to learn. It takes you to a completely higher and more expansive level of understanding. After my interview with Rita, we realized that even though our paths are different, we shared a common love for plants, their teachings, and the intricate relationship between nature, ourselves, and our animal friends.

The health of an individual ecosystem includes the emotional, physical, and spiritual connection to nature, nutrition, and wellness. Since most of us share continual space with our pets, our entire environmental picture needs to be considered, focusing on the cause of disease instead of solely the symptoms. Vibration is the key to health, and when we focus on the symptoms, it causes us to worry and obsess about our beloved pets.

Rita has created a unique and much-needed guide to knowing and supporting your dog as an individual through herbs. She also gives you the basic knowledge you need to understand your dog as an ecosystem. *The Herbal Dog* takes you on a different journey of individuality and root causes within the context of individual plants, energetics, and suggestions for health and resiliency. It will help deepen your relationship with nature and help you get to know your dog through observation and reflection.

A saying goes, "Animals do speak, but only to those who know how to listen." I'd say this is true for all we are a part of, including plants. They are speaking, calling to us, and offering their medicine. Rita helps us speak their language so we can utilize their medicine more effectively and intuitively. She says there is an herbalist in all of us, and I couldn't agree more.

ISLA FISHBURN, PH.D., has a bachelor's of science degree in zoology and master's and doctoral degrees in conservation biology. She is the founder and owner of Kachina Canine, a center focused on supporting canine health, wellness, and longevity through plant intuition and shamanism. Isla is passionate about ecosystem health and works to promote the human connection with nature and animals through ritual, workshops, courses, energetics, and plant therapies.

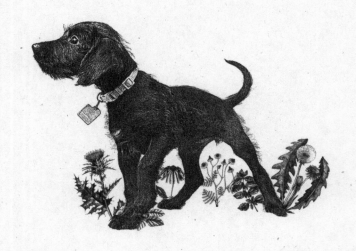

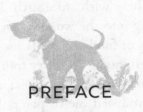

PREFACE
My Herbal Beginnings

A Dog's Prayer: *I pray you who own me, let me continue to live close to Nature. Know that: I love to run beneath the sun, the moon, and the stars; I need to feel the storm winds around me and the touch of rain, hail, sleet, and snow; I need to splash in streams and brooks and to swim in ponds, lakes, and rivers; I need to be allowed to retain my kinship with Nature.*

JULIETTE DE BAIRACLI LEVY,
*THE COMPLETE HERBAL HANDBOOK
FOR FARM AND STABLE*

When I was growing up in rural Michigan in the early 1970s, I spent most of my time outside with my best friend, Cathy, on my horse or hanging out with my dog Susie. We would play in the water of the roadside stream, hang from the trees in the apple orchard, and explore the pine woods.

When I was around seven or eight, I saw my first lady's slipper (*Cypripedium arietinum*). It was magical. I sat there gazing at it like it was a faerie. Though I wanted to pick it for my mother, she had taught me that lady slippers were rare and had a bigger purpose than her love for beautiful flowers.

My maternal grandmother was an "unknowing" herbalist. She never considered herself a healer; herbalism was simply a way of life for low-income families. She raised sixteen children during the Great Depression with only a midwife to help with childbirth. I love my mother's stories of my grandmother going into the woods with her basket and returning hours later with a bounty of food and medicine.

In the time of my childhood, "country folk" knew the plants around them—which ones to avoid, which ones to eat, and which ones to use for medicine. My father introduced me to plants by gardening and by caring for our cows, chickens, horses, and pigs. Describing them by color and shape, he would tell me to go out into the field, pick a particular plant, and bring it back to him. My dad loved his garden and grew beautiful vegetables without pesticides or herbicides, using the principles of companion planting. I would kneel beside him, asking if every plant was a weed and if I could pick it.

We had many dogs growing up, but the one I remember best is Susie. She was a shepherd-collie mix. My dad loved her and ensured she was well cared for. Susie was intact (unspayed) and only minimally vaccinated, and she ate a varied diet of raw milk, butter, eggs, and table and meat scraps, including organ meat. She would nibble on grass, berries, apple peels, and self-selected plants. I know this sounds fancy now, a raw-food proponent's dream, but back then it was just how you fed your dog when you lived in the country.

Susie loved the outdoors like I did; she stayed outside except when it was raining or cold. My dad let her choose at night, leaving the garage door ajar so she could sleep inside if she wanted. Susie died when she was twenty-four. That is a long time to live, for a dog, and in my memory it wasn't all that uncommon back then. My adult self wishes I had paid more attention to the details of her upbringing, but I was a busy kid and didn't know that I would be knee-deep in the all-natural dog world when I grew up.

Eventually I left home and settled in Minneapolis, Minnesota, where I embraced my twenties and expanded my consciousness. In college, I studied Eastern religions, anthropology, feminism, and an Eastern herbal medicine practice called ayurveda. My favorite book on the subject was *A Life of Balance* by Maya Tiwari. I loved how ayurveda looked at the body as an individual, and instead of seeking outside yourself for answers, you were taught to look within. This started me on the path of introspection, learning about the importance of diet and working on my emotional and spiritual self. Eventually, I fell in love, got my first pug, and reluctantly moved south.

My partner and I bought a thirty-two-acre hilly parcel in the unincorporated town of Elmwood, Tennessee, about an hour east of Nashville, at the end of a dead-end road. What I loved about our "farm" was that it was mostly a deciduous forest where the dogs and I could walk around, sit in silence, and commune with the flora and fauna, which included beech, elm, and many of the plant friends I learned about when I was young.

In my late twenties, I realized that I didn't want to pursue Eastern medicine even though I loved it; I missed the plants I had grown up with. Our new farm helped me reconnect to the land and my love for animals. We decided to board dogs for a living and opened Almost Home Pet Farm, a kennel-free boarding facility on five acres surrounding our home.

I started noticing straight away the declining health of the dogs we boarded and making the connection to their poor diet of cheap kibble and pills. Luckily, I befriended a brilliant woman who owned an all-natural dog food store in the city. She helped educate me on alternative diets for dogs, the kibble hierarchy, raw food, home-cooked food, and healthy treats.

After finding out about the excellent dog food options available in the Nashville area (where most of our clients came from), I implemented a dietary requirement for dogs that wanted to board with me. This included a pre-boarding interview where I would ask potential clients what types of food they were feeding their dog, gently educate them on the power of a better diet, and then give them a list of acceptable foods. Then I would send them to my friend's store to get food from my list. This might sound drastic, but it resulted in calmer, healthier dogs. It wasn't long before clients were calling me to tell me how improved their dogs were after just a few months of their new diet.

During the early years of Almost Home Pet Farm, a friend and I started a holistic pug rescue organization called Music City Pug Rescue. We were one of the first holistic dog rescues in the country, and we found homes for hundreds of pugs over six years. Doing this type of work taught me so much about dog behavior, the roots of disease, the importance of the nervous system, and the pitfalls of allopathic veterinary care.

Blending rescue and kennel-free boarding was a blessing that allowed me to study herbalism and work with sick dogs and clients desperate for answers. I started putting health puzzles together and seeing the difference diet and herbs could make. Behind the scenes, I started making my own herbal medicines and founded a company called Farm Dog Naturals to sell them.

Around 2005, *The Complete Herbal Handbook for the Dog and Cat* by Juliette de Bairacli Levy found me. Juliette was an English herbalist, skilled animal herbalist, and pioneer of holistic medicine. Reading her book was one of the many transformational moments that guided me toward my practice as a canine herbalist. I learned that I wasn't alone in my thinking. Juliette's bravery in speaking her truth for the world to hear filled me with joy, giving me hope and courage for my own experience.

I began looking for other dog-related health books. I immediately noticed that the idea of individualized care was missing from the field, and plant language was obsolete. I pivoted and focused on herbalism and the plants I knew and loved. Up until this point, the herbalism books I read were general. They taught me to make tinctures, salves, oils, poultices, and infusions. I appreciated the guidance, but something was missing.

One morning, I visited Rhino Used Books in Nashville and found herbalist Matthew Wood's first book, *Seven Herbs: Plants as Teachers*. I had doubted my use of drop dosing with dogs because I kept seeing that books and herbal product labels recommended using large amounts of tinctures. I believed in letting the body speak for itself if higher dosages were warranted. Matthew talked about using "spirit dosages," or very low dosages of a tincture, to stimulate the body to heal itself and, in essence, using plant intelligence. For the first time, I felt validated on my plant path.

Shortly after, a second book, veterinarian Cheryl Swartz's book *Four Paws, Five Directions*, found me. She introduced me to the diagnostic principles of traditional Chinese medicine for dogs and the concept of the body as a connected ecosystem. I knew I didn't want to study Chinese herbs, but I used what I learned and applied those principles to Western herbology.

I studied more and more, saving up for a copy of *Veterinary Herbalism* by Susan Wynn. This massive and detailed textbook helped me fill some gaps regarding practicum and animal veterinary practices. It also provided information on herb-pharmaceutical interactions, which I was lacking.

The moment my world completely shifted is when I read Matthew Wood's third book, *The Practice of Traditional Western Herbalism*. This is where I learned about the system of energetics. It came crashing down on me like a wave of light: finally, a structure for individualized herbalism I could relate to. As I wore out the pages of Matthew's book, one aha moment led to another. I had found my path through the forest and knew my future: helping dogs through holistic canine herbalism. This was not the path of least resistance, but it was the answer to the sickness I witnessed daily at Almost Home Pet Farm.

As the years passed, I learned more and more, sometimes from other herbalists in the area, but mostly I remained reclusive to the farm and my practice. I expanded Farm Dog by taking on a business partner and started writing for *Dogs Naturally Magazine*. I felt grounded in my herbalism practice, and when anyone asked me what I did for work, I proudly answered, "I'm a canine herbalist."

Eventually, the winds shifted, my life opened up an unforeseen path, and after twelve years of kennel-free dog boarding, my partner and I closed Almost Home and moved west to Olympia, Washington, where we could finally find the space for full self-expression.

The trees, moss, and rain in our new home had a lush center that filled me with breath. This was a perfect spot to settle for life's fourth and fifth decades. Early on, I attended the Hawthorn School of Plant Medicine with land-centered herbalist Sean Croke, learning about the local flora and fauna. Quickly, I became acquainted with new tree and plant friends and recognized old ones like cleavers, chickweed, dandelion, and violet. I continued to consult, make herbal remedies, formulate, and help run Farm Dog Naturals, and, with a bit of prodding, I started teaching holistic canine herbalism to a group of thirty women every Thursday. This was a phenomenal opportunity to learn about myself, share my knowledge, and prepare for writing this book. At the same time, I had the privilege of working with Matthew Wood in person over a six-month period, which was a dream come true.

I'm still here in the mossy woods. My life as an herbalist is beyond fulfilling, and the plants are still my best teachers. At the time of this writing, I'm expanding my role as teacher by creating the Ethos School of Holistic Canine Herbalism and looking forward to teaching others about this beautiful nature-based path to healing. Hopefully, others will want to be canine herbalists too.

Acknowledgments

I first want to thank plants and dogs. They are the driving force behind all my work and selfless examples of unconditional love. Thank you to all my mentors who have come in and out of my life exactly when I needed them most. Your patience, guidance, and giving spirits have been an example of how to be with others. I am the accumulation of those who have come before me. I've lit the torch and now carry it forward, bringing forth my own light as light for others.

Special thanks to my acorns. You ladies are the roots of this book, and I'm eternally grateful for your time and energy throughout our four and a half years together. Showing up for you every week cleared a path for these pages.

Thanks to every dog and person who came to Almost Home Pet Farm. You were the first. Thank you for entrusting me and helping me learn.

Much thanks to all of the pugs who came through Music City Pug Rescue and the lovely folks who adopted them. You have all been my mentors, and each pug was so courageous and sweet.

Thank you to Heather, my true north, breath, and fierce defender. I love you. It is a privilege to be your partner and share in the love you have for every animal you meet. Thank you for teaching me the importance of meeting people where they are, nonjudgment, and not holding people to their darkest moments.

Thank you to Maureen Hogan, my late wife, who helped me discover my true identity, a love for the stars, Ireland, the importance of fire circles, whimsical creatures, and my place as an herbalist and healer. Your friendship and love inspired me to rise above my insecurities and take a chance on the person I knew myself to be.

Thanks to my mom, Lilly, whose tenacity, courage, and apple pie have left me awe-inspired and gave me comfort in my darkest moments. You are my guiding star and my hope for the future.

To my father, thank you for taking the time to care for me as I interacted with nature. You gave me soil and a garden to grow in. I am thankful for my introduction to the green and for your patience with my never-ending questions.

Thanks as well to my grandmother. Even though we didn't know each other well, I feel you in my blood. Your capacity for forgiveness is infinite, and your trust in nature foundational. I can't wait to thank you in the life beyond.

Thanks to Cathy, the best childhood friend a girl could ask for. Our adventures were legendary.

To May, you're my rock, thank you for all of your encouragement and unwavering friendship and love. I look forward to a bright future together manifesting our light.

To Lynn, thank you for all of your support, encouragement, mentorship, and friendship over the years. You were with me during some of my darkest moments and continued lifting me up in your own special way. Most of all, thank you for your heart. As hidden as it may be, I've found it to be one of the biggest I've ever encountered.

To Peg, thank you for all of your past guidance, hard work, and pug love.

To my brother Robert, thank you for giving me the space to travel, learn, and explore. You have given me more than I have ever given you.

To Briana, thank you for your selflessness, trust, and kindness. I will never forget all of the sacrifices you made for me, especially when I was dealing with illness. As Brandi Carlile says, "You're nothing short of magical and beautiful to me; I'll never hit the big time without you"—you, my daughter and my friend, my Evangeline.

To Bob and Wave, thank you for being love, extended family, and a light in the darkness. You have given so much and always make me feel special. I adore you both. Wavy, keeper of the plants, your garden is magical. Thank you for loving the flowers and your gift of tears and violets.

To Leslie, Rob, and Doug the Pug, I'm thankful you are in my life! You are two of the most talented, inspiring people I know. Doug, you have been such a mentor and I love all of your pudge.

To Vicky Bowman, thanks for lifting me up and setting me down gently. You are always in my heart and I adore you.

To Carol Trasatto, Cathy Skipper, David Hoffmann, Isla Fishburn, Jim McDonald, Josie Beug, Julia Graves, Juliette de Bairacli Levy, Paul Pitchford, Phyllis Light, Randy Kidd, Sajah Popham, Sean Croke, Sean Padraig O'Donoghue, Susan Wynn, and Swani Simon, thank you for all of your truth, knowledge, space, and wisdom. Your teachings have forever changed me and expanded my own truth more greatly than I could have imagined.

To Matthew Wood, thank you for validating my reclusive practice up on the mountain. Your teaching, words, and ability to channel history have given me structure and purpose. Thank you for solidifying my own process as an intuitive herbalist. You continue to inspire me, and special thanks for being a soul of the green, a Ljósálfar, or light elf.

To Greg Tilford, I'm so glad we have been able to connect and align. You have been holding space and fighting for the validation of animal herbalism for so long. Thank you for being a teacher and guide for all of us.

To Cheryl Schwartz, thank you for looking beyond what is visible. You're a pioneer of integrative care and an inspiration. I appreciate all of your silent mentorship, making difficult concepts understandable and, teaching me how the body is an ecosystem.

To Lorin, thank you for pushing me to share my wisdom with others. I appreciate your belief in me and I am forever grateful.

To Dr. Judy Morgan, thank you for living your truth and being an example of what it means to be courageous in the face of adversity. Your support for the natural dog community is unwavering. I appreciate you.

To Dr. Kevin Brummet, thank you for your love of pugs and all the years of putting up with me questioning everything. You are a such a wonderful vet and a shining example of humility, love, and purpose.

To Dana Scott and the late Julia Henriques, thanks for giving me my start in this community, your support over the years, and saying yes when I sent in my first article for *Dogs Naturally Magazine*.

To Dr. Dee Blanco, thank you for believing in me, respecting my work, and offering beautiful friendship. I look forward to sharing more and collaborating in the future.

Thank you to Rodney Habib and Dr. Karen Becker for bringing natural dog health to the masses, taking a stand against the madness of the standard of care, and writing *The Forever Dog* and *The Forever Dog Life*. Your commitment to this community is astounding and inspiring—now I can simply hand someone your book as an introduction to all-natural dog care instead of going into the long conversation of why. *Forever Dog* . . . forever grateful!

Special thanks to Amy Renz, Dr. Barbara Royal, Dr. Barrie Sands, Becky Kebler, Billy Hoekman, Dr. Brenden Clarke, Cameron Bowery, Carla Antonelli and Don Knarr, Carrie Hyde, Dr. Chris Bessent, Conor Brady, Erica Marie, Jae and Adrienne (Two Crazy Cat Ladies), Jennifer and Dan Foster, Joni Kamlet, Julie Anne Lee, Kailan Hollywood, Dr. Katie Kangas, Katie Woodley, Kelley Marian, Kolt Beringer, Krysta Fox and Bruce, Leith Henry, Dr. Lynda Loudon, Melanie Figg (soul sister), Dr. Odette Suter, Peter Ciancarelli, Poppy Phillips, Regina Beider, Dr. Rob Silver, Ruby Alexis, Dr. Ruth Roberts, Sean Zyer, Sharon Sercombe, and anyone else I've forgotten. I appreciate you!

INTRODUCTION
Using This Book

This book is for you, the dog guardian, caretaker, and best friend. It is also for rescues, dog nutritionists, veterinary technicians, veterinarians, and other canine health and wellness professionals. *The Herbal Dog* provides varying levels of information with two underlying commonalities: dogs and plants.

The best education I've ever received has been from the plants. This book focuses on those that I use most in my practice. I would have liked to include all my plant friends, as well as all the trees and mushrooms, but the subject is too vast, speaking in many volumes.

In these pages you'll find an exploration of plant medicine mapped onto canine health and wellness. It derives from my own herbal relationships, past and present, as well as my mistakes, encounters, and expansion. It centers on plant language—the key to understanding your dog through an herbal lens, as an individual ecosystem. My hope is that you'll finish this book with a better understanding of the interconnectedness of your dog's physical and emotional self, how your dog's body works, and an appreciation for the beauty and effectiveness of holistic herbalism.

Learning herbalism takes time and patience. This introductory book is part education and part application. I recommend that you read this book in order through chapter 6, "Planning Herbal Protocols," and then explore more freely the different canine conditions in chapter 7, learning about the plants that can assist you with your dog's care. Chapter 8, which contains all the plant and fungi monographs, provides the dosage guidelines and detailed information you'll need to effectively use the plants according to the information in this book.

The Herbal Dog will help you begin to make sense of the wide and varied world of holistic herbalism. As is the case for most fields of natural health care, there is a lot of competing and sometimes contradictory information out there about using herbalism with canines. After reading this book, you'll be able to start navigating advice from all the wonderful people trying to make a positive difference through their work in natural pet care. You'll begin to understand the factors at play in their recommendations and determine which are appropriate for your individual dog. I recommend keeping a journal as you begin this herbal journey with your pup. Use it to record your dog's health and symptoms throughout the year, as well as your dog's reactions to different herbs. The body talks; we just need to observe and listen.

My hope is that you'll read and reference this book again and again, finding a place for yourself in its pages. You are such a big part of this journey with your animals. Take things slowly, and work toward a comprehensive understanding of the ways in which small, intentional changes, being present, and holding space for your own and your dog's health can have profound results. You, the guardian and caretaker of these beautiful creatures we call dogs, must take care of yourself in order to care for your dog.

We share space with our pets, and that means we share emotions too. Remember, every day is a new day; leave the past behind, where it belongs. You can't control everything or know everything. You are doing your best. Take what you need but leave enough for others. Make good choices and forgive yourself when you don't. Focus on what you want, not what you don't, and lay waste to guilt, shame, and fear. Worry begets more worry. Your stress is your dog's stress. Breathe. Don't obsess. You are doing the best with the knowledge you have. At the end of the day, all your dog needs is to know you love them.

Nature is all around us but also inside us. Make time daily to connect, seek answers, be still, and listen. You can't hold your dog's health in stasis any more than you can your own; a healthy dog is a way of life.

PART ONE

Dogs and Plants Are Individuals

We believe that the domestic animals were sent here to accept the diseases of humans . . . and to show them how to heal these diseases.

Tis Mal Crow, Indigenous American healer, in *Dr. Kidd's Guide to Herbal Dog Care* by Randy Kidd

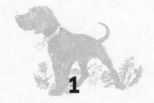

1

Holistic Canine Herbalism

The practice of allopathy is not dependent upon what type of medicine we use but rather upon how we use the medicine.

SAJAH POPHAM,
EVOLUTIONARY HERBALISM

Veterinary medicine has made considerable advancements in diagnostics, surgical methodology, and emergency medicine. Yet it relies heavily on the standard of care approach, in which a set of symptoms denotes specific drug regimens or tests despite a dog's individuality or environmental circumstances. For example, a dog with an itchy skin condition will automatically be given antibiotics and steroids without discussion of the dog's environment, stressors, diet, or supplement regimen.

This same approach is used in what might be called "allopathic herbalism," in which the drugs of traditional veterinary practice are replaced by herbs. Here, too, the standard of care predominates and herbs are prescribed based only on generalizations of which herb is good for what condition.

In contrast, with holistic herbalism, five dogs may present with identical symptoms, but based on their assessment, which includes diet, environment, and stressors, they might be given five different herbs. The standard of care does not apply. Holistic herbalism sees dogs as individuals with unique needs, sensitivities, and energetic patterns. It considers the underlying root cause of symptoms. Why? Because holistic herbalism believes everything is connected.

Let's look at an example of well-intentioned allopathy: Your dog has a cough. You look up herbal remedies for lung health and see a list of herbs. You give a mixture of mullein leaf, echinacea, and plantain. The cough improves. Weeks later, you hear wet breathing, which turns into pneumonia. As it turns out, mullein leaf and plantain are good for the lungs, but both are demulcents (herbs high in moisture) and aren't indicated for moist lung conditions. Even though the cough subsided, demulcent herbs worsened the underlying root cause (moisture).

If instead you are working from a holistic standpoint, first you look at your dog's lifestyle and patterns. What's happening on a deeper level? How's your dog mentally? What stressors does your dog have? What does the cough sound like? Is it moist or dry? What foods is your dog eating? Do these foods contribute to dampness (too much moisture in the body)? Focusing on your dog as a whole organism rather than addressing isolated symptoms is essential. Health ebbs and flows; it is a process, not solely the absence of disease. Almost all holistic modalities embrace a focus on the underlying cause of imbalance or illness, rather than symptoms. Why? The body wants to heal itself; it's always looking to achieve balance.

Key Differences between Allopathic and Holistic Herbalism

1. **Symptoms are only the beginning.** Symptoms are like a warning beacon that something inside your dog is out of balance. You can use drugs or herbs to address symptoms, and the symptoms will disappear. However, that doesn't mean the imbalance disappears. For example, consider a urinary tract infection. Allopathically, you'd treat the infection, and then you and your dog would go about your lives in the same way you did before the diagnosis. Holistically, you'd recognize the infection as a sign that your dog's ecosystem is imbalanced. You'd address the urinary tract infection and then ask, "Why did my dog get an infection?" You'd look at your dog's diet and lifestyle, and you might administer strengthening herbs that support balance in the urinary system to prevent future infection.

2. **Dosage and dosage methodology (posology) are different.** First, dosages vary from herbalist to herbalist. Some practitioners may disagree, but I always teach people to use small dosages for most chronic

conditions, avoiding complete suppression. You can always increase the dose, but you can't go back. Allopathic herbalism gives high "therapeutic dosages" based on weight, without considering your dog's condition, sensitivity, diet, or whether the issue is truly acute or chronic.

3. **Holistic herbalism is based on your dog as an individual**. Your dog is a unique ecosystem with specific physical and emotional requirements. Holistic herbalism understands that what works for one dog may not work for another. For example, your dog's tolerance for an herb may be 1 teaspoon while another dog of the same size may tolerate 2 tablespoons. When looking at food, supplements, and herbs, remember that most general guidelines are based on weight not individuality.

4. **Patience is a requirement in all holistic modalities.** I remember when my cat Bones had a stubborn abscess resulting from a catfight. I decided to deal with the abscess at home with the guidance of a local holistic vet. I gave Bones herbs and homeopathic Silicea to encourage the abscess to drain. However, I had to wait and trust that the remedy was working. On the morning of day three, the wound finally opened and I drained it. I avoided the need for antibiotics by boosting Bones's nutrition and giving immune-supportive herbs. And, even though I've been doing this for a long time, I still had to remind myself to be patient. We have been conditioned to depend on or look for quick fixes, thinking our pets will somehow explode from a torn toenail or a hot spot. With holistic healing, trust and patience are crucial. If healing does not occur (in a nonemergency situation), then the herb choice is incorrect and you simply must try again. Many times, an adverse reaction tells you what direction to take. Rarely is herbalism a one-and-done process.

The Dog as an Ecosystem

Nature teaches us that everything is connected. The dog-as-ecosystem model of canine herbalism centers on your dog as a reflection of nature. Studying how the individual dog relates to its environment is a fundamental component of canine herbalism because the individual is *a part of*, rather than *apart from*, nature. Animals (including humans) and plants have had an innate relationship since the time of our earliest ancestors. Today, holistic canine herbalism works by acknowledging that relationship, using both the tools of measurement given to us by science and the immeasurable aspects of plant intelligence, intuition, and vital force.

While walking the plant path and learning about chronic disease, you'll notice how subtle changes can positively or negatively affect your dog's ecosystem. When herbs enter the body, they clean, balance, support the assimilation of nutrients, balance energetic patterns, support organ health, and strengthen the immune system. The body is always trying to cleanse and balance its ecosystem. A good visual example of this comes from spiders. Yes, you read that correctly, spiders. A spider spinning its web is the perfect example of building, cleansing, and repairing.

When I lived on a farm in the hills of Tennessee, I would sit on my porch at dusk in the fall and watch brown spiders spin their webs. When they were finally done, they'd sit and wait in the middle. I'd throw small pieces of debris into a web and watch the resident spider hurry over, kick it out, patch up the web, and return to the middle. They would do this repeatedly. Luckily for them, I bored quickly. The web-spinning process is similar to how your dog's body functions; it's rhythmic and orderly. When something enters your dog's body—food, medicine, parasite, splinter— either the body recognizes it as building or balancing, or the body works to kick it out, repair the damage, and try to restore balance.

Plants have balance too. They are filled with naturally occurring chemical compounds that can number in the hundreds and even thousands. Each one of these chemicals has a specific function. For example, many plants have constituents that modify the effects of other constituents to reduce their side effects. Even though herbalists and scientists don't understand all plant constituents and how they work, it's apparent that many of them are far from benign.

Whether taken on their own or in combination with other herbs, plants work on the whole body. This is an essential aspect of herbalism because their whole-body effect can work positively or negatively depending on how the body and plant(s) come together. This is one of the reasons why we need people practicing holistic instead of allopathic herbalism; a plant consumed by one individual may produce a completely different outcome for another.

Terrain Theory

Holistic herbalism considers how herbs affect not only the body's physiological processes but also its *terrain*. We can think of terrain as the body's internal ecosystem—all the processes, factors, compounds, microbes, patterns, and energetics that, through their relationships with each other, produce a living, working organism. When we consider the dog-as-ecosystem model, we are in effect talking about your dog's terrain.

Antifungals, antivirals, antibiotics, anti-inflammatories, vaccines, and steroids are allopathy's answers to many dog ailments. Yes, they provide a quick fix, but do they support health in the dog-as-ecosystem? Or do they suppress it?

Germ theory makes us dependent on these pharmaceutical medicines. But the idea that we can keep dogs healthy by controlling bacteria, viruses, and other microbes is maddening. This type of medicine presumes that we have dominion over the microscopic world, but that will never be true. A dog's world is saturated with microbes; working against them isn't the logical answer.

A dog's inner terrain should instead be the focus. We can fortify the terrain without detrimental side effects and without depleting the overall health of the dog-as-ecosystem. Healing from the inside out by supporting balance in the terrain is the key to maintaining a long-term balance with microbes. We do this by focusing on the terrain of the individual dog, including the dog's diet, immune health, mitochondrial strength, and vital force.

Louis Pasteur and Claude Bernard

Terrain theory isn't new; it came about in the same period as germ theory. In the mid- to late nineteenth century, Louis Pasteur and Claude Bernard, French contemporaries in the fields of medicine and biology, came to different conclusions about the origins of disease. Pasteur believed that disease was caused by pathogenic microorganisms. He considered the human body to be a vessel of purity and concluded that it was science's job to eradicate all pathogenic bacteria. He believed humans would not survive without scientific intervention. As we now know, he misunderstood the relationship between the body and bacteria.

Bernard had a different theory: He believed the internal terrain, not microbes, caused disease. Yes, microbes could cause diseases like tuberculosis, but disease wasn't inevitable for every individual carrying those microbes. A deficiency in the terrain, Bernard said, allowed a microbe to become out of balance, initiating the disease process. Like Hippocrates, he believed that good nutrition and immune function were crucial for keeping the body healthy.[1]

The Trouble with Allopathic Medicines

Germ theory believes the body can't protect itself from foreign microbes without scientific intervention.[2] In other words, your dog can't survive without medical intervention, regardless of diet, lifestyle, and immune health, and your dog must be protected against *all* pathogenic microbes. Allopathic veterinary care is very busy controlling microbes! Antibiotics are often overprescribed or given preventively, even though science has verified that the digestive system's microbe colonies are responsible for more than 75 percent of your dog's immune system—and antibiotics decimate them.[3] Yes, antibiotics are lifesavers, this can't be argued, but due to their devastating impact on a dog's internal microbiome they should be given only when all other treatment has failed.

I once took my pug puppy to an emergency veterinary center because he was having unexplained facial swelling. The vet gave him a shot of antihistamine, which I agreed with. Then, after the swelling diminished, the vet recommended a steroid shot and a seven-day course of antibiotics "just in case." What about the consequences of giving a four-month-old puppy antibiotics? Shouldn't we wait to see if he needs them? Giving antibiotics to a puppy can cause issues like fear, food sensitivities, allergies, diarrhea, and autoimmune disease. If the swelling affected my puppy's breathing, I would have agreed to the steroid shot, but his respiratory system was unaffected. I declined both the steroid and the antibiotics. My pup recovered within a day.

Vaccines have improved the quality of life for many, but vaccination as a standard of care, despite the need or risk, has caused more harm than good due to high rates of chronic disease and immune suppression.[4] The vaccination of today isn't the vaccine of the past. Today's vaccines contain hundreds of ingredients, including foreign proteins and heavy metals.[5] And because vaccination falls under the standard of care, I've seen immune-compromised dogs—even dogs with cancer—vaccinated despite the harm the vaccine may cause. Vaccines, like antibiotics, should be administered only when they're necessary (or required by law).

The Power of a Healthy Terrain

In the early twentieth century, Edward Carl Rosenow experimented with what he called "bacterial transmutation": the transformation of bacteria from one strain or form to another based on their environment, and in particular their food source.[6] The inventor of the universal microscope, Royal Rife, replicated Rosenow's work, converting nonpathogenic colon bacteria into typhoid bacteria by changing their food source. Rife discovered a cancer-causing virus, which he called Bacillus X (BX), that could change its form based on the body's terrain and what it was fed.[7] Like Claude Bernard, Rife believed nutrition and the body's terrain were more important than the germs a person is exposed to.

Without germs, life can't exist! Your dog's body is teeming with microbes and is exposed to trillions more each day. But these germs are opportunistic, meaning they wait to take advantage of deficient immunity and vitality. When you help your dog maintain a strong immune system and vibrant vitality by focusing on your dog's toxic load, diet, stressors, and inner terrain, you have control over their health. Pharmaceutical-based veterinary care is helpful if you need it, but only if you do. Medications like antibacterials have helped lower mortality rates, but so have emergency medicine, improved sewage systems, and personal hygiene. Allopathic medicine is great at saving lives with surgery and medication for acute conditions, but it is failing dogs in terms of preventive care and longevity.

A holistic approach to canine health care includes a minimally processed diet, low stress, and support for a balanced terrain. This puts your dog's health back into your care. As I said earlier: A healthy dog is a way of life.

Whole-Plant Medicine

In the late 1800s and early 1900s, herbalism and homeopathy were the mainstays of medical care, including veterinary care.[8] Shortly after 1942, when laws prohibiting the practice of medicine without a license were passed, allopathic medicine and standardized pharmaceuticals took hold.[9] Today, the veterinary industry is chemically dependent, dispensing Big Pharma's antibiotics, anti-inflammatories, immune depressants, and steroids. Instead of focusing on disease prevention, conventional veterinary care emphasizes symptom suppression; instead of seeing the animal as a whole ecosystem, it treats each body system as a separate part. Even many "holistic" veterinarians and practitioners use herbs allopathically and rely on standardized herbs.

Standardized herbs are laboratory extracts of whatever is considered to be an herb's "active" constituents, standardized to a certain level so they can be studied and utilized according to pharmaceutical principles of what has become known as evidence-based medicine. This isn't herbalism; it's just science taking plants back to the lab and creating herbal drugs. Standardized herbal extracts are adulterated; chemically, they don't resemble the plant used to create them. A standardized extract guarantees you, the consumer, a specific amount of a plant's "active" ingredients, but it may contain only one or two of a plant's constituents, rather than the whole plant's chemical profile. Curcumin, for example, is commonly extracted from turmeric root and forms the basis of many commercial turmeric supplements—which makes them lab products, not plant products. Studies have shown that high doses of curcumin can decrease iron levels, leading to anemia.[10] Extracts of the whole root of turmeric, which don't isolate curcumin from the other constituents in the root, don't have this effect.

Standardized extracts do have their place. Exact dosages of specific constituents allow for more accurate measurements, which enables plant extracts to be used in clinical trials and, later, to be marketed as "proven" and "effective." This is the "evidence" required by evidence-based medicine. I always smile when science "proves" the validity of a substance traditional herbalism has known about for hundreds of years. Unfortunately, people tend to gravitate toward the familiar, favoring clinical evidence and statistics, leaving little room in modern veterinary medicine for plant intelligence and human intuition. Standardization offers evidence-based herbal medicine, but this process comes at a cost. Standardized extracts require high dosages and have none of the self-modulation that naturally occurs among the varied constituents in whole-plant extracts. In contrast, whole-plant extracts, with all of a plant's constituents, allows us to use small dosages without much risk of extreme side effects.

Modern evidence-based medicine would have us believe that a plant's medicinal effect comes from just one action or constituent. That is simply not the case. In their whole form, plants have synergy, meaning their constituents are more effective when used together. Synergy allows whole-plant extracts to buffer their own side effects while increasing their effectiveness.[11]

Milk thistle offers a good example of isolating one plant constituent at another's expense. I use milk thistle seed consistently in my practice. If well indicated, it's an effective liver regenerator and protects the liver from toxins. The "active constituent" in milk thistle seed is silymarin. As an isolated standardized extract, silymarin can interfere with the liver's ability to metabolize prescription drugs. This is the opposite of the effect silymarin has when administered in an extract of the whole milk thistle seed. Milk thistle seed preparations, which have high levels of silymarin but also hundreds of other constituents, support the liver by assisting with detoxification rather than interfering with it.

Another problematic aspect of standardization is the plant quantity needed to make the standardized extracts. As is the case for essential oil production, standardized extracts require large amounts of plant material, and so manufacturers tend to focus on quantity, not quality. Plants are sourced worldwide and grown and harvested under different conditions and principles. In contrast, one of the foundations of holistic herbalism is the quality of the plants used as medicine. Organically cultivated and ethically wildcrafted plants are optimal for making effective herbal medicines.

Furthermore, herbalists traditionally use water, alcohol, or glycerin as a menstruum (solvent) for making medicines. Large manufacturers may use more powerful solvents like hexane and acetone, which can leave behind toxic residues and lead to unwanted side effects.

Standardized herbal extracts do have their place in modern medicine. With proper use and guidance, they can be effective when we need to force the body to react because time is of the essence. However, when using plants for everyday medicine or for long-term healing and health, it's best to use the plants in their natural, whole form.

The Trap of Evidence-Based Medicine

By ignoring phenomena outside the scientific realm, a skewed
and incomplete view of the world is offered.

MATTHEW WOOD,
"THE PRACTICE OF WESTERN HERBALISM"
PLANT HEALER MAGAZINE

Holistic healing modalities like Western herbalism, traditional Chinese medicine, homeopathy, and ayurveda are often at odds with science because they don't fit the current evidence-based paradigm. For traditional herbalism in particular, standard methodologies of measurement don't apply because medicinal potency can vary from plant to plant and harvest to harvest, and reactions can vary from person to person. When the principles of pharmacology are applied to herbs, they often lack replicable results because most traditional herbal medicines don't force the body to react like pharmaceuticals do. Instead, herbs stimulate the body's own healing capacities, sometimes taking weeks or months to produce a positive effect.

Most critics don't understand that herbalism is based on methodologies and principles that are completely different from pharmaceutical medicine's "gold standard" of double-blind clinical research. Holistic medicine is more than lab reports and clinical trials. It's individualized medicine, considering the entire person or animal's ecosystem. Evidence-based medicine has been the foundation of modern veterinary medicine. However, as people connect with more natural forms of care, alternative practitioners are experiencing a rift between evidence-based medicine and traditional practices.

We've been conditioned to believe that all forms of medicine must have a strong foundation in evidence-based research. Unfortunately, this leaves any system of medicine other than Western allopathy labeled as pseudoscience, quackery, or unproven. The underlying current of disbelief is so strong that collectively science holds anecdotal evidence and historical use captive until proved valid. I often find myself in the evidence-based research trap, citing studies solely for public appeasement. Don't get me wrong, if I start offering up percentages or statistics or saying that a remedy has a certain amount of a constituent, I need evidence to back up my claims, but if I say turmeric helps decrease inflammation and pain, I've got thousands of years of historical use to back up that statement.

Evidence-based medicine involves statistical analysis of research, clinical trials, and peer evaluation. Its methodology provides standards of practice based on double-blind, randomized studies. I've read more research papers than I can count and have used many as references for this book, but each study must be looked at closely and evaluated for validity and potential bias toward the evidence-based paradigm. There are fundamental concerns with current mainstream, evidence-based research models that should be noticed, understood, and addressed. Here are some considerations.

1. Evidence-based medicine is the foundation for standard-of-care practices; one-size-fits-all guidelines for treatment based on clinical presentations and symptoms. As a result, individuality is overlooked; patients are seen as interchangeable and reduced to statistics despite their complexity.
2. Laboratory settings aren't always representative of real life. Mice, rabbits, and rats are unrepresentative of humans and canines.
3. Psychological, emotional, and generational impacts are seldom tracked due to the use of animal models and the constraints of time.
4. The placebo effect can be as high as 50 percent in human studies.[12]
5. Research must consider the education, background, and views of the researchers themselves. In addition, we must acknowledge that the requirement for most researchers and academics to publish papers consistently can allow for a high error level.[13]
6. Money and greed can undermine good research. Corporate sponsorship of clinical trials is rampant, even in double-blind studies,[14] and food and drug companies can create studies to validate their products. When we assess the results of a study, we must know who paid for the study.
7. Funding is skewed toward pharmaceutical-based research.[15] Many studies are undertaken in service of potential financial gain. Studying an herb in its natural form doesn't have a high monetary return as it can't be patented and is available to the general public.[16]

8. The potential of studies failing to procure the correct outcome can negatively affect research validity due to financial investment and pressure for clinical success.[17] In addition, study results can be affected by political, institutional, and financial concerns.

9. Results need to be verified and consistently replicated. This is often not possible due to funding.

10. Herb studies often use standardized extracts for measurability. These extracts don't represent the herb medicines that are freely available to the people but are instead compounds synthesized in laboratories and derived from hundreds of plants grown under varying conditions. The method of extraction, too, must be considered. For example, studies of the plant constituent berberine sometimes use water-based extracts and sometimes alcohol-based ones. Berberine is an alkaloid, and alkaloids love alcohol.[18] An alcohol extraction used in large dosages will not produce the same effect as water extraction. The results of an investigation into an alcoholic extract of berberine won't apply to all extractions of berberine.

11. Most studies don't consider holistic concerns like energetics, stress levels, toxin burden, and the interconnectedness of an organism's anatomy.

The Principles of Holistic Herbalism

Hippocrates, the so-called father of modern medicine, had two important theories that today's science is currently proving valid: It is more important to know what sort of person has a disease than to know what sort of disease a person has, and all disease begins in the gut.[19] This was more than two thousand years ago!

Evidence-based medicine has a mechanistic view of the body, presuming that parts and systems can be fixed or removed without affecting others. Holistic herbalism views the body as a reflection of nature and functions on the premise that a dog, for example, is an ecosystem in which everything is connected. In contrast to the concerns affecting evidence-based medicine, traditional herbalism can offer four principles:

1. Holistic herbalism matches individual energetics (cool, warm, dry, moist) to a plant's energetics.
2. Holistic herbalism looks at your dog's symptoms as well as diet, stress, life experience, and environment in evaluating patterns of health and disease.
3. Dogs, cats, and people are not mere statistics, nor are any of them like any other dogs, cats, and people. Individualism must be taken into account. Research can be used to guide treatment, but not to create rigid prescriptions we must adhere to. Holistic herbalism considers and looks at the entire picture of health—the ecosystem of the animal or person.
4. Holistic herbalism considers the underlying causes of illness and chronic disease. It dismisses the one-size-fits-all methodology of addressing symptoms and instead focuses on *why* a condition occurs.

Integrative Veterinary Medicine

When performed with integrity, the clinical studies of evidence-based medicine are an excellent method for verifying the efficacy of veterinary care. The same can be said for the centuries of use and documentation of traditional medicinal herbs. Herbalism can provide valuable clinical and field experience along with repeated anecdotal evidence.

Integrative veterinary medicine blends the two paradigms. Yes, there can be differences of opinion, but with mutual respect, everyone can see the validation of experience. Combining clinical experience, anecdotal and historical evidence, and evidence-based medicine provides a powerful platform of support for the patient, which matters most.

Holistic herbalism can help veterinary medicine understand the importance of plant language, individuality, preventive care, and the dog-as-ecosystem. This sort of individualized medicine is the key to longevity, and it's missing from standardized veterinary care. Holistic herbalism and allopathic medicine must set aside their differences and find common ground.

Our Dogs, Ourselves

More important than providing a big house and yard for our dogs is providing an environment of love and joy. This helps keep their heart healthy and in sync with yours. A dog living their best and longest life lies within your very own heart.

ERICA MARIE COSTON,
DOG HERBALIST

What you are putting out into the field around you is being picked up by your dog (because you are emotionally relevant to him or her) and your dog will take that on as if he was expressing that himself. (So, for [your dog's] sake, be mindful of what you think and how you feel.)

BARRIE SANDS, DVM,
"YOUR ENERGY AND YOUR DOG"

Holistic herbalism centers on the mind-body-spirit connection, and that includes the vibrations we share with our dogs. Research has shown that dogs respond to human emotions and even take them on physically.[20] As we know, dogs have heightened senses, making them especially sensitive to smells. When humans are stressed, they give off hormones like oxytocin, and dogs can literally smell them![21] I've observed many cases of this over the years, and it fascinates me and fine-tunes my awareness of how I speak to and speak about my animals.

With their keen senses, our dogs constantly interpret our emotions and our interactions with our environment. Like humans, dogs want to feel safe. When we don't feel safe, neither do they.[22] I once worked with a woman whose dog suffered from anxiety. As it turns out, my client was anxious, and that anxiety was spilling over to her sweet pup. Unintentionally, my client's stress became her dog's stress. We started working with flower essences and body language so that both my client and her dog could become more relaxed and less anxious.

The HeartMath Institute studies the physical and emotional aspects of heart intelligence. One of the things they've discovered is that our emotions affect the manner in which the body harmonizes the heart's electromagnetic output. The heart puts out a strong electromagnetic field; it's approximately five thousand times stronger than that of the brain and can be detected more than two feet from the body in most cases.[23] This is a vibrational field of moving particles, even if we can't see them moving. Like the wind, the heart's field may not be able to be seen, but it definitely exists, and it's one way in which we interact with those around us—including our dogs.

Dogs can physically experience your emotions through their own heart and nervous system. As we will discuss later in this book, the heart is controlled by your dog's autonomic nervous system, which switches between parasympathetic (rest and relaxation) and sympathetic activity (fight or flight) as your dog interacts with their environment. The act of switching back and forth has a profound effect on the heart; we see it in a dog's heart rate variability. Emotions, too, affect the rate at which the heart and nervous system switch back and forth from reaction to relaxation. Prolonged emotional relationships have an even more profound impact on your and your dog's mind-body-spirit connection and can have measurable physical effects.

Science has proven that both positive and negative emotions can affect the heart's electromagnetic field.[24] What we do in our environment directly affects our dog's emotional and physical health, whether we like it or not. I'm reminded of animal behaviorist Temple Grandin's work and how she encourages people to focus on joy around their animals and limit feelings of fear, anger, grief, and panic as much as possible.[25]

I don't share this information to make you feel guilty for being negative or even angry around your dog; it's meant to help you be mindful of your mood and tone. Having a bad day here and there isn't going to harm your dog, but having consistent emotional displays of anger, resentment, regret, or jealousy can eventually take its toll. These feelings can put you into fight-or-flight mode. Your stress directly affects your dog's stress, and as is the case for humans, a dog with chronic stress is at risk of a wide range of health issues, including in the all-important microbiome.[26]

The bond between dogs and owners can be so profound that sometimes dogs take on their owner's illnesses. In her book *Emotional Freedom,* Dr. Judith Orloff shared the story of a woman with a rare kidney disease who became pregnant against her doctor's stern warning. To the doctor's surprise, she made it through the pregnancy and gave birth to a healthy baby. Unfortunately, during the same period, her golden retriever, whom the woman was extremely close to, came down with sudden-onset kidney disease and passed away shortly after the baby's birth.[27] This is just one example of possible emotional transference. This is the subject of much study right now as science learns more and more about the shared energy between humans and dogs. The beautiful takeaway here is that you can have a positive effect on your dog by working on your own physical and emotional health. When you relax and bring down your stress levels, your dog can relax too.

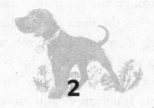

2

Food as Medicine

Over time, the foods we choose to feed our dogs either heal or harm—and the responsibility to choose wisely falls squarely on us, as guardians. To avoid inevitable regrets, we must evolve from pet food consumers to knowledgeable health advocates. . . . Our dogs deserve nothing less.

KAREN BECKER, DVM,
COAUTHOR OF *THE FOREVER DOG*

When I brought my first pug Finnbar home, I did what any uninformed puppy mother would do: I put him on a puppy kibble formula. Over the next year, he developed a stinky face, left a fur-based imprint on everything he touched, and snored like a bear. Various vets and other pug owners told me, "These issues are just a part of being a pug owner." We were at the vet every few months giving Finnbar steroids for chronic phenomena. As he approached three, he started developing arthritis. I was done. I went down the rabbit hole of nutrition for dogs and ended up dedicating my life to holistic canine herbalism.

I quickly changed Finnbar's kibble, then transitioned him to limited-ingredient kibble, dehydrated food, then to freeze-dried food, then to raw. As Finnbar went through each food transition, the changes in his body were phenomenal, and we never made another trip to the vet for pneumonia. His wrinkles cleared up, his snoring went from epic to slight, and his shedding became minimal. The big lesson I learned from all this is that a clean diet is a foundation for health and cellular function.

As you know, this is a book about herbalism. Nutrition is a massive subject, but I've provided some guidelines and helpful observations I've made after working with all types of dogs with different dietary needs. For more information on building a better bowl, all types of diets, and how to be successful in feeding your dog as an individual, visit TheHerbalDog.com.

Facultative Carnivores

Humans are omnivores, which means we eat plants and animals. Though there is much debate on the subject, dogs are carnivores, not omnivores. That said, they are *facultative* carnivores, meaning they can eat both meat and plant matter, but meat-based dietary protein is a must for them to thrive.[1]

Today's domesticated dogs are privy to a more varied diet than their ancestors, including excessive carbohydrates. Yet dogs produce very little to no salivary amylase, which breaks down the starches in plant matter. They also don't produce cellulase, the enzyme that breaks down the cellulose in plant matter. While some dogs do okay on modern dog food formulations that incorporate grains and other plant-based foods, others have a harder time digesting them and can develop food sensitivities.

Canines in the wild eat the plant matter found in the intestines of their prey, which is already partially digested. One way to mimic that arrangement is to make sure that any vegetable matter you serve to your dog is slightly cooked, cooked, or combined with digestive enzymes and chopped in a food processor.

Kibble and Canned Food

Though I believe that a minimally processed diet works best for dogs, I also believe in meeting people where they are, including feeding kibble and canned food. There's a hierarchy, starting at the bottom with ingredients like food dyes, meat by-products, propylene glycol, and GMO corn gluten meal and moving all the way up to ethically sourced, limited-ingredient diets. If you're feeding your dog a highly processed diet, try to make it as high-quality as possible.

Cooked at high temperatures, kibble forces the dog-as-ecosystem into working nonstop because it's dry, lacking enzymes (dead food), and filled with inflammatory ingredients like hydrogenated oils, white rice, corn gluten meal, animal by-products, various forms of sugar and salt, and artificial dyes and flavorings.[2] Kibble makes your dog's liver and digestive system work overtime because it takes approximately eight to ten hours to process.[3] Canned food may look healthy but it has also been cooked at high temperatures and is filled with different liquids to increase moisture. Canning adds endocrine disruptors like bisphenol A (BPA) and polyvinyl chloride. Cheryl Rosenfeld, DVM, PhD, notes "When dogs consumed canned dog food containing BPA for two weeks, it was associated with metabolic and gut microbiome alterations."[4] Like kibble, canned food can range from poor to more healthy formulations. If you choose to feed canned food, make sure to read the labels.

I suggest reading Conor Brady's *Feeding Dogs* and Dr. Karen Becker and Rodney Habib's *The Forever Dog* and *The Forever Dog Life*. These books will educate you in the specific dangers of processed food and give you a good background and foundation in moving your dog toward a more natural lifestyle.

In the meantime, here is a simple support protocol to improve your dog's bowl as you work toward feeding a minimally processed diet. Remember to breathe and take small steps each day for yourself and your pups! Consistent small changes accomplish huge goals.

Basic Kibble / Wet Food Support Protocol

1. Give a low dose of milk thistle seed every other day to help your dog's liver deal with toxins.
2. Add digestive enzymes.
3. Feed a good prebiotic and rotate probiotics.
4. Add a lymphatic stimulant, like cleavers or calendula. (See chapter 4 for more details on the importance of the lymphatic system in canine health.)
5. Add a rotation of mushroom extracts or cooked mushrooms for extra antioxidants.
6. Add rotational herbs to your dog's bowl to increase nutrition, antioxidants, and vitamin and mineral content. Here are some examples: chickweed, dandelion greens, nettle (dried), parsley, plantain, self-heal, turmeric, or violet leaf. (See the monographs in chapter 8 for more information on the herbs that can be helpful for dogs.)

Cooked Food

Digestion, absorption and assimilation of nutrients takes energy. Lightly steaming vegetables and meats can provide a net energy gain because it compromises the structural integrity of the foods, making them easier to digest. This dynamic can be very helpful for dogs as they age, deal with health issues, or transition from ultra-processed foods to raw diets.

AMY RENZ, OWNER,
GOODNESS GRACIOUS PET FOOD COMPANY

Cooked food is a good option compared to kibble diets, and some dogs do better on a cooked diet due to their physical condition, age, or underlying disease. Cooking helps break down foods, especially plant fibers, serving as a form of predigestion. Cooked food is perfect for dogs without a spleen, with a history of pancreatic disorders, or with digestive weakness. For these dogs, cooking allows them to better assimilate nutrients while also supporting their gut microbiome, immune system, and organ health. And the proper assimilation of nutrients is more important than the preconceived notion that raw is better.

The biggest obstacle to a healthy cooked diet is how the food is prepared. Avoid microwaving, broiling, and deep frying. Stick to lightly sautéing on low heat (in grass-fed butter, olive oil, or avocado oil), steaming, low-temperature baking, or using a low-heat slow cooker.

There are many books and even apps that can help you design and prepare a cooked diet for your dog. You can also find many commercial options for lightly cooked, minimally processed dog food. See TheHerbalDog.com for suggestions.

· ·

Tip! When feeding vegetables to your dog, avoid conventionally grown apples, bell peppers, celery, citrus, cucumbers, green beans, peas, peaches, pears, potatoes, strawberries, and watermelon; they are highly sprayed with pesticides and herbicides. Also ensure you are using only organic sources of hemp (CBD), kale, spinach, and sunflower; these plants, known as superaccumulators, remove heavy metals from soil. Using organic sources reduces your dog's exposure.

· ·

Raw Food

There is no easier way to instantly enhance your pet's diet than adding fresh food. You can make healthy, positive changes simply by what you put in their bowl. Every bit of fresh food counts!

KELLEY MARIAN, FOUNDER,
GREEN JUJU CANINE HEALTH
SUPPLEMENT COMPANY

Dogs are a product of evolution, and they, like their ancestors, do best on a 100 percent raw diet of meat, bones, and organs (with the occasional bit of plant matter). A healthy diet of fresh food is important to canine health because food is the raw material of nourishment and overall metabolism. The hormones that govern the stomach, nervous, and endocrine systems all depend on the breakdown and assimilation of nutrients. Research has shown that diet has a great impact on an animal's microbiome (the community of microorganisms that live in the dog-as-ecosystem); you can, for example, change the balance of the bacterial population on your dog's skin from pathogenic to beneficial and vice versa based on what foods you are feeding.[5]

There are many ways to work with a raw diet, from beginner to advanced. Let's look at some options.

Commercial freeze-dried foods can be a part of a raw diet. These foods are cold processed, which removes moisture but keeps enzymes, vitamins, and minerals. These products are shelf-stable until opened. Steve Brown, an experienced animal diet formulator, recommends putting freeze-dried food in the freezer between meals to help keep it from oxidizing.[6] Also, make sure that your dog gets plenty of water to go along with freeze-dried foods, which will help ensure proper digestion.

Commercial raw food is prepackaged and frozen. It generally contains blends of meat and vegetables or blends of meat, bone, and organs. Traditional raw includes different cuts of meat, bone, and organ in varying proportions depending on your individual dog.

When feeding raw food, consider grass-fed raw goat and cow milk. Raw milk is full of digestive enzymes, probiotics, vitamins, and minerals—by itself, it is a whole, beneficial food. Raw milk can give your dog's gut the bioavailable boost it needs to thrive. I recommend raw goat milk for dogs who are more cool, as it is warming, and raw cow milk for warmer dogs (see chapter 3, "Canine Energetics," for an explanation of warm and cool).

Bones

In a raw diet, uncooked bones (never feed cooked bones) can provide your dog calcium, which supports the health of their brain and nervous system. However, too many bones can cause constipation and white, crumbly poops, and large bones can cause cracked teeth. According to Dr. Peter Dobias, dogs should not be given large bones like beef shanks as they can break teeth. He notes: "Small dogs (all the way down to Chihuahuas) do well on raw chicken thighs or chicken wings. Medium and large dogs should get bones such as lamb shanks or legs, lamb necks, and rib bones (cut into medium size pieces)."[7]

Other choices for bone include powdered bone supplements and eggshell calcium, if you're uncomfortable feeding your pup raw bone.

Treats

Be mindful of how many and what type of treats you're giving your dog. Avoid treats with wheat, preservatives, gluten flours, and artificial color and flavors. Treats do not need to be large—only big enough for your dog to feel like they got something. Be mindful of dryness when giving dehydrated treats, especially if your dog is already dry (dryness is an energetic condition; see chapter 3 for details).

Supplements

Whether you feed kibble, cooked food, freeze-dried food, or some form of a raw diet, consider the following supplements as well.

Enzymes

Enzymes are responsible for triggering biochemical processes in the body, and they are particularly key for gastrointestinal and liver function. Dogs rely on both the enzymes created in their bodies and enzymes they receive from the food in their diet. Processing, such as high-heat cooking, destroys the enzymes in food, and food that lacks enzymes—such as most forms of commercial kibble—strains the gastrointestinal system and liver and decreases metabolic function.[8] The lack of enzymes in a processed-food diet can lead to food sensitivities, congested organs, skin conditions, hot spots, and flea infestations. In raw food diets, certain foods such as avocados, meat and organs, kelp, seaweeds, fermented foods, papaya, pineapple, pumpkin, and raw milk and dairy can be a natural source of digestive enzymes.

Tip! Avocado flesh and oil are safe for dogs. Avoid feeding avocado skin, leaves, and pits (seeds). Another common misconception is that garlic is unsafe for dogs; this is true only in large amounts. Garlic is warming and anti-inflammatory. You can use it to support your dog's heart, immune system, and gut and to keep fleas away during the summer. The appropriate dose of freshly chopped organic garlic is 1/8 tsp daily for every 10 pounds of weight.

For dogs who consume kibble, plant fiber, cooked foods, dehydrated foods, or freeze-dried foods, I recommend supplementing with digestive enzymes. Digestive enzymes can also help avoid stomach upset for dogs transitioning from one diet to another. I also recommend these enzymes (temporarily) for conditions including chronic pancreatitis, low absorption of nutrients, allergies, yeast overgrowth, leaky gut, and excessive gas.

A dog taking digestive enzyme supplements may experience problems if the dosage is too high or if the enzymes are not energetically appropriate for them. Signs that a dog's digestive enzymes aren't working include excessive gas, nausea, vomiting, chronic digestive upset, and loose stool.

Prebiotics and Probiotics
Probiotics (beneficial bacteria) and prebiotics (nutrients for beneficial bacteria) support your dog's microbiome. I recommend rotating different

types of prebiotics and probiotics in your dog's diet. If your dog is cooler (see chapter 3), small portions of fermented foods can be beneficial along with raw goat or cow milk.

Testing your dog's microbiome can help you know how balanced it is, which, in turn, can help you decide what pre-and probiotics to give your dog. Visit the TheHerbalDog.com for testing recommendations.

Healthy Fats

Cellular membranes become inflexible when not adequately hydrated through water and fats, resulting in decreased assimilation, elimination, and cellular communication. These vital structures are composed mainly of fats. The quality of these fats helps determine the health of your dog's cells, including those in the brain, heart, and nervous system.[9]

Pet nutrition scientist Billy Hoekman agrees that the healthiest forms of fat come from unprocessed, whole foods. He talks about pastured meats and eggs being healthy because their omega-6 and omega-3 content is in the correct ratio. He shares that "your dog will always get adequate omega-6s through diet, so if you are looking to supplement omega fatty acids it should be something that is basically only omega-3s."[10] Algae oil, wild-caught fish, green-lipped mussels, and other oils extracted from fish like anchovy, sardine, and cod liver are rich in omega-3 fats that help support your dog's lungs, heart, immune system, gut microbiome, nervous system, and overall cognitive function. When adding omega-3 oils to your dog's food, make sure they are purchased in amber glass bottles and stored in the refrigerator to help avoid oxidation. Other healthy oils include coconut and extra-virgin olive oil. These oils are suitable for health conditions like dementia, seizures, yeast, constipation, and as an ingredient in treats or medicinal (food therapy) meals.

Unfortunately, there are numerous sources of unhealthy fats in commercial dog foods and treats, particularly refined vegetable oils. These oils, which are highly processed and inflammatory, promote free radicals, which can congest your dog's liver, decrease omega-3 levels, and damage cellular structures, leading to premature aging and disease. Unhealthy fats include cooked fats like those found in kibble diets, nondescript vegetable oil, hydrogenated oils, and refined peanut, canola (rapeseed), corn, cottonseed, grapeseed, soy, sunflower, and safflower oils.[11] Try to avoid feeding these oils when possible.

Feeding Guidelines

These guidelines can help your dog better assimilate nutrients, live longer, and decrease their toxic load.

1. Never feed your dog cold food. Cold food causes stagnation in the gastrointestinal tract, affecting assimilation.[12] If your dog's food is frozen or refrigerated, let it warm up to room temperature before offering it to your dog. Fully hydrate all freeze-dried and dehydrated food with warm or room temperature water before feeding.

2. Feed your dog just once or twice per day. Feeding once per day is associated with greater longevity and a decrease in chronic disease markers.[13] That said, dogs are individuals, and some dogs may need to be fed twice daily. Feeding schedules can change according to your dog's needs and condition. For those who feed twice per day, try to feed your dog most of their calories in the first meal and make the second meal smaller. The second meal is a great opportunity to feed broths, raw milks, and supplementals.

3. Don't feed your dog the same diet throughout the year. Mix up proteins, vegetables, and supplements for nutritional variety. You may also want to adjust your dog's diet according to their condition, age, and individual situation.

4. Don't overfeed your dog. Overfeeding puts pressure on the liver and causes gas and digestive upset.[14]

5. Avoid storing or serving food in plastic containers. Exposure to plastic increases your dog's toxic load and disrupts healthy endocrine function. Many chemicals found in plastic are fat-soluble, and your dog's food contains fats. Use stainless-steel or glass containers instead. If you use plastic lids on these containers, or canning jar lids, which often have a plasticized lining, cover the top of the container with natural waxed paper before putting in the lid. *There is no such thing as healthy plastic.*

6. Filter your dog's water. Municipal tap water is often contaminated with the chemicals used to sanitize it. Well water can contain environmental runoff, heavy metals, and other unknowns; even our rainwater contains glyphosate.[15] Bottled water is full of plastic-based toxins, and it's an environmental disaster.[16] Have your water tested so you know

what type of filter or system you need to provide clean water for yourself and your animals.

7. Never feed foods that are poisonous or can make your dog extremely sick. These include caffeine, chocolate, grapes, macadamia nuts, onions, raisins, raw potatoes, and anything with artificial sweeteners like aspartame, sucralose, or xylitol.

8. Don't offer any foods or herbs that your dog consistently refuses to eat. Many dogs are capable of self-selection, and when they consistently refuse to eat something, you can interpret their refusal as a warning sign that the food you're offering may be inappropriate for your dog.

9. Avoid salt. Many kibbles, canned foods, and lower-quality commercial "fresh" foods are high in salt. Too much salt can lead to dehydration, edema, stagnation, and kidney and musculoskeletal conditions. Most dogs get enough salt from a minimally processed diet. If they need more, give them a size-appropriate pinch of Himalayan salt or sea salt in their food a few times per week. You can have their salt levels checked by your veterinarian.

10. Get your dog outside playing in the dirt, breathing fresh air, interacting with nature, and getting age-appropriate exercise. This contributes to a more diverse microbiome, aids in digestions, decreases stress, and increases longevity.

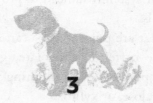

3
Canine Energetics

What is important is that the cure is [on] the same axis as the disease. Suppression occurs when the organism is forced to act in a certain way, according to artificial, external agents, which hide the disease process and symptoms. This, however, does not cure, but sets up a new disease.

MATTHEW WOOD, *THE PRACTICE OF TRADITIONAL WESTERN HERBALISM*

Dogs are born with a unique energy pattern or signature. Plants, too, have energetic signatures, and you can use these signatures to match herbs to individual dogs. When using herbs according to energetics, you'll look at each herb as an individual, know what symptoms it's indicated for, what organ systems it has an affinity toward, and whether it matches the energetics of your dog. This gives you an effective way of figuring out what herbs will work for a particular condition and devising a protocol that gets to the root of a dog's issues.

Working with herbal energetics requires a holistic view of medicine and the body. Let's use the ever popular ginger as an example. We often hear that ginger is good for inflammation. That's true, but the idea that we should use ginger for all cases of inflammation derives from the principles of Western pharmacology, simply substituting an herb for a drug. Instead, we can look at the whole picture. Ginger's anti-inflammatory effect is only one of its many actions. Energetically, it is hot and dry. A dog who is energetically cold and damp will most likely find ginger to be warming and drying and will benefit from its anti-inflammatory action. For a dog who is hot and dry, however, ginger will manifest as hot, reducing circulating fluids and increasing heat. And for a dog who is hot and damp, it can help with drying the damp but at a cost of making your already hot dog hotter and miserable. For these types of dogs, I would recommend rose hips instead because it too has an anti-inflammatory effect but is energetically cool and drying.

The discussion here is only an introduction to energetics, as the subject is vast. However, I hope it expands your understanding of the need for individualized health care. Throughout this chapter, you will see lists of symptoms that match particular energetic conditions. Understand that your dog doesn't have to have all the symptoms on the lists for one of these conditions to exist.

The Five Flavors

Tasting and smelling herbs is an effective way to get to know plants and to determine if an herb is active or potent. Taste involves the taste buds, tongue, and nose (because the sense of smell is a huge part of tasting). But taste and flavor are not the same, though they sound alike. Taste is how an herb feels in the mouth—its sensory effect. You experience taste on your tongue. Flavor is something different. It involves taste but includes smell and energetics. A plant's flavor affects how its constituents are experienced in the body.

For example, consider sage. Most of us know what sage tastes like, but its bitter, pungent flavor has a unique effect on the body. Energetically, sage is warm and drying. I once put a drop of sage tincture under my tongue. The experience was fascinating and awful all at the same time. The tincture had the most intensely bitter taste I've ever experienced. I felt like I couldn't breathe, and I couldn't do anything about it except wait for it to go away. I wouldn't want my dog to experience this type of bitterness! Sage tincture *must* be diluted.

Smell and taste are intimately related, and dogs can tell more about their food than humans can because their sense of smell is thousands of times more sensitive than ours—they can taste aromas. Your dog's olfactory system has tiny hairs called cilia and a protective layer of mucus to help absorb aromas. When their nose begins to smell, the cilia send nerve impulses directly to the brain, where the olfactory bulb processes the smell. Since it's connected to the limbic system, the part of the brain associated with emotion and memory, the olfactory bulb triggers a feeling associated with the scent, helping your dog identify and recall certain smells.

Dogs have more than 1,500 taste buds in their mouth, located on the papillae (tiny bumps) on the tip of the tongue. Their taste buds can detect each of the five flavors: bitter (high sense), pungent/spicy, salty (not so much), sweet, and sour. According to traditional Chinese medicine (TCM), these five flavors are each associated with an organ system. Through the organ-flavor relationship, the flavor of a food carries the "action" of the food to specific areas in the body. Too much or too little of each flavor can put a dog out of balance, depending on its individual constitution. In a parallel manner, we can use the energetics of the five flavors to address imbalances or deficiencies in particular organs. These five flavors can connect us with plant intelligence and herb complexity, especially their action and function.[1] Even though it is a detailed subject, I've included a general overview of working with each flavor.

The Sweet Flavor

The sweet flavor is associated with the spleen, pancreas, and stomach. It can tonify the body. Energetically, the sweet flavor can be cooling and moist, warm and dry, or warm and moist. Many times, sweet herbs are warm to slightly warm, moving energy upward and outward.

The sweet flavor is especially helpful in balancing the spleen. A healthy spleen supports digestion; it also keeps lips from getting dry and gives them their reddish color. Spleen energy helps nourish the body, working with circulation to transport nutrients throughout the body. Weak spleen energy symptoms include craving sweet foods, gas after eating, hypothyroidism, lethargy, and unexplained weight gain. Their nourishing ability makes sweet foods suitable for deficient conditions, but too much can exacerbate conditions of excess.[2]

Warming sweet foods include cabbages, cherries, pine nuts, spearmint, sunflower seeds, sweet potatoes, and walnuts. Neutral sweet foods include carrots, figs, peas, shiitake mushrooms, and yams. Other sweet foods include almonds, apples, apricots, blue potatoes, chard, chestnuts, coconuts, cucumbers, eggplants, lettuces, olives, raw honey, papayas, peaches, pears, sesame seeds, squashes, and strawberries.

The Sour Flavor

The sour flavor governs the liver and gallbladder. It can have a strengthening effect on the lungs. Liver energy is connected to redness in the eyes, blood pressure, hyperthyroidism, aggression, constipation, and insomnia. When there is heat or stagnation in the liver, your dog can be easily agitated and emotionally unstable. Consuming sour flavors can help balance and calm liver energy.[3] Sour fruits and herbs include blackberries, elderberries, decaffeinated green tea, hawthorn berries, lemons, limes, rose hips, and olives. The sour flavor can increase tension, so avoid it if your dog has constipation, a pulled muscle, or a cruciate tear.

The Salty Flavor

Salty flavors are cooling and have an affinity for the kidneys and urinary system. Salt (pure and unadulterated; avoid iodized salt) is ruled by the earth element and helps moisten dryness, bringing life to aching joints and stiffness. It works with the waters of the body and helps soften hardness, pushing through stagnation and supporting detoxification. The salt flavor has a downward and inward movement, focusing on the body's core, where the kidneys reside. The "action" of salt uses minerals to detoxify and soften tissues. Salt's water element helps regulate moisture levels.

Salty foods and remedies can strengthen your dog's body by helping balance electrolytes and supporting kidney and lymphatic health. Too much of this flavor can cause stagnation and stress the kidneys and heart. Avoid in cases of dampness, high blood pressure, or edema.[4] Salty herbs include chickweed, cleavers, nettle, seaweed, and violet.

The Bitter Flavor

Most bitter flavors help clear heat and are associated with the liver, heart, and small intestine. The energy of this flavor moves inward and toward the middle.[5] Many bitter herbs and foods are drying or can be drying when used long-term. Dandelion root is a perfect example of bitter; it can relieve conditions of excessive dampness and heat and has an affinity for the liver, heart, and lungs. Avoid excessive amounts of bitter herbs and foods with deficient, cold, weak dogs. Common bitter herbs and foods include alfalfa, asparagus, burdock root, California poppy, celery, chamomile, echinacea, lettuce, pau d'arco, quinoa, skullcap, vinegar, and yarrow.

The Pungent/Spicy Flavor

The spicy or pungent flavor is associated with the lungs, the large intestine, and the air element. This flavor's warming energy expands and disperses, moving upward and outward. Pungent herbs with an affinity for the large intestine and the lungs can help decrease pathogenic overgrowth. The spicy flavor also increases circulation, supporting the heart, lungs, kidneys, and lymphatics.[6] Pungent or spicy remedies can be hot and dry, warm and dry, or cold and dry. Common spicy or pungent herbs include basil, cardamom, cayenne, cinnamon (Ceylon), cumin, dill, fennel, ginger, mustard greens, oregano, peppermint, radish, rosemary, spearmint, and turmeric.

Energetic Temperature: Heat and Cold

As you can see in the chart below, energetic temperatures exist across a broad range of warm and cool. Hot and cold, at either end of that range, tend to be disease states. A dog's food, herbs, supplements, lifestyle, stress levels, and other factors have energetic effects, keeping them in a healthy range or moving them toward hot or cold, depending on their natural energetic pattern. Note: Dogs rarely go from being naturally cool to naturally warm or vice versa. They are born with a natural energetic signature somewhere between cool and warm.

ENERGETICS SCALE

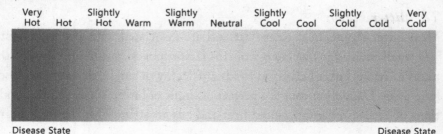

| Very Hot | Hot | Slightly Hot | Warm | Slightly Warm | Neutral | Slightly Cool | Cool | Slightly Cold | Cold | Very Cold |

Disease State   Disease State

Heat

To fully understand the nature of energetic heat in the body, you must understand the fire element. Fire burns and breaks things down. The body mimics nature, and heat in the body moves upward and out. It stimulates, irritates, and increases activity.

An overabundance of fire activity can manifest as redness, swelling, and sensitivity. It can increase metabolic wastes and cause stagnation due to heightened oxidation when allowed to proliferate. Organ function decreases as demand increases. Heated metabolic processes can move too quickly, and your dog's body can have difficulty keeping up. When this happens, warm is quickly moving toward hot. Heat can become acute—for example, an inflamed stomach or gastrointestinal tract.

Elements become patterns, and patterns become energy. When accessing heat, dogs can have a few signs or many signs. The more cofactors (symptoms) your dog has, the likelier it is that your dog is on the warm-to-hot spectrum. The most telling sign is how your dog relates and interacts with the fire element. How do they tolerate heat? Do they seek it out? Do they sit by the fire and bake themselves? Generally, a warm dog does this for only five to ten minutes. Will they choose a cool floor over a warm bed? Do they consistently seek shade in the summer?

What Is a Cofactor?

In my practice the term *cofactor* refers to a blend of symptoms and conditions your dog has, may have experienced, or is prone to experiencing. Looking at the number of cofactors helps determine if what is being discussed pertains to your dog or is well-indicated for your dog.

Cofactors for Warm Energetics

Always "on" behavior	Excessive panting
Doesn't like to lie in the sun	High metabolism
Exercise intolerance	Inability to maintain body
Excessive movement	temperature

Increased appetite

Loud barking

Nervousness, excitability, anxiety

Prone to loose stool

Rapid intestinal transit

Restless, agitated, in-your-face behavior

Seeks out cool places and cold floors

Won't sleep covered up

Excessive Heat

When a warm dog edges slowly toward hot, symptoms of imbalance can manifest. Excessive heat conditions result from a buildup of overactivity and irritation of the tissues.[7] Inflammation may be present, but note that inflammation on its own is not always a sign of a runaway problem. Short episodes of inflammation are needed for healing because your dog's body calls for healing assistance through heat and increased circulation. The problem occurs when inflammation develops past the point of healing, becomes systemic, and causes disease.

When considering energetics, people often confuse heat with inflammation. You might be thinking, What? Inflammation *is* heat. Well, yes and no. Yes, inflammation involves heat, and it's associated with redness, swelling, and pain; however, inflammation can originate from other energetic patterns too, including cold.[8] We'll look at this in the next section of this chapter.

Too much heat is rooted in excess. It can manifest in many ways: excessive oxidation producing free radicals and inflammation, high blood pressure, cardiac stress, hyperactivity, heat sensitivity, thinning of mucosal linings, heightened nervous system responses, and more. Hot energetics often lead to an overactive inflammatory or histamine response. When this happens, it can cascade into hyperimmune activity and autoimmune disease.[9]

Cofactors for Hot Energetics

Acid reflux

Allergies

Aversion to lying in the sun

Aversion to lying on dog beds

Barking in your face; uncooperative

Chronic diarrhea

Dark urine

Excessive immune response

Food sensitivities and allergies

Histamine intolerance

Hot spots (from heat with dampness)

Hypersensitivity (overactive immune response)

Hyperthyroidism

Hypothyroidism (from heat with
dampness)
Leaky gut (though this condition is
not exclusive to hot energetics)
Lipomas (from heat or cold with
dampness)

Pain that worsens with movement
Ulcers in mouth or
gastrointestinal tract
Undigested food in stool
Urination with crying out
Yellow discharge from the eyes

Addressing Hot Energetics

When looking at herbs that can help rebalance energetics falling on the
hot end of the spectrum (hot dogs), you'll find them in action as cooling
or cold. In the case of heat with dryness, a cool/cold and damp herb can
add moisture to put out the fire. When there is heat with too much moisture (damp), you'll look for herbs that are neutral to cool/cold and drying.

Herbs and fungi for warm to hot energetics: blackberry leaf, burdock root, chaga mushroom, chamomile, chickweed, cleavers, couch grass,
dandelion, echinacea, hawthorn, lemon balm, licorice root (neutral temperature), lion's mane mushroom, marshmallow root, maitake mushroom,
nettle, Oregon grape root, passionflower, plantain, poria mushroom, red
clover, rose, rose hips, self-heal, skullcap, Solomon's seal, tremella mushroom, turkey tail mushroom, yarrow, yellow dock

Cold

Cold energetics range from cool to deep cold. Drawing energy inward and
down, cool-to-cold energetics revolve around your dog's core. The cool
spectrum deals with the vital force because the body's energy stores come
from the core. As is the case with warm energetics, you can determine cool
energetics by focusing on the fire element. How does your dog interact
with heat? Do they gravitate toward it and soak it up? Do they like to bask
in front of the fire? Sleep under the covers? Consistently seek out warmth?

Cofactors for Cool Energetics

Chronic shaking
Decreased appetite
Dull fur
Easily fatigued
Frequent urination

Hypothyroidism (though
this condition is not
exclusive to cool energetics)
Inability to gain weight
Lacks thirst

Lacks vital force

Laid back

Likes to be covered up

Loves to be in the sun

Needy and clingy

Pain decreases with movement

Poorly digested or undigested
food in stool

Prone to constipation

Prone to pathogenic
overgrowth

Quiet and shy

Seeks out warmth

Slow pulse

Stresses easily

White or clear discharges

Excessive Cold

Cold builds toxins and thickens fluids. It also affects the elimination channels, causing slow lymphatic drainage, which results in decreased circulation and an imbalance of fat-soluble hormones and vitamins, leading to malabsorption. Cool moves into cold and then into deficiency, contracting, restricting, and slowing everything down. Organ function decreases while energy declines due to a lack of heat.[10] As a result, the vital force diminishes from the body's core. So instead of a dog barking in your face, they lie in the corner, uninterested.

Cool energetics can easily be moved toward cold, such as, for example, by feeding your dog cold food (from the fridge) and subjecting them to too much time in cold temperatures. An energetically cold dog sickens easily, consistently seeks out warmth, and has poor digestion and issues with assimilation. Excessive cold decreases your dog's metabolic functions. As a result, tissue function decreases, including how the body responds to pathogenic attack and immune stimulation. Blood and lymph circulation becomes stagnant, leading to the buildup of toxins. This results in decreased circulation and a lack of cellular nutrition. When toxins build, the immune system is constantly stimulated, eventually leading to a compromised immune system. It's more difficult to balance deficient conditions than those originating from excess.[11]

While too much heat has roots in excess, deep cold is seeded from deficiency, and specifically decreased metabolic function. The organs most affected by deep cold are the heart, vasculature (arteries, veins, blood), colon, immune system, liver, lymphatics, and pancreas.[12]

Cold decreases digestive function, reducing levels of digestive enzymes and beneficial bacteria. When allowed to proliferate, this leads to malabsorption and the buildup of toxins, which causes stagnation and systemic congestion. An energetic pattern moving into deep cold makes dogs more susceptible to malnutrition and pathogenic infection from viruses, bacteria, and fungi. Some of these bacterial pathogens secrete exotoxins (peptides that function as superantigens), which causes cellular deterioration, making waste elimination critical.[13] This results in a downward spiral of effects because pathogens use wastes and unprocessed nutrients to increase their numbers.

Food creates the building blocks of ecosystem function, making digestion a key factor in working with the cold spectrum. Warming both the digestion and the core can help rebalance cold conditions. The goal is to combine warming digestive agents with stimulants that energize and move the vital force. Angelica, cayenne, and ginger are all warming and stimulating.

Cofactors for Cold Energetics

Antibiotic use	Pale tongue
Bladder weakness	Pathogenic overgrowth
Chronic fungal infections	Poor appetite
Dull eyes	Poor circulation
Dull fur	Sepsis (with deep cold)
Heavy metal buildup	Slow pulse
Hypothyroidism	Splenectomy (creates cold)
Lethargy	Swollen lymph nodes
Long-term antibiotic use	Symptoms improve with heat
Low adrenal function	Undigested food in the stool
Low organ function	(chronic)
Malabsorption	Weight gain or severe
Muscle tightness	weight loss

Addressing Cold Energetics

When looking at herbs that can help rebalance energetics falling on the cold to deep cold spectrum, you'll find them in action as aromatic bitters, circulatory stimulants (circulation is critical with cold), urinary stimulants, carminatives (warm digestion), and expectorants (clear mucus). Stimulants are vital for deep cold as the diminished vital force needs circulation and stimulation to gain strength.

Herbs and fungi for cool and cold energetics: angelica, ashwagandha, calendula, cayenne, cordyceps mushroom, echinacea, elecampane, fennel, ginger, goldenrod, juniper berry, reishi mushroom, rosemary, thyme, turkey tail mushroom, turmeric

. . . .

Tip! Spleen removal can cause sudden cold, even in naturally warm dogs. Calendula is excellent in such cases as it warms the core and helps deter pathogenic overgrowth.

. . . .

False Heat from Excessive Cold

Dogs who display signs of exterior heat but aren't actually hot are said to have false heat. This isn't true heat; it comes from too much cold, dampness, or dryness.[14] It's often a secondary pattern, and it can be tricky to figure out. We'll talk about false heat arising from dampness or dryness later in the chapter; here, we'll focus on cold.

Heat arising from cold begins with a lack of warmth in a dog's core. The body builds heat to warm the dog-as-ecosystem. Remember, the body is always trying to get back to a state of balance. When false heat occurs, it seems counterintuitive to give warming herbs, but once you warm the core, the body returns to normal. Herbalist Matthew Wood refers to false heat as a condition of "cellular inactivity."[15] When a dog is deficient, circulation decreases, and so the dog will have difficulty cooling itself as heat rises.

Systemic inflammation increases with heat from cold, which overstimulates the immune system, specifically inflammation in the gut. It causes an increase in free radicals and damaged cellular structures through the generated heat of oxidation. Antioxidants are vital in helping to keep heat in check. Luckily, many herbs and supplements are good sources of antioxidants.

Dry Energetics

Once you understand if your dog is on the warm or cool spectrum, you can move on to figuring out how dry or damp they are. In the dog-as-ecosystem model, moisture rules the environment and it's all about balance depending on how dry or damp your dog is.

ENERGETICS SCALE / Dry - Damp

Very Dry	Dry	Slightly Dry	Neutral	Slightly Damp	Damp	Very Damp

Disease State   Disease State

To understand dryness, you must first understand the water element. Though it is named for water, this element governs all forms of moisture, including all the water and fats inside the body. Question: Are cells made up of water or fat? If you said both, you're right. Understanding this is key when balancing moisture in the body, as it permeates every cell.

Each cell has a fat (phospholipid) layer through which it excretes toxins, communicates with other cells, and absorbs nutrients. Without proper moisture, cells dry up and lose efficiency, causing a cascade of faulty cellular communication throughout the ecosystem.[16]

The water element serves many functions, including allowing other substances to dissolve and flow. For example, water-soluble and fat-soluble components like vitamins, minerals, and hormones all need moisture to nourish tissues and perform their functions. When the body suffers from dryness, a breakdown of both elimination and nourishment begins, leading to stagnancy. Organs and systems weaken; cellular energy is lost. The nervous system is moisture-dependent, and dryness often leads to anxiety.

With dry energetics, you're dealing with a lack of moisture—insufficient water and fats. The first step toward correcting a dry condition begins with diet. Does your dog consume enough moisture and healthy fats in their diet? How much hydration are they getting? Are they eating too much dried, freeze-dried, or dehydrated foods and snacks?

Cofactors for Dryness

Anxiety	Dry elbows and paw pads
Conjunctivitis	Dry nose (not
Cracking of joints	pharmaceutical-related)
Dandruff	Dry skin and nails

Dry stools

Dry tongue

Endocrine conditions

Excessive heat or cold

Excessive thirst/increased
water consumption

Irritated mucosal linings
(dry cough)

Itchy skin

Lethargy

Nervousness

Nutrient deficiency

Prone to allergies

Rapid pulse

Rough coat

Sensitive skin

Skin crusts

Stiffness in joints

Undigested food in stool

Weakness or exhaustion

Excessive Dryness

Heat slows the circulation of fluids, which can cause dogs to be both hot and dry. Determining dryness and heat is important because bodily fluids are cooling, and when their circulation is deficient, heat increases. Water and fats form the delivery system for all nutrition; without them, the body can't function and heat builds. Dryness leads to low levels of digestive enzymes, bile, and pancreatic secretions. This can cause poor digestion, food sensitivities, hyperimmune function, indigestion, malabsorption, hard stool, constipation, and anal gland conditions.[17] The endocrine system is especially sensitive to moisture balance because many hormones are fat-soluble, meaning they dissolve in fat so they can be distributed throughout the body.

Excessive dryness is referred to as dry atrophy. Looking up atrophy in the dictionary, you'll see a few different explanations, such as "tissue and organ wasting," "cell degeneration," and "decreased tissue size." Merriam-Webster's online dictionary describes atrophy as a "progressive decline." In the context of the dog-as-ecosystem, dry atrophy is dryness causing a lack of function.[18] The body's tissues, organs, and systems are compromised when the cells are compromised. When cellular membranes (the phospholipid layer) start drying up, cellular communication decreases, which interferes with elimination. Important fat-soluble hormones like thyroxine and cortisol depend on fats. When dryness occurs, they can't reach their destination at the rate required for normal endocrine function. Both hyper- and hypothyroid conditions can fall into the category of dry atrophy.

The nervous system is extremely important when working with chronic diseases or imbalances. The myelin sheath is a conductive insulating layer that forms around nerves, and it is composed primarily of lipids (fats). Without adequate fats, the nervous system can't work correctly, and the body suffers from nervous exhaustion. A dog in this situation is unable to recover from exercise or stress. Dogs in constant stressful situations—for example, working dogs who are always "on the job" or rescue dogs—can suffer from excessive dryness due to adrenal exhaustion and excessive adrenaline. This, in turn, can affect the kidneys and immune system by drying out mucous membranes (found in the digestive tract, lungs, and urinary tract).

In the gut, dryness can cause inflammation and affect nutrient absorption, resulting in decreased organ function through lack of fluids (low moisture and fats) and insufficient secretions. Total digestion declines, promoting poor absorption and elimination. The dry atrophy pattern starts with dryness and moves through many levels until atrophy settles in. This tissue state occurs in a range with dryness being obvious and atrophy a bit more elusive.

Tip! The dry atrophy pattern is prevalent in geriatric dogs, so keep it in mind if your dog is older.

Fluid circulation feeds your dog's tissues. When fluids aren't circulating, tissues aren't being fed and things start to slow down. The lack of fluids in the dry atrophy pattern leads to poor fluid circulation and dryness in mucus throughout the mucous membranes of the body. Mucus helps protect your dog against infection; it's also critical to the health of the digestive system, as it governs the release of digestive enzymes. Mucosal dryness can affect your dog's ability to break down food and assimilate nutrients.

Cofactors for Excessive Dryness

Arthritis with stiffness

Brittle nails

Chronic constipation

Chronic infections

Chronic stress response
Cracking joints
Cranial cruciate ligament
(CCL) tears
Dehydration
Dry eyes
Dry mucous membranes
Endocrine disorders
Excessive gas
Excessive tension
False heat
Gallstones
General weakness
Hard stool
Hypothyroidism
Insomnia
Joint stiffness

Kidney stones
Lack of appetite
Lack of bile
Lack of saliva
Malabsorption
Nervousness
Pacing
Red or pale tongue
Rough coat/fur
Severe anxiety
Skin crusts
Stiffness
Is abnormally thin or
overweight
Weakened recovery
Weak pulse
Withered ear skin

False Heat from Dryness

Dryness can produce a condition of false heat, in which the primary condition is dryness manifesting as heat. Dryness can amplify heat because it reduces and slows circulating fluids, so the body can't cool itself. With true heat, you would employ cooling herbs. With false heat from dryness, you would turn to moisturizing herbs to put out the fire.[19]

Addressing Dry Energetics

Most herbs are drying to some degree, leaving us with a limited selection of moisturizing herbs. These moisturizing herbs are referred to as demulcents. All of the herbs in the list below have demulcent actions. Remember, though, that diet is an important part of combatting dryness. Make sure that healthy fats are a consistent part of your dog's diet.

Herbs and fungi for dry energetics: aloe, astragalus, burdock root, chickweed, cleavers, licorice root, lion's mane mushroom, marshmallow root, milky oats, mullein leaf, plantain, red clover, slippery elm, Solomon's seal, tremella mushroom, violet

Damp Energetics

Water shows two imbalances in nature and in the dog-as-ecosystem: It overflows or it slows down and stagnates. Too much water, especially slow (swampy) water, has a cascading effect on the entire dog-as-ecosystem, with the liver and lymphatics taking the biggest hit. Yet recognizing dampness can be difficult because it mimics other energetics.

The pattern of dampness arises from an excess of moisture that affects metabolic processing. It decreases circulation and digestive functioning and encourages lymphatic stagnation and swelling. Excessive moisture builds up mucus and water in the body's elimination systems. As a result, you'll see excessive internal and external bodily fluids in one of two patterns: damp stagnation (slowness and sluggishness) or damp relaxation (overflow and dilution).

Dogs can have heat with dampness. Damp heat is associated with an aversion to humidity and a need for balanced heat and dryness in their surroundings. This condition can start with true heat and be exacerbated by antibiotics, pharmaceuticals, vaccines, and higher-fat diets. Dogs with damp heat usually have difficulty digesting fats and have an unsupportive microbiome.

Cofactors for Dampness

Acid reflux	Eye drainage
Acne	Fungal infections
Allergies/sensitivities	Greasy skin
Arthritis	Gut flora depletion
Bacteria overgrowth	Hot spots
Chronic skin irritation	Hypothyroidism
Chronic vomiting	Inflamed joints
Cloudy urine	Leaky anal glands
Constipation	Leaky gut
Decreased circulation	Lipomas
Difficulty digesting fats	Loose stool
Dull eyes	Lung congestion
Ear infections	Mucus in stools
Eczema	Panting when ambient
Excessive mucus	temperature is above 65°F

Poor assimilation	Stinky stool (on a fresh food diet)
Runny nose	Swellings (non-acute)
Sebaceous cysts	Swollen lymph nodes
Sensitivity to humidity	Water retention
Slow wound healing	Waxy ears

Damp Stagnation

Moisture (water and fats) makes nutrients and hormones solvent and transports them and waste products throughout the body. You can't have healthy cells without balanced fluids. Balance is the key word here. With excessive dampness that leads to stagnation, the body's metabolic processes and circulation slow. Nutrient absorption slows; toxins accumulate.[20]

As damp dogs move down the spectrum toward excessive dampness and stagnation, elimination through the skin is common, resulting in hot spots, itchy skin, and eruptions, including sebaceous cysts and lipomas. The liver pushes toxins to the skin instead of moving wastes through the bowels and kidneys.

Unlike dry atrophy, where tissues become brittle and weak due to a lack of circulating fluids, excessive dampness creates an environment in which tissues get loose and weak, lacking tone due to fluid buildup. The main difference is that there is a backup of fluids instead of a lack of fluids. Damp stagnation can take over as toxicity builds and stagnates. This is usually a result of a blocked organ or pathway. Vitality is a product of healthy assimilation and elimination; when something goes wrong with elimination, everything starts to slow down in a cascade of stagnation. Elimination is a *huge* factor in damp stagnation. Organs of elimination include the colon, kidneys, liver, lungs, and skin. When stagnation is present, the liver pushes out toxins via the skin and eyes. The kidneys eliminate toxins via the ears and urine, while the gastrointestinal tract empties into the colon and forms stool. The lungs empty to the colon and the mouth, excreting toxins through carbon dioxide.

Cofactors for Damp Stagnation

Acne	Constipation
Bacteria overgrowth	Dull eyes
Chronic infections	Eczema

Excessive mucus	Sensitivity to cold
Fluid retention	Sensitivity to dampness
Food allergies	Slow wound healing
Lack of vital force	Swollen joints
Leaky gut	Swollen lymph nodes/glands
Lipomas	Thickening of fluids
Low urine volume	Undigested food particles in stool
Poor assimilation	White discharges
Poor elimination	White tongue coating/cold
Sebaceous cysts	Yellow tongue coating/heat

Damp stagnation can be caused by any of the following:

- Antibiotics
- Blocked elimination channels
- Flea and tick medications
- Hypothyroidism
- Liver malfunction
- Low metabolism
- Overvaccination
- Stagnant lymphatics[21]

Hypothyroidism can be caused by deep cold but can stem from other energetic patterns like damp stagnation. With depressed liver function and low metabolism from dampness, the thyroid becomes sluggish, creating nutrient and elimination depression cycles. If you suspect hypothyroidism is caused by damp stagnation, check your dog's T4 levels, which are usually higher, because T4 isn't converting to T3. Randy Kidd, herbalist and DVM, mentions this pattern and explains that the liver might be involved.[22] Therefore, you'd address the thyroid and the liver.

False Heat from Damp Stagnation
Damp stagnation can cause false heat. In this case the heat isn't the root of a pattern but most likely arises from increased metabolic wastes, which increase the body's inflammatory response.[23]

Damp Relaxation

Damp relaxation is a dilution from too much moisture. Dilution causes flaccid tissues that are unable to contract. Processes of nourishment and elimination are diluted. There is an outpouring of dampness; fluids leak and flow, and the dog-as-ecosystem begins to lose moisture. Often dilution leads to a loss of minerals and electrolytes, eventually causing bone and teeth decalcification as well as arthritic deposits, swellings, bone growths, and kidney stones.[24]

Damp relaxation lacks stagnation and is now overflowing and thin. The skin is usually moist, and you don't see much inflammation. Instead, you see undernourishment, depletion of minerals, and a taxed nervous system.

As is the case with damp stagnation, the dilution of damp relaxation affects both organs and pathways. For example, when the portal vein that feeds the liver becomes too relaxed, nourishment decreases. The portal vein communicates with the small intestine and liver, helping deliver digested nutrients from the small intestine. What happens when there's too much relaxation in the system? The portal vein loses shape and slows its delivery rate. Imagine if the tires on your car lost their circular shape; you wouldn't get far. The portal vein is gravity fed; without a solid structure holding its shape, it must fight gravity. When nutrients don't reach the liver as they should, the liver becomes congested and stagnant.

Damp relaxation is the pattern least prone to inflammatory conditions because of the dilution of the water element. However, it's prone to undernourishment through the depletion of minerals, especially trace minerals, which the body needs to function to build healthy tissues, including the kidneys and the nervous system. For this reason, kidney weakness is associated with damp relaxation.

Damp relaxation may result in organ prolapse because connective tissues support the organs, keeping them in place. When fluids dilute, you can get calcium depletion, thus breaking down connective tissues and causing muscle twitching. (Note: Both dampness and dryness can cause muscle twitching and nervous system depletion.)

Cofactors for Damp Relaxation	
Anal gland leakage or congestion	Anemia
	Clear mucus

Diarrhea

Excessive drooling

Excessive menstrual bleeding

Loose tissue

Low white blood cells

Musculoskeletal weakness

Panting even when dog is not hot

Poor dental health

Profuse diarrhea

Prolapsed uterus

Pronounced nervousness

Runny nose (excessive)

Systemic yeast infection

Twitching muscles

Addressing Damp Energetics

When seeking to address dampness, first figure out if your dog is warm or cool. This way you will be able to look up herbs that either cool and dry or warm and dry. For example, in the list below rose hips are cool and dry and turmeric is warm and dry. Try to feed a balanced diet that is predominantly drying so you can balance out the damp. Some nutrient-rich foods like raw milk are slightly dampening, but you only need a small amount for the nutritional value. If feeding something damp, balance it with drying proteins and herbs. Once you dry up the damp, you can find a balance to avoid an excessive buildup of damp.

Herbs and fungi for damp energetics: angelica, artichoke, ashwagandha, astragalus, cayenne, chaga mushroom, chamomile, dandelion, echinacea, elecampane, fennel, ginger, gotu kola, hawthorn, juniper berry, nettle, Oregon grape root, poria mushroom, red root, reishi mushroom, rose, rose hips, rosemary, skullcap, St. John's wort, thyme, turmeric, usnea

Energetic Tone: Tension and Relaxation

Tone describes the relative tension or relaxation of tissues. Are they tight or loose? Are they constricted or do they lack structure? A dog who pulls their cruciate ligament—that's tension. In contrast, a dog having issues with their anal glands leaking—that's relaxation. Often you can identify issues related to relaxation or tension in your dog's connective tissues. Think about it; your dog's organs and bones would float inside their body without connective tissues.

When you begin putting tone together with all the energetics we've discussed so far, from hot and cold to dry and damp, you will start seeing patterns. For example, relaxation is related to dampness and tension to dryness.

ENERGETICS SCALE / Tension and Relaxation

Excess Tension		Neutral		Excess Relaxation

Disease State   Disease State

Tension

Tension can have both physical and emotional origins. Lack of movement can cause excessive inflammation and acid buildup, resulting in tight tissues, jumpy nerves, and spasms. Emotionally, it can lead to anxiety and restlessness.

The normal function of your dog's nerves involves contraction and relaxation as a continuous alternating mechanism. The nervous system runs through the entire body, especially in the musculature. Muscles are connective tissues that keep organs and bones in place. Voluntary and involuntary nerve contractions cause muscle movement. As examples, a voluntary contraction is your dog lifting its leg for a paw shake; an involuntary one is the simple act of your dog's heart beating or eyes blinking.

A state of extended nerve contraction, such as might occur during vigorous exercise or with extreme stress, can cause muscles to spasm and tighten, and tension results. Tension in the tissues can prevent the circulation of bodily fluids; energy becomes stagnant and unable to flow. Tension can be expressed physically, behaviorally, or both. As a result, you might see lethargy, a decrease in bodily fluids, dryness, alternating constipation and diarrhea, vomiting, shaking, and/or high-strung nervous behavior.[25]

Tension causes tightness in the connective tissues, which can lead to decreased flexibility and constriction in the blood supply. Many times, with tension, you get heat. Since everything is connected, the heart and its connective tissues, meaning the entire cardiovascular system, can become involved. Tension tends to affect the nervous system and cause dryness (though not always). Many times, symptoms of tension get worse when dogs are stressed and better when they can work out their energy and then relax.

Cofactors for Tension

Acid reflux	Inability to deal with stress
Acting as if always "on the job"	Low bile
Aggression	Muscle tears
Alternating constipation and diarrhea	Nausea
	Nervousness
Anger	Picky eater
Anxiety	Poor circulation
Asthma	Poor digestion
Chronic digestive upset	Reverse sneezing
Constipation	Tightness in the abdomen, ligaments, or tendons
Decreased appetite	
Decreased fluids	Shaking
Epilepsy	Spasms
Heat	Uncontrollable movements
High blood pressure	

Relaxation

Relaxed tissues are too loose. When the smooth muscles that line your dog's organs and blood vessels are too relaxed, the fluid flow rate decreases. When the anal glands or the large intestine are too relaxed, they become flaccid; they can't squeeze like they need to. This may cause your dog to have fluids backing up or to become constipated.

Relaxed tissues can't hold secretions. Instead, they open and give off fluid. Like an aboveground pool that has lost its poles, the liner gets wobbly and collapses, spilling out the water. When the tissues are too relaxed, the container fails. Relaxed tissues might help cool the body, but like too much water, they may erode a surface.

Cofactors for Chronic Relaxation

Anal gland stagnancy with leakage	Fluid stagnancy
	Leaking anal glands
Diarrhea	Leaky gut
Excessive eye discharge	Lethargy
Excessive secretions	Megaesophagus
Excessive urination	Nutrient malabsorption

Pale urine
Prolapse of organs
Runny nose

Secretion of clear fluids
Yeast overgrowth

Addressing Tension and Relaxation

You can use herbs to address issues of tension or relaxation. Moisturizing herbs help with stiffness and tightness in the musculoskeletal system; they work well for tension. Astringent herbs bind together or constrict tissues; they work well for relaxation. However, before you consider which herbs to use for tension or relaxation, first consider energetics. Is your dog warm or cool? Dry or moist? Then consider the effect of the herbs you're considering on organ systems, such as the kidneys. Many of these herbs have a diuretic component, while others have an astringent component, and as we've discussed, the balance of moisture is critical to ensuring the dog-as-ecosystem is working efficiently. This is especially important in the musculoskeletal system, where joints and muscles need the correct lubrication; otherwise, stiffness or tension can occur.

Herbs and fungi for tension: aloe, ashwagandha, astragalus, burdock root (balancing) California poppy, chamomile, chickweed, cleavers (use short-term for tension), cordyceps mushroom, goldenrod, licorice root, lion's mane mushroom, maitake mushroom, marshmallow root, milky oats, mullein, passionflower, red clover, rosemary, skullcap, slippery elm, Solomon's seal, St. John's wort, violet, wood betony

Herbs and fungi for relaxation: agrimony, blackberry leaf and root, burdock root, calendula, chaga mushroom, elecampane, goldenrod, gotu kola, hawthorn, meadowsweet, nettle, parsley, plantain, reishi mushroom, rosemary, turmeric, uva-ursi, wood betony, yarrow, yellow dock

Energetic Guidelines

The cause of a disease will vary from dog to dog because of their individual energetic patterns and the patterns of their imbalances. Yes, imbalances and diseases have energetics too. This takes energetics a step further.

When an herb is chosen for its energetics, less of it is required for a medicinal effect, and the chance of side effects decreases. Herbs are individuals. They have intelligence and interact with the spirit of your dog.

You won't be able to tell if an herb is right until you try it. Build an energetic profile for your dog. Then compare your dog's profile to the herb's profile. Always consider the spectrum for both animals and plants as a range. Every herb you consider is somewhere on the spectrum.

Here is an example: One of my canine clients suffers from inflammation and has trouble regulating his body temperature. His mom was giving him turmeric, thinking it would help. Instead, it made him miserable. Violet worked better because violet is energetically cooling, and its cofactors include the inability to control one's temperature. In this case, the symptoms and energetics together helped pinpoint an appropriate herb. The more specific and well-matched a dog's profile is to the herb's set of indications, the less medicine is needed for correction and the better your chances of restoring the body's natural balance.

Let's look at another example: Stella, a warm and damp golden retriever, suffers from a chronic liver imbalance. She is a sweet dog who is prone to gaining weight and constantly seeks out cool places. Her symptoms include fluid retention, agitation, sensitive stomach, vomiting, muscle pain, and constipation. Dandelion root and milk thistle seed are two herbs to consider for her liver imbalance. Dandelion is indicated when there is indigestion, stomach pain, constipation, high blood pressure, muscular pain, fluid retention, and aggression. Milk thistle seed is indicated for a hot and swollen liver, general cleansing, constipation, chills, diarrhea, and drug-induced liver congestion. While both herbs are energetically appropriate, dandelion is better indicated for Stella's specific symptoms because dandelion is bitter and stimulates stomach enzymes, bile flow, and urine production.

I recommend writing down each symptom to help you see the bigger picture. Then, for each herb you are considering, ask these questions:

- Why is the herb helpful for these symptoms?
- What are the herb's actions?
- What are the herb's energetics—warm, cool, damp, dry?

It's important to consider plants individually. Yes, they have synergy when blended together, but premade formulas are designed with herbs for a specific condition, not for your individual dog. A premade formula may contain herbs that your dog doesn't do well with, which could be detrimental to your dog's condition. I'm not against premade formulas, but you should consider each plant in the formula, and in particular how energetically balanced it is for your individual dog. This is especially relevant for dogs with chronic illness or extensive sensitivities.

Considering energetics helps you understand premade formulas. For example, if you want to give a cool dog a cooling formula, you would need to make sure you also give enough warming herbs to balance it out. That said, this sort of approach may not work if one of the herbs in the formula is strong or weighted (meaning it makes up a large proportion of the formula) and your dog takes issue with it. This is especially important when your dog is on the hot or cold end of the energetic temperature spectrum or if your dog is extremely sensitive.

Dogs can have acute issues that don't coincide with their main energetic pattern—for example, a naturally damp dog could have a dry, hacking cough. In this case, you would address the acute symptom first and just keep their core energetic pattern in mind. Energetics is all about consistency; short-term care (meaning roughly one to two weeks) for an acute condition should not throw off your dog's energetic balance, even if the regimen works against their natural energetic pattern. When the acute symptoms resolve, you can return to your regular diet and herbs. If acute symptoms don't balance out after a couple of weeks, you must look at different herbs or herbal combinations.

Any long-term use of herbs requires consideration of energetics because you don't want to push your dog down the energetic spectrum toward imbalance. If your dog has any chronic conditions, work with a consistent protocol of energetically appropriate foods and remedies. If you must give a substance you know isn't energetically appropriate, offer a countermeasure; for example, if you must give ginger to a warm dog, give it along with something cooling, like marshmallow root.

Working with an herb's energetics and your dog's energetics can bring about true healing. It will put you on the right path to an effective healing regimen. Minimize the use of energetically incompatible remedies and foods unless you are providing short-term care for an acute condition or working in dietary variety in the case of a healthy dog.

You may have to review this chapter more than once to fully comprehend the material covered, but just figuring out if your dog is warm or cool can help you begin to understand your dog as an ecosystem.

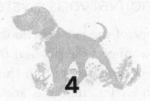

4

Everything Is Connected

*By developing a deep understanding of the ways in which
the patterns, rhythms, and cycles of nature intimately affect
the human body and its internal processes, you can pinpoint
what needs to be balanced and which herbs will do the best
job doing so.*

SAJAH POPHAM, FOUNDER,
SCHOOL OF EVOLUTIONARY HERBALISM

I'm always surprised when I'm told to see a specialist for my eyes, teeth, bones, skin, nervous system, intestines, liver, kidneys, and so forth. Logically, one would think that all of these doctors would like to speak to one another and see how an issue with one system is related to the other, but this is rarely the case in Western medicine. Unfortunately, the same is true for Western veterinary medicine. Nobody is talking to one another and trying to figure out where the disease originated. Your dog's systems, like mine, are treated as entirely separate when they are, in fact, part of an intricate ecosystem and depend on one another for thriving health. When one part of the ecosystem has issues, it puts pressure on all the other parts. Nowhere in your dog's body is there a benign component. Everything is connected. The following pages go through some of the ways in which your dog's key bodily systems work and how they are connected, depend on one another, and form a working ecosystem.

The Nervous System

The nervous system is one of the most overlooked aspects of disease prevention, even though it connects the physical body with the brain. It's a component of almost every other system in the body, including the cardiovascular, digestive, endocrine, immune, and musculoskeletal systems. When you feed and nourish the nervous system, it cascades and supports the whole body.

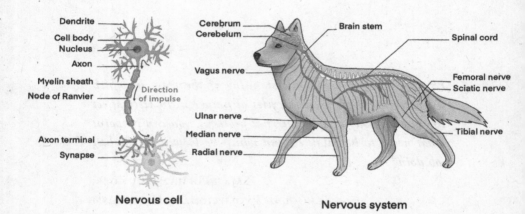

Nervous cell

Nervous system

Nervous System Mechanics

Your dog's nervous system has two parts: the central and the peripheral nervous systems. The central nervous system consists of the brain and spinal cord. It helps dogs interact with the world, perceive threats and act on them, and it governs involuntary movements like muscle contractions, breathing, and beating of the cardiac muscle. The peripheral nervous system involves motor and sensory neurons, and it branches out from the brain and spinal cord through nerve fibers.

The peripheral nervous system is divided into the somatic and autonomic nervous systems. The somatic system helps coordinate your dog's movement and musculoskeletal function. The autonomic system runs in the background, controlling smooth muscle tissue in your dog's digestive system and monitoring stress.

The autonomic system is itself further broken down into the parasympathetic and sympathetic branches. The parasympathetic branch originates in the spinal column (part of the central nervous system) and controls your dog's relaxation, rest, and digestion processes. It's the stress-reducing component of the nervous system and interacts with the endocrine, cardiac, and musculoskeletal systems and the gastrointestinal tract. The sympathetic nervous system is your dog's fight-or-flight mechanism and interacts with the adrenal glands, which releases adrenaline when the brain perceives a threat. This sympathetic response increases your dog's heart rate and gives them access to energy stores that activate the musculoskeletal system so they can react quickly.

The parasympathetic and sympathetic branches of the autonomic nervous system balance unconscious function. They manifest a natural opposition to each other that is complementary and necessary. Essentially, the parasympathetic response turns off your dog's sympathetic response.

The Parasympathetic Nervous System: Rest and Relax

All of your dog's organs except the adrenal glands are under parasympathetic control. Unlike the sympathetic response, which is controlled by adrenaline and cortisol, the parasympathetic response makes your dog feel safe and has a soothing effect on the heart. The parasympathetic system regulates glandular and organ function while the body rests. Think of it as your dog's zen master, monitoring internal relaxation, digestion, and breath.

The parasympathetic nervous system stimulates or downgrades the following functions:

- Blood pressure
- Breathing
- Detoxification
- Digestion
- Elimination (defecation and urination)
- Heart rate
- Production of tears in the eyes
- Salivation

The parasympathetic system works with the sympathetic system to regulate automatic functions like heart rate and digestion while adjusting and conserving energy. After a significant stress response, it helps return your dog's body to a balanced, calm state.

The Sympathetic Nervous System: Fight or Flight

The sympathetic nervous system strengthens your dog's internal workings. This is one of the reasons why the nervous system almost always needs to be addressed when you are dealing with disease. One of the most important aspects of holistic healing is looking at sympathetic dominance, which characterizes the condition in which the body is stuck in or constantly activating the fight-or-flight mode. This type of chronic sympathetic state can be a foundational or root cause of illness. This is especially true of digestive patterns, such as irritable bowel disease, gastrointestinal inflammation, or chronic vomiting, diarrhea, or nausea.

The sympathetic nervous system controls the body's fight-or-flight response. It manages the nerve and hormone reactions needed for this response by releasing adrenaline and noradrenaline from the adrenal glands. Both perceived and real threats can activate the sympathetic nervous system, including constant stress. Even our own stress can trigger a sympathetic response in our dogs; they can smell it.

The sympathetic response can trigger the following:

- Constriction of blood vessels
- Dilation of blood vessels for muscle response
- Dilation of pupils
- Decreased motility in the large intestine
- Increased heart rate and blood pressure
- Increased strength
- Peristalsis of anal sphincter
- Raising the hair on a dog's back

All these functions prepare the body for a fight-or-flight situation. But this quick systemic activation takes a lot of energy. Unfortunately, the body can get used to this response because "always at the ready" creates a mind-body disconnect, resulting in high cortisol levels and depleted adrenals.[1] It also has a negative effect on the digestive system, causing the gallbladder and liver to slow down and interfering with your dog's ability to digest fats.

The more your dog's sympathetic nervous system is activated, the harder it can be to switch back and forth, leading to tension. Keep this in mind when working with any suspected tension; you'll have to address stress to balance your dog out, which sometimes means dealing with your own stress.

Expressions of Sympathetic Excess

Adrenal fatigue*	High prey drive
Aggression	High arousal
Always "on" behavior	Hyperadrenalism
Barrier aggression	Hyperthyroidism
Chronic anxiety and stress	Leash aggression
Chronic barking or whining	Resource guarding
Constantly on the job	Seizures (stress induced)
Feeding off your emotions	

The Vagus Nerve

The vagus nerve was first described by the Greek physician-philosopher-scientist Galen in the second century. A part of the parasympathetic branch of the autonomic nervous system, it is the longest nerve in your dog's body. This intricate nerve, dividing into left and right sections, travels down the sides of your dog's neck, chest, and abdomen, connecting the brain with the ears, esophagus, gut, heart, kidneys, larynx, liver, lungs, pancreas, spleen, and tongue. From the esophagus, the vagus enters the abdomen via the opening of the diaphragm. Then it enters the stomach and intestines.

Common Causes of Vagus Nerve Dysfunction

Abuse and trauma	Reflux
Anxiety and stress	Small intestinal bacterial
Chronic fatigue	overgrowth (SIBO)
Digestive issues and sensitivity	Vitamin B$_{12}$ deficiency
Irritable bowel syndrome (IBS)	

---

*Adrenal fatigue can cause faulty pituitary function, which increases sympathetic excess.

Vagal Tone

The vagus nerve helps regulate your dog's heart rate, which naturally varies with inhalation (increasing) and exhalation (decreasing). In particular, it is responsible for activating key aspects of the relaxation response of the parasympathetic nervous system. After a stressful event, the brain uses neurotransmitters, like GABA and acetylcholine, to trigger vagal activation and induce a calming physiological response in the heart and other organs.

Vagal tone characterizes the effectiveness of the vagus nerve in regulating heart rate and the stress response. For example, you might identify poor vagal tone in dogs who are "always on"—jumpy, reactive, and seemingly filled with a low hum of constant excitement and anxiety. Another example might be your worriers—dogs who startle easily and whose muscles are tight and stiff.

In addition to restoring normal heart rate patterns, lowering blood pressure, and inducing relaxation after a stress response, the vagus nerve is responsible for calming bodily organs like the stomach, intestines, heart, lungs, liver, spleen, and kidneys and reducing inflammation. Low vagal tone in dogs is associated with high levels of chronic disease because the inability to switch off the stress response leads to chronic stress, anxiety, and inflammation.[2] Chronic inflammation can damage organs and blood vessels. Good vagal tone can reset the system and switch off the production of proteins that fuel inflammation.

Chronic stress can create a self-perpetuating cycle: The more stress a dog has, the lower their vagal tone, and the nerve gets used to this state. This issue can occur in dogs who come from a traumatic situation, like many dogs in rescue homes. This is why we must always consider the nervous system in any healing regimen.

. . . .

Tip! Dogs have mechanisms for shaking off stress, like literally shaking it off. You'll often see them do a head-to-toe shake after stressful encounters or events.

. . . .

Vagal Tone Observations

The key to assessing vagal tone is understanding that the vagus nerve works concurrently with a dog's heart and breath. A dog with poor vagal tone will reveal the persistence of their sympathetic nervous system response in the following ways:

- Erratic breathing (you may often see the dog panting)
- Fixed rather than soft eyes
- Hard, always "on" facial expressions rather than calm and relaxed
- Perked up ears rather than relaxed
- Excessive swallowing
- Difficulty eating or disinterest in food; low appetite
- High-pitched bark (most dogs with good vagal tone have an even, deep bark)[3]

The Gut Brain

The vagus nerve travels through the gastrointestinal tract and has a direct effect on what is known as the "gut brain," or the enteric nervous system, a network of neurons inside the digestive tract that regulates digestive functions, monitors the microbiome, plays a key role in emotional responses, and communicates directly with the central nervous system.[4] Herbalist Guido Masé talks about how cells of our microbiome and our "mobile immune cells" can speak to each other. The nerves and mucosal layer tie in together in the digestive tract, and your dog's immune system fights pathogens through this mucosal communication.[5]

The gut brain coordinates with the vagus nerve to calm a dog. Parasympathetic activation slows your dog's heart rate, regulates respiration and digestion, and supports their organ function. It interacts with the spleen and promotes the filtering of blood and flushing of fluids through the kidneys. All these processes occur after stress, so a healthy gut and organs are directly related to a healthy nervous system.

The vagus nerve links the brain to the gut, relaying changes in the gastrointestinal tract through the enteric and central nervous systems. When it malfunctions (sends out the wrong signals), the vagus nerve can slow digestion, creating a domino effect with the endocrine system by slowing hormonal responses.

The gut and brain can both be supported by improving the health of the microbiome. A heightened sympathetic state can alter hormone levels, leading to adrenal fatigue, behavioral issues, and stress that depletes the microbiome. Research is beginning to show that vagal tone is positively influenced by beneficial bacteria and negatively affected by pathogenic bacteria in the gut microbiome.[6] (And since that's the case, think about the effect of the overuse of antibiotics on vagal tone.) Research also shows that probiotics like *Lactobacillus rhamnosus* and *Bifidobacterium longum*, which can help stabilize the microbiome, lower anxiety levels and improve mood and brain function.[7]

The vagus nerve is key to the gut-brain axis, meaning the communication between a dog's gut and brain—and I would add the vagus nerve and heart to that communication network. Herbs with the highest affinity toward the vagus nerve also have an affinity toward the heart. Therefore, these remedies don't pressure the heart but support overall cardiac function.

The vagal nerve regulates many of the functions that are vital to not just digestion but overall health. For example, it stimulates parietal cells in the gut to produce intrinsic factor, a glycoprotein that enables the absorption of vitamin B_{12} in the stomach. Low vagal tone can lead to a B_{12} deficiency, which in turn can lead to inflammation, dementia in older dogs, muscle weakness, alternating constipation and diarrhea, and weight loss.

The vagus nerve also prompts cells in the stomach to release the acids that break down food. And it's responsible for stimulating enzymatic secretions that help combat dryness, positively affecting the microbiome and the nervous system. Dogs with acid reflux often have low vagal tone and food sensitivities due to low stomach acid levels, a leaky gut, and a depleted microbiome.[8]

Digestive Factors Regulated by the Vagus Nerve

Appetite	Digestive enzyme production
Bacteria and yeast populations	Gut microbiome
Blood glucose balance	Inflammation
Bile release from the liver	Motility
Communication between the gut and the brain	Parasite proliferation
	Stomach acid levels

Stress, Stress, and More Stress

Herbalist Jim McDonald points out the relevance of distinguishing between internal and external stress. Internal stress refers to how organisms respond to the stress, while external stress happens to organisms.[9] For our dogs, sometimes that external stress comes from us, their humans. They feed off our reactions. Stress for all of us is detrimental; we must manage it for ourselves *and* our dogs. Be mindful of the media you watch, the people you hang out with, the responsibilities you commit yourself to, and your overall stress load. You and your dog both need rest, relaxation, and gentle, age-appropriate activity in order to manage stress in a healthy way.

Strategies for a Healthy Nervous System

When devising a strategy for supporting your dog's nervous system, first consider stressors, diet, and environment. Consider cofactors, too, and don't forget about dryness, which can negatively affect the myelin sheath that covers nerves, facilitating and protecting the nervous system.

Flower Essences

Five-flower essence, known commercially as Rescue Remedy, is a synergistic blend of cherry plum, clematis, impatiens, rock rose, and star of Bethlehem flower essences. This blend is typically used to relieve panic and fright, and in my experience, it's highly effective for moving dogs out of sympathetic excess. Give three drops three times per day in the mouth.

Flower essences prepared from bitter plants, such as burdock root, gentian, and skullcap, are a good solution for dogs with low vagal tone because they bring energy (and fluids) downward from the head toward the core and heart center. Other essences that support the nervous system include borage, comfrey, fireweed, marshmallow, Oregon grape, Scotch broom (especially for dogs who are aggressive), St. John's wort, vervain, violet, and yarrow.

Nervines, Relaxants, Sedatives, and Tonics

Nervines act on the nervous system, specifically by relieving tension. Relaxants act on the musculoskeletal system, relaxing your dog's muscles while decreasing or preventing spasms. Some relaxants address physical tension, while others work on a dog's emotional and spiritual centers. Sedatives help calm the nervous system and relieve anxiety and restlessness. Tonics strengthen and nourish the nervous system; most act slowly, over a period of months. Sedatives should be used only for short periods of time; tonics can be used long-term.

Make sure you consider the following herbs as individuals, looking at their energetics and your intention when choosing them or combining them in blends. Much like your dog, each herb has a range in each energetic category. Remember that dryness can be an issue with nerve dysregulation; your dog may need a demulcent, such as marshmallow root or licorice root, along with some of the herbs below to help moisten them.

Stimulating nervines: black currant (phytoembryonic), rosemary
Relaxants: agrimony, catnip, chamomile, lemon balm
Sedatives: California poppy, lemon balm, passionflower, valerian
Nerve tonics: alfalfa, ashwagandha, burdock root, fig (phytoembryonic), lion's mane mushroom, milky oats, passionflower, reishi mushroom, rosemary, skullcap, wood betony

• •

Tip! Catnip is indicated for dogs with a nervous stomach and a tendency toward vomiting, nervous pooping, and gagging. Prepare it as an infusion, steeped for less than five minutes.

• •

Adaptogens

Adaptogens provide slow and nourishing support for tissues and systems, including the cardiac, endocrine, immune, and nervous systems. Make sure to consider energetics when picking out adaptogens for your individual dog.

Adaptogens for the nervous system: ashwagandha, gotu kola, holy basil, linden, lion's mane mushroom, milky oats, nettle, reishi mushroom, rhodiola

Alteratives

Alteratives help your dog deal with stress but in a different way than adaptogens. They support the adrenals and elimination organs, including the kidneys, immune system, liver, and lymphatics. In addition, they help with overall body function (metabolism), which includes how nutrition and wastes are handled within the dog-as-ecosystem. Alteratives can have different affinities and energetics; look at each herb as an individual. For example, one of my favorite herbs, cleavers, is cooling and has an affinity toward the lymphatic system. In contrast, another cooling herb, dandelion root, is geared more toward the liver and intestines. Many alteratives can help your dog deal with stress but don't fall into the nervine category.

Alteratives: burdock root, cleavers, dandelion, nettle, Oregon grape root, red clover, reishi mushroom, violet, yellow dock root

Bitters

Bitters can help regulate dogs in sympathetic excess by activating the vagus nerve and increasing digestive enzymes and other compounds, including gastrin, hydrochloric acid, pancreatic enzymes (amylase, lipase, protease), and bile. In fact, dogs have bitter receptors in not only their digestive system but also their heart, lungs, and veins. I learned this from herbalist Guido Masé, who wrote, "The entire GI tract is a sensory organ and not just a digestive one."[10] Brilliant. I love the concept of communicative nourishment and function—the blend of chemistry, emotion, mind, body, and spirit working together for metabolic balance. The gastrointestinal tract provides nourishment for *all* cellular activity. Perhaps that's why Hippocrates believed that all disease starts in the gut.[11]

Caution: Bitters should be avoided in dogs with chronic acid reflux, kidney or gallbladder stones, ulcers, severe gastrointestinal inflammation, or pregnancy.

Bitters: angelica, artichoke, burdock root, chamomile, dandelion, ginger, milk thistle seed

Trophorestoratives

Trophorestoratives are herbs that help restore function to specific areas of the body. For example, milky oats, lion's mane mushroom, and St. John's wort help slowly restore nervous system function. The effectiveness of these types of herbs will depend on your dog's condition. Herbalist Jim McDonald makes a good point about their restorative range:

[Trophorestoratives] act restoratively on both the structure and function of an organ, system or tissue, and provide a lasting effect that remains after discontinuation of the herb (provided, of course, that a reasonable time of administration was given . . . tonics generally take weeks to months to manifest their effects, and no one is likely to experience the full potential of a tonic herb if it's taken short term or too sporadically). It's important, as well, to have reasonable expectations about what is implied by "restoration." If an organ, system, or tissue has degenerated to an extreme, that certainly limits the potential of any medicine to act restoratively if we think that means we'll end up as good as new or close to that. As an example of this, David Winston, who introduced the use of nettle seed as a trophorestorative for the kidneys, tells us of one client who was at 16% kidney function and slipping and who, after nettle seed was added, improved to 28%.[12]

Trophorestoratives can gently help restore function, but as you can see, the severity of the condition can determine the range of healing.

Trophorestoratives for the nervous system: burdock root, chickweed, dandelion, gotu kola, hawthorn, horsetail (phytoembryonic), licorice root, lion's mane mushroom, meadowsweet, milk thistle seed, milky oats, mullein, nettle, St. John's wort*

Essential Fatty Acids

Essential fatty acids are fatty acids that are essential to the health of dogs (and humans) but not manufactured in the body; dogs (and humans) must get them from their diet. (See "Healthy Fats" on page 27.) In particular, essential fatty acids are necessary for a well-functioning nervous system, good parasympathetic response, and good vagal tone.[13] These fatty acids help relieve anxiety, inflammation, and nervousness and support brain function by increasing dopamine and serotonin.

Massage

A simple massage can make a big difference in your dog's vagal tone. Massaging your dog decreases their heart rate and blood pressure by

---

*St. John's wort shouldn't be used in combination with pharmaceutical medicine because it interferes with the liver's P450 detoxification pathway.

releasing acetylcholine. This is also true of acupressure, reflexology, and acupuncture. These methodologies can help dogs who are predisposed to sympathetic excess or live with a low hum of worry.

Pre- and Probiotics

Pre- and probiotics are essential to a healthy microbiome. They help boost immune and digestive function.[14] Rotate strains to give your dog variety; give small amounts of veggies or herbs or opt for raw milk.

The Lymphatic System

The lymphatic system is the vehicle through which the immune system acts.

MATTHEW WOOD, *THE PRACTICE OF TRADITIONAL WESTERN HERBALISM*

Almost every modern-day chronic disease can be attributed to a stagnant lymphatic system.[15] It's a popular belief that one must detox and then detox some more, but no one can effectively detoxify without a well-functioning lymphatic system. If the lymphatic system is not operating as it should, the body will circulate waste without opening the proper elimination pathways.

Diet Is the Foundation for Elimination

Before focusing on detoxification, you must first look at lifestyle and stress, environmental toxin exposure, and diet. In other words, before addressing what's going out of the body, address what's coming into the body. It's so important to support healthy cellular reproduction, mitochondria, and interstitial fluid with anti-inflammatory foods high in amino acids, antioxidants, carotenoids, flavonoids, trace minerals, and natural vitamins and minerals. Diet is the foundation for healthy elimination!

The lymphatic system is a one-way intricate pathway of nodes and vessels filled with lymph, a translucent liquid containing white blood cells called lymphocytes (B cells, T cells, and macrophages), emulsified fats, hormones, nutrients, oxygen, and wastes. It moves in your dog's physiological background, maintaining fluid levels, nourishing cells, fighting infection, and eliminating wastes through the colon, kidneys, liver, lungs, and skin. The only time most people ever think about the lymphatic system is when there is a problem with it. This needs to change!

There are more than one hundred lymph nodes in your dog's body, and they can swell when your dog is fighting an infection or if there is a backup of stagnant fluid. Lymph nodes absorb toxins in the digestive system and neutralize them into harmless wastes. Think of them as little checkpoints along the way. Nodes contain lymphocytes that work with the immune system to determine what type of threat or pathogen your dog is dealing with. When the lymphatic system is stimulated, the nodes produce more lymphocytes, increasing your dog's ability to fight infection. Herbalist Betsy Costilo-Miller notes, "The majority of our immune system resides in the lymph—it facilitates the formation of immune cells, is the site of acquired immunity, and plays host to various immunoglobulins and macrophages that are poised to mount an immediate immune response."[16]

Remember, your dog is an ecosystem; the cool thing about an ecosystem is that it adapts. This is true of your dog's lymph system. It works with the immune system, imprinting incoming stimuli, learning to overcome certain pathogens, and creating antibodies with the spleen. The spleen is the largest part of the lymph system, and it helps keep circulating fluids moving while it (along with the liver) holds blood. When it's swollen, this usually indicates an issue with lymphatic drainage.

Key Lymphatic Functions

Cleans and defends the immune system	Removes cellular wastes and transports them to the liver
Collects toxins from the body	Returns circulating fluids to the blood
Filters out harmful wastes	Slowly drains the ecosystem

The lymphatic system produces white and red blood cells (with bone marrow), developing B cells (lymphocytes) and phagocytes. After this process is complete, it ties in with the thymus gland (which is both an endocrine organ and a lymphatic organ), where lymphocytes mature into thymus cells (T cells). The lymph transports T cells to the rest of the body. These T cells help program your dog's immune system against pathogens.[17]

System Connections

The key to a healthy lymphatic system is the assimilation of nutrients and fats. In the gastrointestinal tract, the intestines absorb the emulsified fats and process them into the lymph via Peyer's patches, which are clusters of lymphoid tissue in the wall of the small intestine that help filter out any toxins found in food while transporting fats and nutrients into the blood plasma. When the intestinal lymph isn't moving, gut functions can stagnate, slowing down the Peyer's patches' ability to filter pathogens and assimilate fats. This can easily lead to leaky gut and chronic disease. The term "leaky gut" refers to the condition in which undigested food and toxins move across the intestinal lining and into the bloodstream. This hyperstimulates your dog's immune system, causing a cascade of negative reactions, including an imbalance in gut bacteria.[18] Peyer's patches depend on good gut health. Everything is connected!

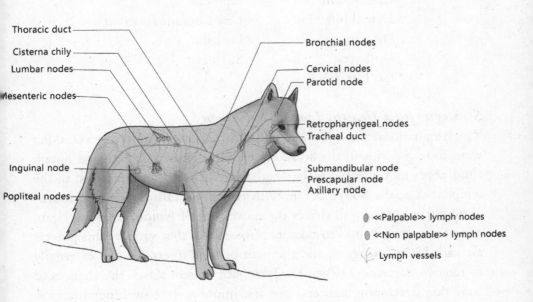

Lymphatic System

Circulation

Blood and lymph are the two major circulation systems in the body, and they depend on each other. As your dog's heart beats, it moves blood through the blood vessels of the body. As blood flows, it pushes plasma, proteins, and wastes into the tissues and into the lymphatic capillaries. The lymphatic system—which can be seen as a drainage system for the blood—recirculates fluids back into the blood, while at the same time transporting nutrients and eliminating metabolic wastes.

Yet blood pressure is not the only process responsible for lymph circulation. Breathing, exercise, and temperature contribute to lymphatic circulation as well.

Stagnant Lymph Cofactors

Allergies	Edema (swelling)
Arthritis	Eye drainage
Asthma	Food sensitivities
Chronic pain	Hot spots
Congestion	Itchy skin
Constipation	Lethargy
Crusty skin	Lipomas
Dental infections	Low immune function
Dryness	Parasites
Dull eyes	Stiffness
Ear infections	

Strategies for a Healthy Lymphatic System

The lymphatic system is the key to healthy elimination because you don't want to trap toxins in the body. For effective lymphatic drainage, lymph fluid needs movement. The late herbalist Michael Moore referred to the lymphatics as the body's ocean, with rising and falling tides. That synchronous push-and-pull drives the movement of lymph, allowing clean, nourishing lymph fluid to take its place. Herbs that support this process are called lymphagogues, and they can be used internally and externally to remove stagnancy. When the lymphatic system slows, the chances of your dog developing cancers, tumors, lipomas, and swellings increase. Lymphagogues stimulate the lymph system to keep your dog's ecosystem clean, send waste to the elimination organs, and nourish tissues simultaneously.

Alteratives gradually restore function in the elimination organs, including the lymphatic system. They support the gastrointestinal tract, liver, lungs, kidneys, and your dog's largest organ, the skin.

In my practice, the two herbs I recommend most for stimulating lymphatic movement are calendula and cleavers because they are gentle and effective at moving lymph.

Cleavers for Warm Dogs

Cleavers has a cooling effect on the dog-as-ecosystem, flushing out toxins, pushing through stagnation, and bringing down swelling in the lymph nodes. Energetically, cleavers is moistening and cool. It works on the lymph fluid, blood, circulatory system, liver, and stomach, making it a superb tonic for the entire system. In the spring, it pushes through winter stagnation and supports the immune system during sudden weather changes. Cleavers works with the tides of your dog's lymphatic "ocean," cleaning and moisturizing tissues. It is safe for long-term use.

Calendula for Cool Dogs

Calendula is a lymphatic alterative for cool dogs, gradually restoring healthy functioning to the lymphatic system, as well as the blood, intestines (nutrient assimilation), and liver system. It brings warmth to the lymphatics and thins the fluids so they can pass more easily through the lymph nodes for processing. Calendula is safe for long-term use.

Other Lymphatic Herbs

Other lymphatic herbs include chickweed, echinacea, ginger, mountain pine (phytoembryonic) nettle, red clover, red root, rosemary, and violet.

The Liver System

The liver connects the breathing and circulation operations of the chest with the digestive functions of the abdomen.

CHERYL SCHWARTZ, DVM,
FOUR PAWS, FIVE DIRECTIONS

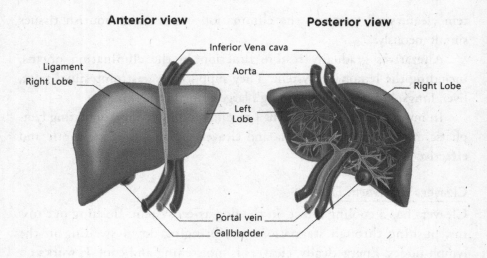

Anterior view

Posterior view

Inferior Vena cava
Ligament
Right Lobe
Aorta
Left Lobe
Right Lobe
Portal vein
Gallbladder

Liver system

Many people think the liver is a toxin-storage organ; this is a fallacy. The liver allows for passive filtration of the blood within two phases of detoxification. Regenerative liver tissues break down and build up metabolic substances, playing a significant role in your dog's metabolism and body temperature. Metabolism encompasses breathing, cellular production, digestion, elimination, repair, and organ function. A balanced liver nourishes your entire dog through assimilation, producing cholesterol and hormones, supporting immune function, storing vitamins and minerals, and producing proteins.

Liver energy touches everything, including the nervous system, as it deals with circulating fluids that can add or deplete moisture. It's important to support the liver and nervous system when working with imbalances because they govern all diseases, including autoimmune cascades, digestive dysfunctions, inflammation, musculoskeletal imbalances, food sensitivities, skin conditions, and blood disorders.

Liver Energy and Connection
In traditional Chinese medicine (TCM), the liver is associated with anger and aggression, it governs the body's ligaments and tendons, and its meridian (energy channel) opens to the eyes. Cataracts, conjunctivitis, glaucoma, eye redness, dry eyes, and chronic tearing are all related

to liver function. The liver is most active between 11 p.m. and 3 a.m. If your dog consistently wakes up during this time, look to the liver for answers.[19]

. . . .

Tip! If you are assessing an organ based on the TCM energy clock, if you are in a region observing daylight saving time, adjust for the forward clock time.

. . . .

Negative Influences on the Liver

Aggression and anger
Anxiety and stress
Eating quickly
Flea, tick, and heartworm
    medications
Heart weakness
High toxic load
Kibble/dry food

Kidney weakness
Overeating
Pharmaceuticals
Poor-quality fats
Tumor load
Unfiltered water
Vaccines

Liver Stagnancy

The liver stores approximately 10 percent of your dog's blood, filters the blood (along with the kidneys), and helps move fluids. When blood circulation slows, you'll see dryness, constipation, poor vision, brittle nails, and lethargy. Poor circulation affects the kidneys, spleen, and pancreas, leading to digestive upset, diarrhea, and vomiting. When blood isn't filtered correctly, it feeds inflammatory conditions like arthritis, lipomas, heart disease, and cancer.

When the liver isn't working well, kidney function increases to help cool down your dog's body. The heart needs support when the liver is stagnant, which helps take the stress off the kidneys and the entire system. The stomach, spleen, and pancreas all wane when stagnation occurs, decreasing circulating fluids and increasing inflammation and weakness.[20] Dogs will show gastrointestinal inflammation, irritable bowels, and possible loose stools (stomach heat). This is especially prevalent when dogs are overfed, as it causes excess liver heat and congestion.

Liver Stagnancy Cofactors

Aggression/agitation
Allergies
Anemia
Arthritis
Cancer
Constipation with straining
Diarrhea
Digestive disorders
Dryness
Eating grass or dirt
Excessive gas
Excessive heat
Excessive thirst
Eye redness or dryness
Food sensitivities
High blood pressure
Histamine intolerance
Hunger paired with refusal
   to eat
Impatience

Inability to stay asleep
Indigestion
Irregular menses cycle
Kidney weakness
Lethargy
Lipomas
Loose stool
Mucus in the stool
Muscle spasm
Obesity
Panting (excessive)
Physical and emotional
   inflexibility
Poor vision
Restlessness
Skin conditions
Sleeping in, hard to wake up
Tight musculoskeletal system
Vomiting bile or water
Weak legs

The Gallbladder

Your dog's gallbladder stores bile and blood for the liver. It contains ducts that send bile to the small intestine for digestive functioning. Bile is an emulsifier that breaks down fats and transforms them into fatty acids, which is vital for healthy assimilation and elimination. (Note: The bile duct also interacts with your dog's pancreas.) Bile is made from liver cells (hepatocytes), bile acids or salts, bilirubin, water, sodium, copper, trace minerals, potassium, and cholesterol. It helps lubricate your dog's stool, activates peristalsis, and gives your dog's poo its brown color.

Gallbladder Weakness Cofactors

Changing positions often
Cool ear tips and paws when
   they should be warm

Numbness in the legs and
   paws
Poor circulation

Scratching first thing in the morning	Stiffness improved by motion
Stiff hind end	Twitching
	Inability to digest fats

The Portal Vein
The portal vein carries blood from the digestive system to the liver, bringing nourishment and toxins for processing. On the way, it connects with the spleen and pancreas, providing oxygen to the liver through blood flow.

Liver Enzymes
Liver enzymes are the enzymes responsible for specific jobs inside the liver. If the liver is the hive, the enzymes are the worker bees. Many clients call me in complete panic because their dog has high liver enzymes. And I'm glad they do; if testing shows that your dog's liver enzymes are high, definitely speak to your vet about it so they can help you interpret those results. In this situation, it's essential to look for the root issue, which might be diet (including treats), energetics, supplements, pharmaceutical use, vaccine history, air and water quality, environmental factors, and stress levels.

. . . .

Tip! The environmental factors that can lead to high liver enzymes include the pesticides, insecticides, and other chemicals used in your own yard, your neighborhood, and nearby golf courses or other venues. If your dog has high liver enzymes, check around to see if they are picking up toxins from chemical exposure outdoors.

. . . .

A dog's blood work will generally show results for the following liver enzymes:

- ALP (alkaline phosphatase) predominates in the liver, bones, bile ducts, intestines, and kidneys.
- ALT (alanine aminotransferase) is found in the intestines, kidneys, and liver. When elevated, it can indicate liver inflammation or cell death.
- AST (aspartate transaminase) enzymes are found in the bile, heart, muscles, pancreas, red blood cells, and liver.

- GGT (gamma-glutamyl transferase) is found throughout the body but predominantly in the liver. High levels can indicate liver disease.[21]

Many indicators of liver imbalances can be seen *before* liver enzyme levels become elevated. As well, many dogs can have good liver enzyme values and still have liver disease, so it's essential to look at other chronic signs of liver malfunction, including allergies, arthritis, autoimmune disease, bowel inflammation, constipation, cysts, eye discharge, digestive issues, hypothyroidism, lipomas, nausea, obesity, poor appetite, skin conditions, and tumors.

Phase I Detoxification

The liver has two phases of active detoxification. Phase I happens through the cytochrome P450 pathway, which filters your dog's blood and neutralizes toxins, using enzymes to convert them into water-soluble metabolites. In particular, it breaks down herbal constituents, nutrients from portal blood, and fat-soluble toxins—including glyphosate, heavy metals, herbicides, hormones, and pesticides. Phase I can release toxic by-products like free radicals, damaging essential DNA, mitochondria, and essential proteins. Your dog needs an antioxidant-rich diet to help them balance free radical production and exposure.

Phase I detoxification is all about limiting free radicals. The liver uses antioxidants, cysteine, choline, CoQ10, flavonoids, folate, glycine, glutamine, glutathione, lipoic acid, methionine, magnesium, pantothenic acid, taurine, selenium, vitamin A, vitamin B complex, vitamin C, vitamin E, and zinc for healthy phase I detoxification.

Phase II Detoxification

Phase II processes and neutralizes water-soluble toxins through the bile. This detoxification pathway helps keep toxins from recirculating in the bloodstream, which can happen if things back up in phase I. Thankfully, these two processes occur at the same time. Through phase II detoxification, the liver breaks down compounds like alcohol, heavy metals, histamines, hormones, and pharmaceuticals. It does this using nutrients including glutathione, glycine, selenium, sulfate, and vitamin E.

Stagnancy in phase II results in a toxin accumulation in your dog's fat cells, which can cause imbalances and disease. Issues arise when phase I detoxification is faster than phase II. Phase II depressants include anesthesia, antibiotics, benzoates, BHA, BHT, BPA, food dyes, fungicides, glyphosate, herbicides, mycotoxins, NSAIDs, overcooked meats, perfumes, pesticides, petroleum-based products, pharmaceuticals (many), plastics, toxins reabsorbed from the small intestine, vaccine preservatives, and vitamin and mineral deficiencies.[22]

The above list is long, but don't worry, because there are many foods, herbs, and supplements that stimulate phase II liver detoxification. These include apples, asparagus, astaxanthin, bee pollen and propolis, blessed thistle, burdock root, chlorella, cruciferous vegetables, dandelion, dill, eggs (from pastured chickens), fennel, glutamine, glycine, grass-fed butter, green tea (decaffeinated), licorice root, milk thistle seed (speeds up phase I detox too), moringa, nutritional yeast, olive oil, phytoplankton, probiotics, red clover, rosemary, sesame, spirulina, taurine, turmeric, vitamin B_{12}, wheatgrass, and yellow dock. And that's not an exhaustive list!

Strategies for Liver Health

In our current toxic world, the liver needs to be supported through continuous gentle cleansing. This can be achieved through diet and supplementation. Foods high in chlorophyll, antioxidants, fiber, and prebiotic fibers help support your dog's immune system, decrease oxidation and free radical formation, bring down inflammation, and promote healthy cell formation.

Foods for the liver: almonds, apples, asparagus, avocado, broccoli, broccoli sprouts, beets, black currants, bok choy, Brussel sprouts, cabbage, cauliflower, celery root, dark leafy greens, eggs, kale, kelp, liver, mushrooms, spinach, squash

Supplements for the liver: astaxanthin, b-complex vitamins, beta-carotene, betaine, choline, digestive enzymes, fiber, folate, glutathione, l-methyl folate (folinic acid, not folic acid), magnesium, nac (n-acetylcysteine), omega-3 fatty acids, phytoplankton, prebiotics, probiotics, quercetin, resveratrol, sam-e, selenium, vitamins (B_{12} (methylcobalamin), C, D, K, E), zinc

Herbs and fungi for the liver: artichoke, burdock root, calendula, chamomile, chickweed, cleavers, dandelion, echinacea, ginger, green tea (decaffeinated), licorice root, marshmallow root, milk thistle seed, nettle,

Oregon grape root, poria mushroom, reishi mushroom, rosemary, St. John's wort, turkey tail mushroom, turmeric, yarrow, yellow dock

Note: Liver herbs can cause temporary itching and excessive eye drainage. Start out with one-quarter of the suggested dose to avoid symptoms. If hair loss occurs, stop the herb, wait two weeks, then start at one-quarter of the dose and make sure the herb is well indicated for your individual dog.

The Skin

The skin is your dog's largest organ and is part of the integumentary system, which includes the anal glands, ear flaps, fur, lymph, sweat glands, and tail. It provides an elemental barrier holding muscles, internal organs, bones, and connective tissues inside the body, giving your dog its shape. The skin is composed of three layers: the epidermis, dermis, and hypodermis. It makes up an estimated 12 to 24 percent of your dog's weight[23] and has a variable pH of approximately 6.2 to 7.4, depending on your dog's breed, color, and stress levels. Nutritionally, the skin stores electrolytes, fats, proteins, and vitamins. It prevents dehydration, regulates temperature, and excretes water, salt, and organic wastes. Ninety-five percent of a dog's skin is covered in fur (give or take some hairless breeds).

Suppression vs. Holism

Traditional allopathic care of the skin focuses on the suppression of symptoms. This approach tends to confuse the immune system, pushing any imbalance deeper into vital organs, like the kidneys or liver, or into the nervous or digestive system, and produces heat, congestion, and inflammation.[24] A cycle of sickness may occur.

The standard of care for most skin issues, acute or chronic, involves administering antibiotics, antifungals, immunosuppressants, and/or corticosteroids. Steroids turn the body off and keep it from responding so the skin can heal, but often, as soon as the steroid is gone, the body goes right back to what it was doing before the steroid was introduced. There is a complete disregard for how the body works and what it's trying to tell us.*

---

*While steroids are typically overused and not always needed, they are certainly useful if your dog is having an acute health issue. They saved my pug Finnbar's life when he couldn't breathe. Sometimes you need a hammer, and allopathic medicine has many to choose from.

The body heals from the inside out, and skin conditions show us that the body is pushing imbalances to the outside. Itching, scratching, biting, and gnawing are all reactions to skin afflictions. Unfortunately, these types of issues can make you feel desperate to find quick solutions. Often you can find something to quell the symptoms, but for proper healing, you must look inside.

Herbal medicine can help by acting as a catalyst to encourage your dog's body to adjust and heal itself. Once the imbalance creating the symptoms is addressed, the body will begin to correct itself; this includes opening your dog's elimination system. Chronic skin issues will require consistency and time, often six months to a year, for proper healing.

From a holistic perspective, the skin functions as a complex, integrated organ that communicates with the rest of the body through systemic pathways, including the digestive, renal, liver, lymphatic, and nervous systems. When you look at how logical the body is, how it functions with its own checks and balances, it makes sense that the body would protect itself by sending toxins to the periphery when the bowel, liver, and kidneys are sluggish. With herbal medicine, we can minimize symptoms with palliative care, but we should not wholly suppress skin reactions unless there are extreme circumstances like a severe infection.

The argument that the skin is an isolated system is infuriating, especially when standard-of-care approaches keep dogs in a cycle of sickness. Releasing toxins through the skin is the body's way of trying to rid itself of disease. When you pay attention, the skin can be an early warning system that alerts you to chronic illness and imbalance.

Strategies for Healthy Skin

When discussing skin concerns, unless a dog has an acute issue like an abrasion, bite, or wound, the underlying problem is almost always a chronic condition. I can't emphasize enough that healing takes time; the body doesn't work on hyperdrive. Trying to get the body to heal too quickly isn't how it works, and pushing it only leads to frustration for everyone involved. This is why pharmaceuticals have so many side effects; they force the body into submission and don't support the innate healing response.

To begin, ensure that your dog's diet is a healthy one, with adequate protein, fats, minerals, vitamins, and trace elements. Pay special attention to vitamins A and E, the B-complex vitamins, amino acids, essential fatty acids, and zinc. Poor absorption of nutrients can be a factor in skin conditions, so the gut must be assessed and healed if necessary.

Thyroid imbalances are epidemic in American dogs and often go undiagnosed.[25] You'll see symptoms like thinning hair, thickened skin, and poor muscle tone. Always request a full-panel thyroid test when you suspect a chronic skin condition.

Supporting the liver and lymphatic system helps clear skin toxins because the liver is directly connected to many skin diseases. With environmental pollutants and the state of our food supply, our dogs are bombarded by toxins. The heightened toxic load can be the reason behind many chronic skin conditions.

Massage and Chiropractic

Investigate your dog's musculoskeletal system for any underlying causes of skin maladies. For example, blocked energy in the spine and misalignment can cause tightness in the muscles, which in turn causes dogs to get on a biting, chewing, and licking cycle. Chiropractic adjustments and massage can be extremely beneficial because they release blocked energy and increase circulation.[26]

Crab Apple Flower Essence

Whenever skin issues are present, I give crab apple flower essence. Crab apple is well-indicated for dogs with any chronic skin condition. It helps cleanse and balance your dog's system and emotional state by supporting the liver, calming obsessive behaviors, and breaking the biting, chewing, and itching cycle.

Herbs for the Skin

The selection of herbs that are helpful for the skin is vast, but almost all of them support liver and elimination health. As you look through the monographs of healing plants in chapter 8, you'll notice that many of them have liver and skin connections. When the liver pushes out to the skin, causing chronic skin eruptions, you can be assured that your dog's elimination systems are congested.

Alteratives for the liver-skin connection make positive changes because they *slowly* open the elimination systems, gently stimulating detoxification. Most alteratives are cooling and draining through their cleansing action. If your dog is dry, be careful with alteratives and ensure that your dog gets proper hydration and healthy fats. Don't give cooling alteratives to cool dogs that are moving toward cold. These dogs need warming nourishment and energetic focus before you begin looking at any detoxification. Again, herbs are individuals, and your goal is to match the herb to your individual dog. There isn't a one-size-fits-all solution in holistic herbalism.

Herbs and fungi for the skin: alfalfa, aloe, ashwagandha, burdock root, calendula, chamomile, chickweed, cleavers, dandelion root, echinacea, horsetail (phytoembryonic), milk thistle seed, nettle, parsley, plantain, poria mushroom, rose hips, rosemary, tremella mushroom, turkey tail mushroom, turmeric, yarrow, yellow dock

The Gastrointestinal System

The gastrointestinal (GI) tract runs from the tip of the tongue to the last layer of anal tissue exiting the body under the tail. The "upper" GI includes the mouth, esophagus, and stomach, while the "lower" GI includes the small and large intestines and the anal sphincter. The primary function of the GI tract is turning food into fuel and separating it from unneeded

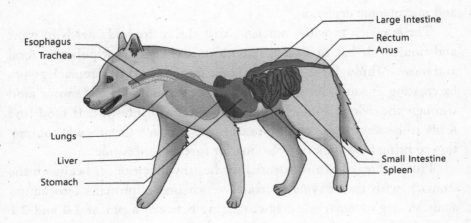

Gastroinestinal tract

wastes, otherwise known as poop. The term for this process is *digestion*. Acute ailments, like constipation, diarrhea, nausea, and vomiting, are all directly related to improper digestive tract functioning. When the digestive system functions correctly, all organs are balanced.

The Upper GI

The upper GI starts in the mouth, including a dog's lips, teeth, tongue, and saliva. Unlike the human mouth, a dog's mouth lacks digestive enzymes. A dog makes up for that in saliva, which lubricates the food, facilitating its passage down the esophagus and into the stomach. Most dogs have a set of forty-two teeth and lack molars. Since dogs can't effectively chew their food (their jaw can't move from side to side), sometimes they swallow it and almost immediately regurgitate or throw it up again. This process is normal and easy for them. It's their esophagus's way of saying, "Chomp these portions into smaller pieces, please." When food reaches a dog's stomach, it's quickly met with an onslaught of hydrochloric acid, pepsin, and other strong digestive enzymes that break down the food into a liquid called chyme.

The stomach is ruled by the water element and is sensitive to dryness. It has dual movement, as it both stimulates saliva in your dog's mouth and helps move food into the small intestine. Your dog's stomach is integral for the proper function of the dog-as-ecosystem. When your dog's stomach is low on acid and enzymes, it won't digest food correctly, resulting in poor nutrient absorption, food sensitivities, pathogenic bacteria overgrowth, and microbiome depletion.[27]

The stomach provides nutrients that the entire body needs to grow and flourish. It has two thick smooth muscle layers that pulverize food and move it through the stomach. These muscles help the stomach empty by creating pressure. As food mixes, the pressure builds and moves food through the pyloric sphincter and into the small intestine. If food isn't ready to be sent to the small intestine, the stomach uses muscle contraction to bring food back into the mix for further processing.

Protein breakdown is essential for healthy digestion. It begins in the stomach with the enzyme protease, which breaks proteins into amino acids. A dog's stomach is acidic, ranging between a pH of 1.0 and 2.1 (though it's usually between 1.5 and 2.1). This is how a dog can process a high-protein diet and even solid bones. Stomach pH is at its lowest an hour after eating a meal. However, the higher the protein in the diet, the more acidic the stomach environment will be.[28] Most pathogenic bacteria can't survive in this harsh acidic environment.

Dogs depend on strong stomach enzymes to kill pathogens, help break down foods into chyme, and transfer those nutrients into the small intestine, where they're absorbed. The stomach is lined with a thick layer of lubricative mucus, which is alkaline, helping it protect your dog against the acidity of the digestive process.

In the mix of your dog's digestive "juices" is intrinsic factor, a protein-based glycoprotein made by the parietal cells in your dog's stomach mucosa (the mucus lining). It's needed for the absorption of vitamin B_{12}. As food is broken down in the stomach via pepsin and acids, B_{12} binds to gastric proteins and travels to the small intestine, where it binds to intrinsic factor. Receptors in the small intestine mucosa allow B_{12} absorption by the portal blood. B_{12} is super important for the dog-as-ecosystem as it ensures critical metabolic functions.[29]

Critical Functions of Vitamin B_{12}

Energy production	Red blood cell formation/maturation
Eye health	
Iron absorption	Serotonin regulation
Musculoskeletal support	Healthy skin and coat

The Stomach and Histamine

Histamine is more than bee stings, reactivity, mast cell tumors, and sensitivities; it's vital to your dog's immune system and gastrointestinal health. Histamine governs capillary permeability, blood vessel dilation, bronchial contraction, gland secretions, and white blood cell production.[30] It causes smooth muscle contraction, stimulates hydrochloric acid production, and alerts your dog's immune system to possible threats.

Your dog's body (and yours) has multiple histamine receptors that activate the histamine response. When out of whack, histamine levels can remain high, and inflammation can become systemic. Histamines are found throughout your dog's tissues, including the lungs, mouth, skin, and stomach mucosa. You can find histamine in blood platelets, brain and spinal column neurons, and the gastrointestinal tract.

Produced with the help of enzymes from the amino acid histidine, histamine is manufactured by the stomach and provided through diet. Breaking it down further, it's released by basophils (white blood cells) and mast cells, among other types of cells. The mast cells in your dog's gut release the most histamine.

Histamine Function

Appetite regulation	Nervous system support
Blood pressure regulation	Pain controls
Circadian rhythm regulation	Pathogen control
Inflammation (for healing)	Serotonin regulation
Memory retention	Swelling

Things go wrong when your dog's body doesn't break down histamine. It causes systemic, out-of-control inflammation leading to anxiety, arthritis, cognitive decline, fear-based behaviors, food sensitivities, insomnia, leaky gut, and pain. Undigested proteins lead to higher histamine in the blood because the amino acid histidine interacts with pathogenic intestinal bacteria and transforms histidine into histamine. High histamine levels can cause many issues, including mast cell tumor disease.

For discussion of histamine intolerance, see chapter 7.

Gastrin

Gastrin is a histamine-dependent peptide hormone found in the stomach and small intestine and responsible for gastric acid—that is, digestive fire. It controls acid secretion and helps with smooth muscle contraction in the stomach. When the stomach expands and moves, gastrin stimulates the release of gastric acid, which is responsible for breaking down proteins. Gastrin helps stimulate the release of hydrochloric acid, which activates the pancreatic enzyme pepsin, starting a protein-digesting frenzy. (The vagus nerve plays a part in this process as acetylcholine, gastrin, and histamine combine to stimulate hydrochloric acid and intrinsic factor. Everything is connected.)[31]

Through neurotransmitters, gastrin tells the pyloric sphincter to limit the amount of chyme coming out of the stomach, thus regulating digestion and peristalsis through the gastrointestinal tract.

The Pancreatic Role in Digestion

The pancreas produces both hormones and digestive enzymes, including amylase, chymotrypsinogen, lipase, and trypsinogen. These substances help break down fats, proteins, and carbohydrates, allowing nutrient absorption. The pancreas also stores sodium bicarbonate, which decreases the acidity of food as it travels from the stomach into the small intestine.

When food arrives in the stomach, the pancreas releases an inactive form of the enzyme pepsin called pepsinogen. Why is the pepsin inactive? If pepsin traveled from the pancreas to the stomach in its active form, it would digest the tissue of the portal vein, causing extreme pain, dehydration, and sickness. This condition is known as pancreatitis.

Digestive Enzymes

Digestive enzymes convert fats into fatty acids, glycerol (glycerin) proteins into amino acids, and complex sugars into simple sugars. If these substances aren't converted through enzymes (and bile), they cause bloodborne allergies.[32] Nutritional deficiencies, inflammation, kibble, cooked food, liver stagnation, and other factors can interfere with bile and enzyme production. When your dog has gas with an odor, it can indicate bacteria feeding on undigested foods, a hallmark of insufficient digestive enzymes and poor absorption.

Digestion Antagonists

Antibiotics	Overvaccination
Fight-or-flight activation	Stagnant lymphatics
Low digestive enzymes	Stagnant portal vein
Low hydrochloric acid	Stress and trauma
Low bile flow	

The Lower GI

The lower GI starts with the small intestine, which is divided into three parts: the duodenum, ileum, and jejunum. The duodenum is the first and shortest section of the small intestine, and it prepares the chyme for absorption by further breaking it down. This nutritive matter then passes to the ileum and the jejunum, which store it and process it still further.

The small intestine is filled with bile acids (produced by the liver) that break down fats. The pancreas provides the enzyme lipase, which digests starches. The enzyme trypsin breaks down proteins and bacteria. Lymphatic tissues (Peyer's patches) lining the small intestine help protect against pathogens. If this process isn't working correctly, it can result in stagnation and inflammation due to toxins entering the bloodstream, referred to as leaky gut. Leaky gut is the number one cause of food sensitivities, malabsorption, and allergies.[33] (See page 207 for more on leaky gut.)

As particles move through the small intestine, assimilation increases and digestion decreases until the digestive matter finally reaches the valve separating the small intestine from the large intestine. Up to this point, the digestive tract is sterile, mainly due to the low pH of hydrochloric acid, which kills microorganisms. However, this changes when waste is passed into the large intestine, where millions of beneficial bacteria are located, ready to finish breaking down digestive matter and process waste. Through the power of competition, these beneficial microbial communities also minimize the presence of pathogenic bacteria.

The large intestine, the last stop in the gastrointestinal tract, includes the cecum, colon, rectum, and anal canal. The ascending colon absorbs water, leftover nutrients, and electrolytes from the stool body, firming things up for evacuation. From a dog-as-ecosystem perspective, the large intestine is the main route of elimination, and most dogs should have two bowel movements per day.

Some issues manifest as slow transit time through the large intestine, including digestive upset in the stomach and small intestine, low digestive secretions, overfeeding, high bone content in the diet, leaky gut, and too much relaxation. Fast peristalsis can cause disruption, too. When stool doesn't have time to absorb water, your dog can have excessive gas, mucus in the stools, and painful diarrhea. Balance is your goal.

For healthy digestion and elimination, dogs require indigestible fiber to build bulk in the stool and support beneficial bacteria.[34] In the whole-prey feeding model, animals ingest small amounts of hair, an excellent fiber source. Depending on your dog's needs, you may have to adjust their diet when feeding commercial raw or home-cooked foods to include extra fiber. I use plantain seeds, mushrooms, and organic raw and lightly cooked apples with their skin. Other sources of fiber include chia seeds, freshly ground flax, greens (including fresh herbs), vegetables, quinoa, nuts, coconut, wild rice, and fruit.

Bile

Bile is produced in the liver and stored in the gallbladder. It is formed predominantly of water and bile acids, with some cholesterol, lecithin, minerals, pigments, and sodium bicarbonate. The bile acids are produced in the liver from cholesterol, which is itself a component of cell membranes, hormones, and vitamin D. That cholesterol—and the constituents used to make it—comes mainly from animal protein in your dog's diet.

Bile breaks down fats and allows the absorption of fat-soluble vitamins like A, D, E, and K, so it is essential to your dog's digestion. It flows from the gallbladder into the small intestine when your dog's stomach needs it. When a dog consumes a low-protein diet, bile production wanes, causing a decline in fat and vitamin absorption and leading to issues like anemia, constipation, vitamin and mineral deficiencies, and weak bones.[35] As well, undigested fats prevent enzymes from interacting with proteins and carbohydrates, which decreases their assimilation, and pathogenic bacteria increase because they feed on the undigested fats, coating the undigested food mass.[36] As a result, your dog's microbiome releases excessive amounts of gas and histamine.

Vitamin E is important for gallbladder health as it keeps your dog (and yourself) from developing calcification inside the gallbladder in the form of stones. Normal to high levels of vitamin E can help dissolve gallstones or keep them from forming.[37]

The Microbiome

Though the large intestine is mainly a storage house for wastes, it plays an important role in absorbing water and electrolytes before sending wastes to the exterior. It houses millions of bacteria that comprise a considerable portion of your dog's microbiome. The gut microbiome, in turn, is responsible for not only processing waste but also manufacturing vitamin B_{12} and K and bolstering the immune system, among many other functions.[38]

Functions of a Healthy Microbiome

Absorption of minerals	Manufacture of serotonin and GABA (gamma aminobutyric acid)
Absorption of nutrients	
Deterrence of autoimmune disease	
Deterrence of food sensitivities	Manufacture of vitamins, including B-complex
Detoxification of heavy metals	
Digestion of food	Minimization of pathogens
Maintenance of balanced glucose levels	Production of enzymes
	Reduction of liver toxicity
Maintenance of immune system	Reduction of stress and anxiety
Maintenance of healthy emotional balance	Reduction of systemic inflammation
Manufacture of anti-inflammatory proteins	Support of good oral health

When your dog's gut bacteria are out of balance, digestion, assimilation, and absorption decrease. The gut microbiome significantly impacts the immune system's overall effectiveness because the various bacteria strains either trigger or suppress the immune system.

Many factors can affect the microbiome, including enzyme levels, diet, pharmaceuticals, and stress.[39] Antibiotics, for example, destroy gut health and disrupt the balance between healthy and pathogenic bacteria. Sometimes they're lifesaving, but when given, knowing how to reestablish microbiome health is an integral part of recovery.[40]

Strategies for a Healthy Digestive System

Supporting your dog's digestive system is multifaceted and, most importantly, it involves a diet that includes whole foods, herbs, and supplements. Below are some strategies to help prime your dog's digestive system and give it what it needs.

Support for the Glycocalyx and IgA

Glycocalyx is the protective coating that lines the gut's epithelial cells, helping beneficial bacteria adhere to the gut lining. Glycocalyx supports a healthy microbiome, allowing for the colonization of beneficial bacteria. IgA production is dependent on glycocalyx levels. IgA (a blood protein) is an antibody found in the mucosal layer of your dog's gut. It helps the immune system fight infection, toxins, pathogenic bacteria, and viruses. Low levels of glycocalyx and IgA can set the stage for pathogenic overgrowth. You can give your dog all the super-powered probiotics they can consume, but without the proper IgA and glycocalyx levels, they'll be excreted in your dog's poo.[41]

One of the best ways to increase glycocalyx and IgA production is by treating the gut with *Saccharomyces boulardii*.[42] This probiotic yeast supports the microvilli (cellular hairs) of the epithelium by decreasing inflammation and increasing digestive enzymes. *Saccharomyces* also increases levels of polyamines that support healthy metabolic functions like cellular growth and survival, which are key to disease prevention.

Supplementation with *S. boulardii* can help beneficial bacteria colonize, support, and repair the gut mucosal layer and increase glycocalyx and IgA production. Regimen duration is usually four to eight weeks, followed by giving pre- and probiotics.

Saccharomyces help rid the body of heavy metals and may cause lethargy. It also can cause constipation and itching if introduced too quickly. Start slow, and work up to five to ten billion organisms.

Probiotic Soil-Based Organisms

Our ancestors—and our ancestors' dogs—spent much time digging in the dirt, filling their bodies with many beneficial microorganisms. I remember eating carrots, peas, and beans straight out of my dad's huge, organically grown garden. My dog Susie would nibble on them too, and we both got a good dusting of healthy soil with our veggies. My dad's soil was a source of pride and nourished the plants and surrounding ecosystem. His garden teemed with life because he used companion planting instead of pesticides and herbicides. He utilized fish waste and horse manure in his compost pile to avoid chemical fertilizers. It turns out humans and animals aren't the only ones with a microbiome; the soil has its own, called a microbiota.

Our soils support the plants and animals grazing on them. We are all soil caretakers, and taking care of this precious earth is important for all our bodies. Clean soils are full of healthy microorganisms. Exploring soil-based organisms (SBOs) as a supplement can help improve gut health especially if your dog suffers from gastrointestinal stress, antibiotic damage, or low immunity. I highly recommend trying them for dogs with food sensitivities, leaky gut, or vaccine damage or for those exposed to environmental toxins.

The difference between regular probiotics and soil-based organisms (SBOs) is that most probiotics move through the colon, while soil-based organisms (*Bacillus coagulans, Bacillus indicus,* and *Bacillus subtilis*) work by colonizing the large intestine. Regular probiotics are easily destroyed by stomach acid and enzymes.[43] This is why high levels (billions) of probiotics are needed in your chosen source or formula, or why many companies put probiotics in special pill cases to help them survive the stomach's harsh conditions.

When SBOs find their environment inhospitable, they curl up and hide, going dormant, which allows them to travel safely through the gut. Once they reach their happy place, they reawaken and flourish.[44]

· ·

Tip! Before you start any probiotic supplement, get your dog's gut biome tested so you know what their gut needs. This helps prevent dominance by any certain species. If you can't afford testing, rotate, rotate, rotate.

· ·

Fulvic and Humic Acid

Fulvic acid contains humic acid but not all humic acid contains fulvic acid. Both humic and fulvic acid help support the work of the microbiome and probiotics. Fulvic acid is sourced from decayed organic matter and has high levels of antioxidants, electrolytes, and trace minerals. It helps balance your dog's microbiome, increases assimilation of nutrients, and helps rid the body of heavy metals and glyphosate.[45] Research shows that fulvic acid balances electrolytes and improves a dog's cellular access to nutrients and oxygen, strengthening your dog's immune response.[46]

Humic acid is also sourced from earth. Like fulvic acid, it has high levels of trace minerals, and it has a pulling nature, helping rid the body of foreign toxins like pesticides and herbicides. When purchasing supplements, I focus on fulvic acid knowing I'm getting humic acid too.

You can naturally incorporate fulvic acid into your dog's diet by feeding different types of organically grown root crops, such as dandelion root and out-of-the-garden, dirt-on carrots and parsnips. If you plan on using fulvic acid supplements, make sure you go slow and don't give too much, as they can cause loose stool or stomach upset when too much is given too quickly.

Gastro Herbs

The selection of herbs that support the digestive system is vast and wide. As always, consider energetics and cofactors when choosing any herb. Below you'll find a list of the herbs I use most often for gastrointestinal conditions in my practice. Review their monographs in chapter 8 to see which ones might be helpful for your dog.

Herbs and fungi for gastrointestinal health: agrimony, aloe, artichoke, blackberry leaf, burdock root, calendula, chaga mushroom, chamomile, dandelion, ginger, gotu kola, lemon balm, licorice root, lion's mane mushroom, marshmallow root, meadowsweet, milk thistle seed, parsley, plantain, poria mushroom, reishi mushroom, rosemary, slippery elm, tremella mushroom, turkey tail mushroom, turmeric, violet, wood betony, yarrow, yellow dock

The Cardiovascular System

The cardiovascular system isn't a pump and tubes—it's a rhythm and communication system. Just like the nervous system and immunity.

GUIDO MASÉ, "A NEW TAKE ON
CARDIOVASCULAR RISK," *HERBAL CLINICIAN IV*

Your dog's heart is interconnected within its ecosystem, functioning like a conductor of life. It works with the blood to feed and nourish cellular structures and keep your dog connected to its surroundings, including you. Heart flow is governed by the nervous system's electrical impulses and the matrix's holding space, the interstitial fluid surrounding your dog's cells.

Heart Energy

According to traditional Chinese medicine, the heart is most active in the summer. Like the sun is the center of our planet's ecosystem, the heart sits at the center of your dog's body. Summer helps calm the nervous system, support vitality, and strengthen the immune system and organs.[47] This is the heart's responsibility, which it carries out through its relationship with the blood, endocrine system, lungs, lymph, nerves, and kidneys. Holistically, your dog's heart reaches out, connecting with you through your dog's heart-generated electromagnetic field, which radiates outward, syncing up with your own heart center.[48]

Joy activates the heart as it radiates and supports parasympathetic activity. Over a twenty-four-hour cycle, the heart is most active between 11 a.m. and 3 p.m., and the heart's protective membrane, the pericardium, between 7 p.m. and 11 p.m.[49] If you suspect your dog is having heart issues, observe them during this window of time, checking for discomfort. Heart conditions can get more severe in summer, but it's the best time for heart support and strengthening.

Heart Function

Your dog's heart has four sections: two atria (*atria* is the plural of *atrium*) and two ventricles. The atria draw in blood, and it exits through the ventricles. The right side of your dog's heart takes deoxygenated blood and disperses it to the lungs, where it's saturated with oxygen. Oxygenated blood returns to the left side of your dog's heart, where it is again dispersed for cellular nourishment.

The autonomic nervous system controls the heart, perfectly orchestrating your dog's heartbeat. The heart feeds every cell through the blood, distributes hormones, and supports the nervous system. To make this happen, cardiac vessels constantly expand and contract, creating movement through veins, arteries, and capillaries. Capillaries are tiny but mighty because they allow chemicals and constituents in and out of the bloodstream. Depending on where they are found in the dog-as-ecosystem, they can be more structured, sturdy, or permeable.

Heart Weakness Cofactors	
Agitation	Diarrhea
Constipation	Discerning appetite
Crack down the center of the tongue	Dry energetics
	Easily tired

Excessive panting after
exercise
Excessive sleep paddling
Excessive thirst
Focal seizures
Hot energetics
Inability to gain or
maintain weight
Lethargy

Nausea
Nervous diarrhea
Nervous peeing
Overheating
Poor appetite
Restlessness
Sensitivity
Vomiting (chronic)

System Connections

The heart center is a foundational organ because your dog's body depends on specific oxygen levels and detoxifying toxins, including carbon dioxide. Hormones in the blood and those from the heart mix with nutrients, helping support musculoskeletal and brain integrity. For example, the heart helps protect your dog's brain from the effects of stress by producing hormones.

The heart's endocrine component is far-reaching through its production of ANF (atrial natriuretic factor), which interacts with your dog's adrenal glands, brain, eyes, kidneys, liver, lungs, pineal and pituitary glands, reproductive system, and small intestine. Heart blood cycles, eventually moving through the kidneys, stimulating red blood cells, and supporting immune health, while extracting toxins from the liver through the urine once released from the blood.

The liver can affect blood movement when it becomes overactive in phase I detoxification, as it stores and circulates blood as part of its overall function. When the liver isn't working correctly, it can influence your dog's heart rate and blood flow. According to Dr. Andrew Armour, the heart has more than 35,000 neurons that form a specialized network that communicates with the rest of the body. This brings new meaning to the idea of "heart intelligence." Armour's team of researchers has essentially discovered that the neurons in the heart act similarly to the neurons in the brain.[50]

Strategies for Heart Health

As a clinical canine herbalist, rather than a veterinarian, I don't deal too much with heart disease. Instead, I work to support and prevent cardiovascular disease, using primarily herbs and diet. With preventive medicine, you get into a support mind-set rather than a reactive one. Applying energetics, stress management (for you and your pup), and the cardiac system's interconnectedness, you are ensuring that your dog's heart has what it needs to flourish and maintain the integrity of physiological systems.

Holistically, one of the best ways to support heart function is to reduce systemic inflammation because the cardiac muscle is one of the most concentrated hubs for cellular mitochondria, the energy-producing centers of cells.[51] Inflammation is a complex issue in the heart and its vasculature. Through interaction with the liver, the heart encounters oxidative stress. This process affects your dog's cellular structures, including mitochondria. The effects of inflammation are systemic and damaging to the heart's network of veins and arteries by increasing heat production. This can slow down circulation—and every organ needs good blood volume to keep them moist and nourished.

The heart nourishes the entire liver system, including the pancreas and spleen. Heart disease puts pressure on the pancreas and spleen, directly affecting the gastrointestinal system, and ends up decreasing liver and immune functions.[52]

Foods for heart support: artichoke, arugula, asparagus, avocado, blueberries, bok choy, celery, chard, collards, eggs, grass-fed raw dairy, butter or ghee, grass-fed meats and organs, green tea (decaffeinated), kale, lettuce, mushrooms, seaweed, strawberries, string beans, sweet potatoes, wild salmon

Supplements for heart support: CoQ10, digestive enzymes, lecithin, taurine, ubiquinol, vitamins (B-complex, C, D, K, E)

Herbs and fungi for heart support: astragalus, burdock, calendula, dandelion, ginger, gotu kola, green tea (decaffeinated), hawthorn, maitake mushroom, milk thistle seed, milky oats, red clover, reishi mushroom, rose, rosemary, turmeric

The Respiratory System

The Lung serves as mediator between the inner and outer world. This Organ is the first line of defense.
KAT MAIER, *ENERGETIC HERBALISM*

The lungs are where the outer world meets your dog's immune system. Your dog's respiratory system includes the throat, back of the mouth (nasopharynx), windpipe (trachea), voice box (larynx), air passages (bronchi), and lungs, as well as the sinus passages below the eyes. The larynx, a network of muscle, cartilage, and soft tissue, ensures your dog doesn't get food into their trachea and covers the opening when your dog swallows. The trachea opens into the lungs and then splits into the two bronchi, one on the left and one on the right. Inside the lung cavity, these bronchi branch off again into bronchioles, the smallest airways in the lungs, which themselves conclude in small sacs known as alveoli, where the lungs exchange oxygen and carbon dioxide through breathing.[53]

Breathing

The lungs are deeply connected to the rest of your dog's body. They combine in the act of breathing, intertwined with the central nervous system, musculoskeletal system (which protects and grounds the lungs), and circulatory system. By the simple action of inhaling and exhaling, your dog not only exchanges carbon dioxide for oxygen but also protects their body from pathogens.

Oxygen is needed for cell energy; every system in your dog's body depends on oxygen-rich blood. Respiration brings oxygen into the body and disperses it. Deep, full breaths are needed for a balanced ecosystem. Depending on the size of your dog, respiration rates can vary from ten to thirty-five breaths per minute.[54] As it can in humans, respiration rate can increase when a dog exercises or has a frightening experience. Panting while resting is also normal, as this is how dogs cool their bodies; however, chronic panting or high respiratory rates are abnormal and should be brought to the attention of a vet.

. . . .

Tip! Make sure you know your dog's baseline respiration rate by counting the number of breaths per minute when your dog is relaxed. This will give you an idea of how much their respiration rate has increased or decreased if your dog has any type of emergency or breathing issue.

. . . .

As your dog breathes, the respiratory system filters the air through the mucus that lines the passages through their nose and lungs. This mucosal lining works with the immune system to remove toxins in the air, isolating them so they can be removed or neutralized via immune modulation. The lungs moisturize and warm incoming air, trapping inhaled pathogens. Most particulates are trapped in their mucosal membranes, coughed up, and/or swallowed.

Mucus

Most people look at mucus with some disgust. When it is imbalanced, mucus can cause many issues, including lung congestion, digestive upset, and thick, gooey stools (yuck). But this is because your dog's internal tissues are covered in mucus, which is an integral part of their immune system, sense of smell, and pathogen protection system.[55] Mucus is a balance: not too much, not too little.

Lung Energy and Connections

According to traditional Chinese medicine, the lungs and colon are linked because the lungs work with the large intestine, sweeping wastes and fluids downward, while moisturizing the skin. The lungs work with the heart (via circulation and blood exchange) and the kidneys for balance.[56] When the kidneys call for aid, the lungs respond with moisture. The kidneys can borrow moisture from the lungs when they experience dryness. This works fine for acute situations, but chronic moisture removal will result in lung dryness, with conditions like a dry cough or more severe conditions like asthma. The large intestine helps rid the body of wastes by extracting metabolic wastes, which in turn helps keep the skin healthy and a dog's coat shiny.

Josie Beug, a veterinarian and traditional Chinese medicine practitioner, teaches that the lung and large intestine meridians (energy channels) run down a dog's front leg and through the dew claw to the first digit of the paw.[57] Lung energy peaks between 3:00 and 5:00 a.m., with large intestine energy following between 5:00 and 7:00 a.m. If your dog consistently wakes up at this time, look to the lungs and large intestine for answers.[58]

In traditional Chinese medicine, the lungs are said to process the emotions of grief and sadness (yes, dogs can feel grief). If grief isn't processed, it can settle in the lungs and affect the smooth muscles, decreasing oxygenation.[59] I experienced this with my pug Francis who died of a broken heart in 2017. In late December of the previous year, my first pug Finnbar had passed away, shortly before his eighteenth birthday. Finnbar and Francis were bonded pugs and had spent most of their lives together. After the day Finnbar passed, Francis's tail never went up again. At the beginning of January, I brought Francis in for her bi-yearly X-ray to see how she was doing, and her lungs looked great. By the beginning of March, however, her respiratory rate increased to the point that it was noticeable. I assumed it was heat or congestion and didn't think much of it since her X-ray just two months earlier had been clear. We kept moving forward. Two weeks later, Francis passed away. A final X-ray had shown tumors in her lungs. I thought, how could tumors grow so quickly? Unprocessed grief was my answer. My vet was dumbfounded. Little Fran was so heartbroken over Finn's passing that she never recovered.

I learned a valuable lesson from Francis. She was my heart dog, and I had to do a deep dive into grief's function, its relation to the lungs, and how to effectively deal with the grief of a loved one while moving forward. Lesson? Stuck energy (grief) festers and can manifest in the physical body. Yes, this example is anecdotal, but more and more I hear stories of dogs and people who have chronic lung conditions like tumors, asthma, and pneumonia and have suffered deep loss and grief. It's definitely something to consider.

Respiratory Weakness Cofactors

Allergies	Heartworm disease
Diabetes	Chronic constipation
Elbows out posture	Poor microbiome health
Exercise intolerance	Kennel cough vaccine
Gagging	Periodontal disease
Grief	Wheezing
Heart disease	

Inflammation

Inflammation that runs amok may cause short- or long-term lung conditions, like airborne allergen reactivity, chronic coughing, and/or wheezing.

It can make your dog more susceptible to lung-based bacterial and viral infections. Indoor air pollution is a big issue because most dogs spend so much time inside. Paint, upholstery, carpet, mold spores, household chemicals, fire retardants . . . the list of vectors goes on and on. Outdoor air pollution can also affect your dog's lung health, of course, but due to its insidious and ever-present character, indoor air quality has proven to be worse for dog health. One of the best things you can do for yourself and your dog is to invest in high-quality whole-house or room-specific air filtration systems.[60] Another good strategy for lung health is making sure to get outside often, where you and your dog can breathe the fresh air. You will both benefit from (age-appropriate) gentle walking and exercise.

Dry Lung Conditions

Lung tightness is a common symptom of dryness, especially when the lungs are imbalanced. Dried-out mucus can be a concern. Usually mucus is considered a damp symptom; in dry conditions, mucus becomes thick and solid. Dogs might cough this up and then spit it out or swallow it. (I know: gross.)

When dealing with a dry cough, most people focus on stopping the cough. The goal instead should be to heal and clear the lungs; for this to happen, expectoration must occur. The gunk needs to come out. Many herbs will temporarily increase coughing because they have an expectorant quality. They can soothe your dog's lungs and throat, reducing inflammation and irritation.

Increasing moisture is also essential so the dryness doesn't lead to fluid loss and deeper infection levels. If your dog has dry energetics, you'll see systemic improvement by adding moisture through herbs and foods. The herbs to look for are demulcents, which add moisture.

Herbs and fungi for dry conditions: licorice root, lion's mane mushroom, marshmallow root, mullein leaf, plantain (balancing), slippery elm, tremella mushroom, violet

Damp Lung Conditions

Wet lung conditions can have different degrees of moisture, especially in the lower respiratory tract. Dampness can cause labored breathing and discomfort due to stuck fluids. Usually this is an energetically cold condition that needs warmth and warming herbs like ginger. With dampness in the lungs, you would want to avoid dairy because it causes more congestion, including clogged sinuses. The goal is to dry these conditions and move mucus up and out. When wet conditions settle in, they can lead to inflammation, bacterial infections, and pneumonia.

Herbs and fungi for damp conditions: angelica, cordyceps mushroom, elecampane, ginger, osha root, plantain (balancing)

Strategies for Healthy Lungs

Some simple measures to improve lung health include the following:

- Increase oxygen levels through exercise.
- Invest in a high-quality air purification system.
- Make sure your home has proper ventilation.
- Supply adequate natural anti-inflammatory and immune-boosting vitamins like A, C, and E.
- Supply essential fatty acids, antioxidants, and quercetin, whether through diet, herbs, or whole-food supplementation. These substances help decrease inflammation and free radicals that attack healthy lung cells.
- Utilize acupuncture, chiropractic, or massage if needed. These practices relax muscles, improve diaphragm function, and activate the vagus nerve helping your dog with stress and tension.

Herbs to Support the Respiratory System

As a canine herbalist, I mainly deal with bronchial conditions (inflammation from various conditions like allergies), collapsed trachea (a marker of excessive relaxation), coughs, excessive sneezing, mild colds, mold exposure, nasal cavity inflammation, and pneumonia support. Almost all these conditions are either viral or bacterial based. Herbal support starts with determining if the lungs are too dry or moist and then focuses on stimulating and modulating the immune system, supporting the lymphatics, and opening elimination channels. Another consideration is stress. Excess stress can tax the nervous system by activating your dog's fight-or-flight system (sympathetic nervous system), which can cause rapid breathing, lung spasms, and excess gagging.

Herbs for spasmodic cough: angelica, bee balm, chamomile, elecampane, licorice, mullein, passionflower, red clover, skullcap

Herbs and fungi for immune support: astragalus, cordyceps mushroom, echinacea, ginger, goldenseal, Oregon grape root, reishi mushroom, turkey tail mushroom, turmeric, usnea

The Renal System

The kidney acts like the roots of a tree carrying water and nutrients into the body and filtering toxins out. It aids the lungs in extracting moisture from the air and the spleen/ pancreas in extracting moisture from food.

CHERYL SCHWARTZ, DVM,
FOUR PAWS, FIVE DIRECTIONS

Your dog's renal system consists of the kidneys, bladder, ureters, and urethra. The kidneys, like the liver, filter blood and preserve, process, and balance chemicals like amino acids, glucose, phosphorus, potassium, and sodium. In addition, they help maintain balanced fluid levels while secreting hormones that regulate blood pressure and communicate with bone marrow when red blood cell counts are low. In filtering blood, the kidneys reabsorb glucose, salts, and water into the bloodstream, leaving urine (comprising toxins and other substances) as waste. The urine flows from each kidney through a ureter into the bladder and then into the urethra for evacuation.

When dryness is allowed to proliferate, the body dehydrates, weakening cells and causing organ tension. This can negatively affect the kidneys' ability to regulate electrolytes and eliminate wastes.

Kidney Mechanics

Your dog's kidneys keep them alive through active filtering—they filter the totality of your dog's entire blood volume in less than an hour! How? Through nephrons, or filtering units—close to 400,000 of them. Each nephron has a small blood filter (glomerulus) and a tube-shaped transport responsible for reabsorption and waste removal. So, first blood gets filtered, creating urine; then fluids go through the tubules for redistribution and excretion.

Urine is a collection of ammonia, inactive hormones, proteins, salt, urea, and water. The kidneys are directly connected to your dog's liver, and urea is one of the by-products of the liver doing its job. Your dog's liver produces ammonia, a nitrogen-rich waste product, from protein synthesis. It mixes with carbon, hydrogen, and oxygen to form urea, which forms urine through the nephron filtration system.[61]

Kidney Energy and Connections

In holistic herbalism, traditional Chinese medicine, and Ayurveda, the kidneys are said to govern the musculoskeletal system, generate circulation, and cool and heat your dog's body. Wintertime is the season of the kidney; this is when you will see more arthritis, bladder infections, incontinence, stones/gravel, and kidney disease than in any other season. In winter, kidneys may get dry. In this situation, you might notice your dog groaning when they lie down or having difficulty getting comfortable, constantly readjusting their position.

According to traditional Chinese medicine, the kidneys are most active between 5:00 p.m. and 7:00 pm and the bladder between 3:00 p.m. and 5:00 p.m.[62] If you suspect any kidney dysfunction, observe your dog during these times, noticing if they are having any exaggerated symptoms of discomfort, such as incontinence, urgent urination, moaning, groaning, or excessive weakness in the back end.

When I work with fearful dogs, the first thing I do is add nourishing kidney herbs. Fear can manifest as noise sensitivity or fear of thunderstorms, car rides, vet visits, and going on walks. Excessive fear and trauma can cause kidney weakness and become a draining or even dangerous cycle due to the damaging effects of stress on the entire dog-as-ecosystem. Sympathetic excess can slow your dog's kidney function, increase tension, and reduce fluid levels, drying the entire system, especially the nervous system. In a time of stress, the sympathetic response (fight or flight) dominates the system, slowing kidney filtration to reserve energy for the musculature. This can cause a backup of uric acid and, over time, increase the kidney load.

Another aspect of kidney energy, according to traditional Chinese medicine, is that the kidneys rule the bones and open out to the ears. Kidney health affects your dog's musculoskeletal system through blood and circulation. The kidneys stimulate bone marrow production while signaling for marrow-based red blood cell production.[63] Look to the kidneys if your dog's red or white blood cell counts are unbalanced.

An excellent example of the musculoskeletal influence of the kidneys is cruciate ligament tears. Cruciate tears need good blood circulation, lymphatic stimulation, and elimination mechanisms due to the presence of excessive metabolic waste from the injury. When a dog tears their cruciate ligament, you can be assured that their kidneys need moisture and support.

Tip! Dogs tend to injure their cruciate ligament after winter, the season in which dryness tends to build up in the musculoskeletal system. Working with your dog's kidneys, dryness, and tension over the winter is a great way to prevent cruciate tears.

So far, we have looked at the kidneys' interaction with the liver, immune system (red blood cells), musculoskeletal system, and nervous system, but the connections don't end there. The kidneys are related to the circulatory system through their influence on blood pressure, circulation, and volume. In her book *Holistic Anatomy*, Pip Waller points out that the kidneys are connected to the endocrine system through hormone signaling and balancing fluids and minerals. The kidneys also interact with the liver and its influence on the digestive system.[64] Everything is connected.

Talking Kidneys

When kidneys are unbalanced, function declines, leading to high sodium levels, blood pressure issues, low-volume blood filtering, and fluid imbalance. If you pay attention to your dog's daily living patterns, you'll see the subtle symptoms of kidney weakness well before your dog's kidneys become impaired to the degree that their issues show up in blood work.

Yes, getting blood work done for your dog annually or biannually is essential, but looking at body language can help you be proactive instead of reactive. There are obvious signs of kidney weakness, like excessive urination, incontinence, and urinary tract infections, but there are more subtle indications, too, some of which are seemingly unrelated, but all pointing to an unbalanced renal system. Remember, these symptoms are generally chronic, not acute.

Kidney Weakness Cofactors

Arthritis

Aversion to touch (on the lower back)

Cold energetics

Constipation

Cruciate ligament tear

Dandruff

Dental caries

Diarrhea

Drinking more than they pee

Dry cough

Dry paw pads

Dry stool

Dry tongue

Ear infections

Edema (water retention)

Excessive itching

Excessive salivation

Fear-based behaviors

Groaning when lying down

Hot paws

Lethargy

Muscle twitching

Nausea

"Off" smell

Poor appetite

Poor digestion

Redness between the toes

Rolling on back

Sensitivity to noise

Spinal conditions

Stiff joints

Vomiting water

Weakness in the back end

The Kidney-Spine Connection

Many holistic veterinarians believe that the kidneys are directly related to a healthy spine, especially around the third lumbar vertebra. Vets Cheryl Schwartz and Peter Dobias both advocate for skeletal health, with Dr. Schwartz calling for acupuncture and acupressure and Dr. Dobias for acupuncture, chiropractic manipulation, and physiotherapy. These methodologies all release muscle tension, including tension in the spinal muscles, resulting in increased energy flow. When you understand the body holistically, it makes sense that these spinal considerations would improve kidney health as well.[65]

Kidney Heat

When kidney function declines, dryness proliferates and heat rises. Moisture, or lack thereof, is related to arthritis, joint pain, weak connective tissue, and other musculoskeletal conditions. Conversely, strong kidney function leads to healthy bone marrow, solid teeth, and strong bones. Kidney heat (congestion) can quickly cause imbalances because heat doesn't stay confined to the kidneys; it quietly travels down to all the parts of the urinary system. Some symptoms include fever, infections, urination with crying out, and blood in the urine. Serious complications include kidney and gravel stones. When a dog has a congested liver and heat in the liver, it can sometimes lead to wet, hot skin conditions with a kidney component.

Herbs and fungi for kidney heat: couch grass, licorice root, marshmallow root, plantain, tremella mushroom

Symptoms of Kidney Heat	
Gravel and stones	Rubbing kidney area across
Kidney stones	the floor
Pain and crying	Warmth in the kidney and
out	bladder area

. . . .

Tip! Use yarrow for blood in the urine and mullein root for associated incontinence.

. . . .

Cold Kidneys

When dogs hold their urine, it can get ugly. When urine is stagnant, it thickens, making your dog uncomfortable. When I first moved to Olympia, Washington, which is wet, cold, and rainy in winter, my dog Francis refused to go outside when it rained; the combination of cold and wet created anxiety and fear around potty time. Francis was a cool dog, but as she aged, she would move toward cold in winter. Her fear increased, as did her irritation and constant drive to seek warmth. I gave Francis calendula to warm her core and Rescue Remedy flower essence for fear, and I wrapped her up in a sweater and raincoat when she went outside to help keep her warm. Her urinary issues quickly cleared up as she retained warmth and lessened her fear of the cold rain.

Renal stagnation means that blood isn't getting filtered as it should, and it causes increased energetic cold as well as toxicity and possible pathogenic overgrowth. Cold decreases circulation, causing edema (water retention), especially with age or when female dogs are spayed. Bladder tissues and nerve impulses weaken due to organ trauma and aging. After all, the nervous system is directly tied to the kidneys and lets your dog know when it's time to pee (autonomic control). This pattern of energetic coldness needs stimulation to clear.

Herbs and fungi for kidney coldness: calendula, cordyceps mushroom, ginger, goldenrod, gravel root, juniper berry, reishi mushroom

Kidney Dryness

Dryness in the renal system can cause heat that weakens the kidney and decreases filtration. Heat can reduce lymphatic function and circulating fluids. This can lead to poor fat absorption in the small intestine. In addition, as dryness bakes and proliferates, it can cause gravel and stones, especially calcium oxalate stones, a sign of dry atrophy. Other signs of kidney dryness include bladder weakness, low urine output, and nervous system exhaustion.

· ·

Tip! The nervous system should be addressed in any pattern of kidney imbalance, and especially dryness. Look for signs of nervous exhaustion, hair-trigger reactivity, and fear.

· ·

Herbs for this pattern are like an expanded selection of herbs for heat, focusing on their mucilaginous action, meaning they promote moisture.

Herbs and fungi for kidney dryness: burdock root, cleavers, couch grass, licorice root, horsetail (phytoembryonic), marshmallow root, mullein root, nettle, plantain, tremella mushroom

Kidney Dampness

Kidney dampness occurs much more often in humans but can happen in dogs, resulting in stagnation. Recalling the damp energetic pattern, it affects the entire dog-as-ecosystem due to fluid viscosity. Think slow, thick, and stagnant fluids. You may see candida overgrowth and/or a decline in beneficial bacteria and increase in pathogenic organisms. Cold with dampness is common, and stimulation is needed to boost circulating fluids while drying the dampness.

Herbs and fungi for kidney dampness: blackberry leaf, dandelion leaf, cowberry phytoembryonic, goldenseal, juniper berry, reishi mushroom, uva-ursi

Kidney Relaxation

Too much relaxation causes dilution of fluids and excessive mineral loss. This can throw off your dog's mineral balance, including sodium levels. As a result, you might see bubbles, mucus, or protein in your dog's urine, high blood pressure, and incontinence.

Herbs and fungi for kidney relaxation: agrimony, ashwagandha, blackberry leaf, horsetail (phytoembryonic), nettle, plantain (balancing), reishi mushroom, yarrow (balancing)

Kidney Disease

Kidney disease was once found only in geriatric dogs. Today, it's being diagnosed much earlier—even in dogs under five years of age. It's almost always diagnosed in the later stages of the disease, when blood values indicate decline, because dogs can function with less than 30 percent of total kidney capacity.[66]

When kidney function declines, it leads to slower filtration, kidney stones, high sodium levels, and high blood pressure. These types of malfunctions are the beginning of kidney disease. You might notice excessive drinking and urinating. More advanced symptoms include constipation, dark urine, lethargy, nausea, poor appetite, rapid heart rate, vomiting, and weight loss. In addition, if left untreated, kidney disease can quickly lead to kidney failure through rapid scarring, which occurs as blood vessels (glomeruli) in the kidneys harden, causing proteins to leak into the urine instead of remaining in the blood.

. . . .

Tip! Lyme disease can cause kidney disease and protein in the urine. If your dog has been diagnosed with Lyme or is exposed to ticks, it's important to have your dog's urine tested yearly. Early detection is key for Lyme-based kidney disease (nephritis).[67]

. . . .

Strategies for Kidney Health

Diet is critical when it comes to healthy kidneys. Whether raw or lightly cooked (with added enzymes), fresh food provides highly beneficial nourishment and kidney support. Kibble is dry and depletes the body of water. It's full of ingredients that aren't bioavailable, so the body spends an inordinate amount of time digesting it. Poor diets low in minerals can challenge the kidneys' ability to excrete wastes, maintain salt and water balance, and stabilize blood pH.[68] Your dog's diet and kidneys need minerals to help filter waste.

Dryness is a kidney antagonist. Water is life, and it's the key to healthy kidneys. Again, dryness proliferates, and heat rises and dries kidney energy. Dry kidneys will pull moisture from your dog's lungs, eventually resulting in a dry cough. A healthy volume of circulating fluids is important for proper kidney function.

A fresh-food diet helps the kidneys maintain optimal blood volume, which rids the body of water-soluble toxins. Dogs and cats on kibble can have depleted kidney energy due to the dryness of their food. This includes dehydrated raw food and treats. But don't panic; dehydrated products are okay to feed so long as you ensure that your dog is getting extra moisture when eating these types of treats and foods.

Foods for kidney health: asparagus, beets, berries, broccoli, brown rice, carrots, celery, chlorophyll, cod, cranberries, cucumbers, eggs, kale, kidney beans, kidney glandular (dried kidney), mackerel, pasture-raised meats, peas, phytoplankton, sardines, spinach, string beans, sweet potatoes, watermelon, wild rice

Herbal support can be beneficial in preventing and addressing kidney disease, especially when the disease is caught early. The herbs listed below help support the kidneys, increase elimination, and slow disease progression. As noted above, making sure dogs with kidney weakness get adequate hydration is important, so I often recommend preparing these herbs as infusions or decoctions and pouring them over your dogs' food. (See chapter 5 for more information about preparing herbs.)

Herbs and fungi for the kidneys: agrimony, angelica, astragalus, bee balm, blackberry leaf, burdock root, chickweed, cleavers (cold infusion), cordyceps mushroom, couch grass, echinacea, goldenrod, gravel root, green tea (decaffeinated), horsetail (phytoembryonic), juniper berry, marshmallow root, milk thistle seed, mullein root, nettle leaf and seed, Oregon grape root, plantain, reishi mushroom, tremella mushroom, uva-ursi, yarrow

PART TWO
Herbal Practicum

Keep in mind that plants live in the earth. We need to take care of the earth so that the plants are taken care of, so they can take care of us. Life is truly a big circle.

MARGI FLINT, HERBALIST,
IN *THE HERBALIST'S WAY*
BY NANCY AND MICHAEL PHILLIPS

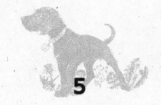

5

Remedies

*Each herb is an individual, and each lends itself better to
certain kinds of preparations, which can be fine-tuned to the
situation, taking into account the constitution of the patient.*

RICHO CECH,
MAKING PLANT MEDICINE

Like Richo Cech says, plants are individuals too. When you take them
into your body or give them to your dog, know that a plant doesn't have
just one action or purpose. The goal is to work with plants and seek to
understand the best ways to use their medicine. There are many ways
to take plant medicine into the body. Remedies are prepared according to what the plant has to offer, its constituents, and if and how those
constituents need to be extracted.

Tinctures and Glycerites

A tincture is an alcohol extraction of an herb's constituents. They're concentrated and quickly absorbed into the body when given orally (in the
mouth). In canine herbology, tinctures are medicinal, supporting your
dog's healing ability. Not only are they quickly absorbed into your dog's
bloodstream, they're easy to use. Often, I choose them over dried herbs
because dried herbs must be broken down and assimilated before their
medicine is absorbed.

Alcohol is an effective menstruum (solvent) for extracting plant constituents, except for minerals and mucilages. It extracts alkaloids, bitter compounds, essential oils, flavonoids, glycosides, resins, saponins, tannins, simple carbohydrates, and volatile oils.

Fresh vs. Dried Herbs for Tincturing

For the most part, I prefer using fresh herbs for tincturing. However, that choice depends on the herb. Some herbs have different properties when they're dried versus fresh. For example, stinging nettle is better dried if you need to access its minerals. Another example is chamomile, whose alcohol-soluble constituents disappear when the herb is fully dried. Many commercial tinctures are made from dried herbs due to availability.

Concerning Alcohol

Many folks have read that alcohol is poisonous to dogs. Yes, this is true, but only for large amounts. I use tinctures in very small dosages unless an acute situation warrants increasing the dosage. Research indicates that the lethal dose of alcohol for a dog is between 5.5 and 7 grams of 100 percent ethanol (200-proof alcohol).[1] One milliliter of 100 percent ethanol is equal to 1 gram. The average tincture for a dog is made with 80-proof (40% alcohol, 60% water) brandy or vodka. To equal the lethal dose, you would need 13.75 ml of 80-proof alcohol for a small dog. This is equal to fourteen full standard droppers of 80-proof brandy or vodka—much, much more than the amount of tincture you'd ever give your dog!

Furthermore, the alcohol percentage that goes into tinctures is *not* the alcohol percentage that comes out afterward. Making tinctures involves macerating (soaking) plants in the alcohol for four to six weeks. Everything breaks down, and plants are 80 to 95 percent water! The water content in the plant material dilutes the alcohol content in the brandy or vodka substantially. In most cases, you'd need six drops of tincture to equal the same amount of alcohol found in one drop of the brandy or vodka that you made the tincture with. In tinctures made with glycerin, alcohol, and water, like the phytoembryonics we'll discuss later in this chapter, the ratio is even higher, with approximately ten drops of tincture equal to one drop of brandy or vodka.

You don't need to worry about the alcohol in drop dosages of tinctures that you might administer for medicinal purposes. When you see warnings about giving your dog alcohol, they are referring to dogs drinking or licking beer, wine, or cocktails. This should never be allowed.

. . . .

Tip! If you're still worried about alcohol, give your dog a low dose of powdered milk thistle seed in their food. It helps protect the liver from alcohol damage.[2] You can also evaporate some of the alcohol by pouring your dog's tincture dose into a shot glass, placing the glass in a cup of hot (not boiling) water, and letting it sit for fifteen minutes. Another way to do this is to mix hot water and tincture and let the hot water evaporate the alcohol. For every drop of tincture, add five drops of hot water. And, if you are still worried about the alcohol in tinctures after reading this, just don't use them. There are other options for administering herbs to your dog.

. . . .

Purchasing Tinctures

When purchasing commercial tinctures, you'll want to know where the herbs came from and to ensure that they are free of pesticides, herbicides, and fertilizers. Choose organic when possible. Some medicine makers do not have certified-organic products, but they wildcraft and grow their own herbs for medicine, which is acceptable. My own garden is organic, but not certified organic; I can't label my products as organic because I haven't undertaken organic certification.

Common names of herbs can be different from region to region and person to person. Be sure you know a plant's Latin name to ensure that you're getting the right plant tincture.

Factors affecting the quality of tinctures include whether they're made from fresh or dried herbs, production practices (cultivated or mass-scale farmed, wildcrafted, or organically grown), solvent-to-plant ratio, and the type of menstruum used. When you purchase tinctures, they should come in a dark (preferably amber) glass bottle with a dropper top. Never buy tinctures in clear glass, plastic, or metal bottles. Tincture color may vary from bottle to bottle and doesn't indicate potency.

Guide to Using Tinctures

I recommend mixing tinctures with a small amount of water and dropping or syringing them into your dog's mouth. I always taste my dog's tinctures so I know what they taste like and how much I need to dilute them. You can mix a tincture with a treat or your dog's regular food, but they don't work as fast or effectively this way, as the gut must digest and assimilate them.

Avoid giving tinctures to dogs with diabetes, kidney failure, or liver failure except under the supervision of a holistic vet.

. . . .

Tip! When administering a tincture, never come at your dog, moving toward their face. Come around from behind, if you can. Squirt the tincture from a dropper into the side of their mouth, on the inside of the cheek, hold for four or five seconds, and gently release. If your dog is mouthy or likes to bite down hard, make sure you have a plastic dropper or syringe. Glass droppers can break if your dog bites down hard enough.

. . . .

Tip! Dogs with histamine intolerance can be sensitive to the histamines in alcohol. To remedy this, give a dose of homeopathic Histaminum 12C or 30C after giving them a tincture.

. . . .

Glycerites

Glycerites are herbal extractions made with vegetable glycerin, a thick, clear, odorless liquid manufactured by the saponification of fixed oils like soy, coconut, corn, and palm oils.* Glycerin is energetically neutral. Glycerin is a humectant, meaning it draws in moisture. It extracts acids, some alkaloids, bitter compounds, enzymes, glucosides, stem cells, mucilage, saponins, tannins, and trace minerals. It's sweet but doesn't contain sugar or raise blood sugar.

Glycerin is best at extracting constituents from fresh, high-moisture plants, such as horsetail. It's not especially good at extracting

---

*Glycerin can also be made from animal fat and synthetic sources like petroleum.

constituents from dried plants unless they're water-infused first. There are many plants for which glycerin isn't an effective menstruum even though you may see them sold commercially as glycerites—for example, calendula and most mushrooms. Glycerin can't extract resin or the chitin in mushrooms. Mushrooms are best extracted first in water and/or alcohol (after which the alcohol is evaporated) and then preserved in a solution that is at least 50 percent glycerin.

Glycerites can be used in large dosages and long-term, depending on the herb. They're great for dogs with organ imbalances like kidney failure, liver disease, and diabetes.

Glycerin-friendly fresh plants: bee balm, burdock root, cleavers, corn silk, dandelion, echinacea, fennel, German chamomile, ginger, goldenseal, hawthorn berry, horsetail, lavender, marshmallow root, milky oats, mullein leaf, nettle, peppermint, plantain, rose, skullcap, turmeric, uva-ursi, yarrow

Glycerin Side Effects

Glycerin is the main alternative to alcohol tinctures, but just because glycerin is nonalcoholic doesn't mean it can be used with abandon. Too much glycerin can cause nausea, vomiting, and diarrhea. Glycerin has found its way into many treats and foods, creating issues for dogs with difficulty digesting fats or simply getting too much glycerin in their system. If your dog reacts to a glycerite, ensure they aren't getting additional glycerin in treats and food. If reactivity continues to be an issue, discontinue the glycerite or try giving it along with powdered burdock root, which helps the body process fats and stimulates the gallbladder to release bile.

Guide to Using Glycerites

Glycerites absorb slowly compared to alcoholic tinctures because they're absorbed through your dog's lymphatic system and gluconeogenic pathway.[3] Whenever I recommend glycerin extracts, I either double or triple the dose I would suggest for an alcoholic extraction.

Alcoholic extracts can keep for years, but most glycerites have a shelf life of eighteen months or less. Mixing a small amount of alcohol (80 proof) with glycerin can help extend its shelf life.

Infusions and Decoctions

Infusions and decoctions are two types of water-based extractions. An infusion requires steeping plant material in water, and it's generally used with more delicate plant parts like leaves and flowers. A decoction involves simmering plant material, and it's generally used with more fibrous plant parts such as berries, seeds, barks, and roots. These water-based preparations extract the nourishing components of plants, such as minerals, vitamins, mucilage (a slippery, gooey, polysaccharide-based protective substance found in plants), alkaloids (weak), bitter compounds, flavonoids, glycosides, polysaccharides, saponins, tannins, and volatile oils. Fresh herbs are generally best for infusions and decoctions, but dried herbs can be used too.

Making Infusions

Below are standard schedules for making infusions from the herbs profiled in this book.

- **Fresh herb:** 2 tablespoons fresh herb per 8 ounces of water
- **Dried herb:** 1 tablespoon dried herb per 8 ounces water

1. Cut up fresh herbs to expose more surface area. If needed, crumble whole dried herbs or zip them through in a food processor.
2. Put the herbs in a mason jar.
3. Heat water to almost boiling and pour the appropriate amount (see the schedule above) into the jar.
4. Stir with a wooden or stainless-steel spoon or stick
5. Put a small square of natural waxed paper over the top of the jar to protect your infusion from any BPA on the inner sealing of the lid.
6. Seal the jar with its lid.
7. Let the plant material steep in the hot water for 20 minutes or more, depending on the herb.
8. Strain the infusion. You can give the spent herbs to your dog in small amounts or compost them.

Making Cold Water Infusions

Some herbs are sensitive to hot water and need cold extraction. These infusions are usually steeped overnight and used in the morning. Cold water infusions are especially suitable for mucilaginous herbs like cleavers and marshmallow root. You can use the standard plant-to-water ratios provided above.

Making Decoctions

Decoctions are generally stronger than infusions and dosages can vary; see chapter 8 for specific details. Decoctions are made from sturdy plant parts like bark, roots, and seeds, and you can decoct this plant material up to three times.

1. Chop up the herbs to expose more surface area.
2. Combine 1 tablespoon of dried herbs with 1 cup of filtered water in a pan (avoid nonstick). Double the amount of herbs when they are fresh.
3. Bring to a gentle simmer and let simmer, covered, for 20 to 40 minutes, depending on the herb. Stir occasionally.
4. Let cool, then strain and use. If needed, dilute with more water to make the decoction less potent.
5. Store any leftover decoction in a mason jar, covered, in the refrigerator, where it will keep for up to 3 days.

Rinses

A rinse is simply an infusion or diluted decoction that you pour over your dog and massage through their coat. You can use rinses daily to help relieve symptoms. Squeeze the rinse into your dog's hair and work through the coat with your hands. Do not rinse it out. Rinses can help your dog find relief without completely suppressing the system. You can also mix a rinse with natural shampoo for a therapeutic bath.

Let's look at some rinse formulations for common skin conditions.

Dry, Scaly Skin with Heat

Combine the following:

6 ounces goldenrod infusion
2 ounces yarrow infusion
1 ounce St. John's wort infusion

You can use dried or fresh herbs to make these infusions. Yarrow is a specific for hot, dry skin; you could replace the infusion with 15 drops of yarrow tincture if you like. St. John's wort is anti-inflammatory and specific for redness and heat, while goldenrod addresses dry, scaly skin and yarrow helps disperse heat.

❧ Warm, Itchy, Irritated Skin

Combine the following:

      6 ounces chickweed infusion
      2 ounces lavender infusion
      2 ounces yellow dock root decoction

Lavender infusion is specific for itchy, dry skin, with an emphasis on the itch. Chickweed and yellow dock help cool itchy skin.

❧ Red, Itchy Skin

Combine the following:

      8 ounces plantain infusion
      1 ml yarrow tincture

Plantain relieves inflammation, draws heat out of the skin, and quells the itch. Yarrow will help bring down the redness and heat.

❧ Yeast with Odor

Combine the following:

      6 ounces chamomile infusion
      2 ounces coconut water
      1 ounce thyme infusion

Cover mixture and let sit overnight. Thyme and coconut water work as antifungals and help relieve itchiness. Chamomile stops itchiness when used as a rinse.

Poultices

Poultices are an effective way of applying herbal medicine to your dog's skin. It's a primitive and powerful remedy that you can make from dried or fresh herbs. The simplest example of a poultice is chewing some plantain, mixing it with your saliva, and placing it on a wound to soothe the pain and inflammation. Alternatively, you can wrap up herbs in muslin or gauze, providing an absorbent barrier.

Constituents from the herbs you apply in a poultice can enter the bloodstream through the skin, so use only nontoxic herbs. The water you use to moisten the herbs can be hot or cold. Moist heat will help draw out infection and heal wounds.

Making a Warm Poultice

These instructions are for a warm poultice using muslin, but you can adapt them to use cold water and other wrappings (or no wrappings) as you require.

1. Lay a few squares of muslin, one on top of the other, on a clean work surface.
2. Spoon 2 tablespoons or so of chopped fresh or dried herbs into a bowl. Pour hot water over them and stir to make a paste.
3. Scoop the herb paste onto the muslin and fold it up around them. Secure the muslin with a rubber band or string.
4. Test the temperature of the poultice on the inside of your wrist to ensure that it isn't too hot. Then hold the poultice to the area of the skin that needs healing.
5. When the poultice isn't warm anymore, you can rewarm it as desired by pouring hot water over it and then reapplying it to the area of concern.

Clay poultice: You can make a poultice with dried herbs mixed with powdered clay and warm water. Hold it to the area of concern until it dries. The clay is helpful for drawing toxins out of the skin. Gently wipe the area with a warm washcloth to remove any dried clay before reapplying.

Capsules

Capsules are used to deliver measured portions of dried herbs into the body. They are made of gelatin derived from either animal sources or plants. Animal-derived capsules are better for intestinal conditions because they don't dissolve well in the stomach and will make it through that acidic environment to the intestines. Vegetarian capsules break open in the stomach, making them good vehicles for nutritional herbs. Capsules come in different sizes, ranging from zero to triple zero. Triple zero is the largest capsule, equivalent to about 1/4 teaspoon or roughly 750–1,000 mg of powdered herbs, depending on the herb. Double zero is the most common size for dogs, and it holds between 500 and 700 mg. Size zero holds between 150 and 350 mg.

Essential Oils

Essential oils are volatile oils in aromatic plants. Conversations about essential oils can get ugly due to misinformation and disregard for common sense. Essential oils are *not* separate from herbal medicines. They are the strongest, most potent form of medicine in my practice.

The average aromatherapist spends more than two hundred hours studying essential oil chemistry. Why? Essential oils are complex!

Know Your Healing Tools

Holistic healing affects your dog's physical, mental, and emotional aspects. You must be able to choose the right tool(s) for true healing. This is why essential oil education is so important. Essential oils excel at healing trauma and emotional stagnation. They can either force or stimulate healing, depending on how you're using them. According to Swanie Simon, an animal herbalist and naturopath who worked with the late Juliette de Bairacli Levy, a pioneer in the field of animal herbalism, knowing a plant is not the same as knowing the essential oil; you must know both. She states: "Essential oils are one part of the plant's chemical makeup, and essential oils have their own complex chemical makeup. Since essential oils are extremely concentrated extracts of aromatic plants, they don't contain the constituents found in the whole plant, and many of these constituents are modifying chemicals that work to regulate the side effects of the plant."[4]

Fresh or dried herbs, tinctures, infusions, and essential oils are not meant to be interchangeable. The extraction process differentiates the products. For example, the steam distillation used to extract essential oils can carry only light molecules. Tinctures, on the other hand, use alcohol extraction and so generally contain large-molecule constituents not found in essential oils, such as alkaloids, mucilages, and tannins.

Holistic Essential Oil Use

As is the case for herbs, essential oil use must include regard for constituents and intention. You'll match your dog's needs in an intentional protocol. A comprehensive picture of your dog's lifestyle, diet, emotional state, and medical history must be considered. Here is a question I often hear: What essential oils would help my dog's arthritis? This is a very allopathic question. What type of arthritis? Where is the arthritis, and how is it manifesting in the body? How long has it been happening? How old is your dog? What other health problems are they having? Are they taking any medications? What other remedies have you tried? Using essential oils based solely on what science has identified as their "active" constituents is allopathic herbalism. Remember, your dog's condition is not separate from its being.

I recommend zoopharmacognosy (self-selection) with essential oils. Self-selection is the safest way to use essential oils with dogs. All you have to do is take the cap off the bottle of essential oil and offer it to your dog, or set it near your dog or in the same room. Your dog will let you know if they are interested in the oil or not. Some dogs will actively smell the oil and others will sit near it if they are comfortable with the oil you are offering. Dogs who are not interested will show aversion to the oil by turning their head away or getting up and moving away from it. There is more to this practice, of course; I'm giving you just a simple explanation. I recommend Caroline Ingraham's book *Help Your Dog Heal Itself: A-Z Guide to Using Essential Oils and Herbs* for more in-depth discussion of self-selection.

. . . .

Tip! When using essential oils for flea and tick prevention, make sure to have your dog sit with the oils you're considering for them. Don't use an essential oil that your dog doesn't want to be around.

. . . .

Essential oils are generally used externally. Use essential oils internally only when they're the only option left and only under supervision or as part of a comprehensive protocol. If you purchase an internal remedy that contains essential oils, use self-selection to see if your dog is interested and if the essential oil is well indicated for your dog.

Don't diffuse essential oils in your home unless you have a therapeutic reason and as part of an intentional protocol. When breathed in, essential oils go directly into the bloodstream.[5] Diffusion exposes *everyone* to the essential oil whether or not they need it. The diffusion isn't confined to one room unless it is airtight.

Essential Oil Safety

Essential oils can have a profound impact on the entire ecosystem of your dog, so their use demands respect and a thorough understanding of each oil. Ask: Why are you using an essential oil? What plant does it come from? What does the oil do when it enters your dog's body? How will it affect your dog's organs?

Intention is vital to essential oil use. Our dogs are vulnerable beings needing care and guidance. When used with mindfulness, essential oils can deliver profound healing. But they are not a stand-alone system of medicine; they belong to herbalism. This makes them subject to evaluation like any other plant remedy. If you use only essential oils, your dog's healing might be limited. Your dog may need moisture or mucilage not found in essential oils. Homeopathic veterinarian Dee Blanco makes a good point about essential oil use: "Nothing we do or give is without effect. Some things are more benign, but *everything* has an effect."[6] The dog-as-ecosystem is sensitive, and essential oils are potent. They should always be used with caution.

I've heard many people say that certain essential oils are so pure that they can be ingested, diffused, and used undiluted. Not true! Even the purest essential oil can harm your dog.[7] Different dogs have different tolerances for different essential oils. Also, when a dog has a negative reaction to essential oils, it can be subtle, as the constituents in the essential oils become stored in the tissues.[8] Whatever you put on or in your dog's body either benefits or causes harm. The difference in a drop can move therapeutic effect into toxicity.

Herbalist and French-trained aromatherapist Cathy Skipper has been using essential oils for decades. In her book *Aromatic Medicine*, she makes a profound observation: "The more powerful an essential oil is, the less of it you need, and once effective results have been obtained, it is inutile, even harmful to the organism to carry on taking it. Prescribing large doses over long periods of time is not applicable to aromatherapy."[9]

Essential Oil Safety by Robert Tisserand and Rodney Young is an industry standard for aromatherapists, scholars, and anyone interested in using essential oils. Robert is one of the pioneers of aromatherapy. In 1977 he wrote *The Art of Aromatherapy*, one of the first books on the field, which validated the use and effectiveness of essential oils. Robert founded the Tisserand Institute for Aromatherapy in London and published the *International Journal of Aromatherapy*. I highly recommend having a copy of *Essential Oil Safety* on your bookshelf.

Sustainability

Sustainability is a huge tenet of holistic aromatherapy. Nature isn't ours to use up. One unfortunate aspect of essential oils is that it takes a great deal of plant matter to make a very small amount of oil. For example, it takes more than 18 pounds of peppermint leaves to make 1 ounce of peppermint essential oil. I don't know if you have ever held a peppermint leaf in your hand, but you can barely feel it. To put this in perspective, 1 drop of essential oil equates to 75 cups of peppermint tea! You need 30 pounds of angelica flowers to produce 1 ounce of angelica essential oil. You need 40,000 rose petals to make 1 ounce of rose essential oil. That is approximately 70 roses per drop! For 1 pound of lemon balm essential oil, you need 6,000 pounds of plant material—6,000 pounds![10] You must let a sandalwood tree grow for 30 years before you can harvest sandalwood essential oil—and the harvest kills the tree in the process.[11]

Sustainability also includes issues with the illegal or unethical wild-crafting of plants, which can disrupt delicate ecosystems, destroy native plant communities, and decimate endangered species.

No matter how much we try to ignore the issues of sustainability, they aren't going away. We are using up our natural resources faster than we can replenish them. I wish I could tell you that most distillers and essential oil companies care about the future of plant populations, but this isn't the case.[12] We all want access to these oils for generations to come. So, when you're buying essential oils, look for products from essential oil companies that are already talking about sustainability and ethical sourcing.

. . . .

Tip! Atlas cedarwood (*Cedrus atlantica*), frankincense (*Boswellia carteri* or *B. sacra*), rosewood (*Aniba rosaeodora*), sandalwood (*Santalum album* or *S. paniculatum*), and spikenard (*Nardostachys jatamansi*) are all sourced from endangered plants and trees. Try to avoid or minimize your use of these oils.

. . . .

Deceptive Practices

Part of selling high-quality essential oils is building relationships with distillers and knowing the origin of your oils. What method of distillation is being used? How and where were the plants harvested? How and where were the oils stored before purchase? What types of testing do they use to determine purity?

Most essential oil companies resell bulk oils. Distillers can't guarantee their oils. Why? Plants vary from batch to batch depending on where they grow and the specific growing conditions at the time. Elevation, moisture, water quality, soil conditions, and wind can affect quality.[13]

The marketing world has taken the language of essential oils and rendered it meaningless. Many companies touting their products as *aromatherapy* sell adulterated oils containing very little essential oil. Some are even synthetic and derived from petroleum.[14] Be cautious of products labeled "made with pure essential oils." That statement is subjective. The amount of essential oil could be just a drop. The real question is, what else are these products made of?

Furthermore, essential oils are not regulated. No grades, therapeutic levels, or standards are set by a recognized governing body. Terms such as *therapeutic grade, clinical grade,* and *veterinary grade* are 100 percent marketing.[15] What is confusing is that good companies have adopted these terms in order to sell their products online and compete for top marketing key words. Some people unintentionally use these terms thinking they are a valid way to describe a quality oil according to their niche—for example, "veterinary grade." All essential oils should be the highest quality but due to plant scarcity, greed, and low ethical standards, many are not. Quality comes from the plants, harvesting practices, distillation process, and storage practices. Does labeling an essential oil as medical-grade or veterinary-grade mean it's safe for animal use? No. Its safety would depend on the quality of the oil, the plant, the individual animal, and how you use it.

Using Essential Oils

Using essential oils involves much more than opening a bottle. Essential oils are powerful and need respect. Understanding them as much as possible will help you confidently approach their use.

Before using any essential oil with your dog, ask: Are you using it as part of an overall healing protocol or wellness plan? Are you using it with intention? Is an essential oil what you need for your dog's condition, or are you using it for convenience or ease of use? Are you clear on how long you should use the oil? What steps have you taken to ensure the essential oil is pure?

When using essential oils on your dog, you should dilute the oil. Use a maximum of 12 drops of essential oil(s) to 1 ounce of carrier oil, which gives you a 2 percent dilution. This is also a good dilution ratio for making medicinal salves and oil blends. You can massage diluted oils into your dog's skin and fur, avoiding their eyes and genital areas. Always wash your hands after you are done applying oils to your dog. And, again, always make sure your dog is not averse to the oils that you are applying on them. For more information, read *The Aromatic Dog—Essential Oils, Hydrosols & Herbal Oils for Everyday Dog Care: A Practical Guide* by Nayana Morag.

Flower Essences

Flower essences work with your dog's emotional center. Different types of these energetic essences have been used throughout history, but Dr. Edward Bach brought them to the forefront of medicine in the early 1900s. He offered a system of thirty-eight remedies for emotional health that he believed also positively affected the physical body.[16] His theories were based on how our emotions affect physical disease, as science today is starting to understand.

One of my dog clients had a kidney imbalance and would constantly wake up in the middle of the night. Her parents weren't sleeping, and everyone was stressed. I told them to give their dog five-flower essence formula (Rescue Remedy) before bedtime and again if their dog woke up. After the second night, their dog was sleeping through the night.

Flowers vibrate at certain frequencies, and the flower vibrations contained in flower essences pair with your dog's emotions, thus helping their cells vibrate at healthy frequencies.[17] Think of flower essences as energy manipulators, shifting and releasing negative energy!

Using Flower Essences

Flower essences come in stock bottles and can be diluted according to your needs. Unlike the case for herbal remedies like tinctures and dried herbs, dosing does not depend on the weight of your dog. Essences are so safe that you don't have to worry about overdosing. Some remedies have an immediate effect, while others are slower in building support.

You can give your dog flower essences in various ways. I like to give them in the mouth when possible. You can also spray them around and on your dog's coat, drop them onto their nose, massage them into the tips of their ears, or add a few drops to your dog's water.

Dosing schedules depend on what you're dealing with. For example, with sudden fears, you can dose your dog every couple of minutes. For a chronic condition, you might give three to six drops of essence twice daily.

Homeopathics

Homeopathy uses highly diluted remedies for healing. Like flower essence therapy, homeopathy uses vibrational energy, and it works on the premise of "like cures like." For example, the homeopathic remedy Apis mellifica, which comes from bee venom, is used for stings and swellings. Much like holistic herbalism, homeopathy indicates remedies based on both symptoms and the individual. Homeopathic remedies affect the entire body, even though they are used for acute and chronic illness.

As an herbalist, I love homeopathy because it gives me access to the power of many poisonous plants I wouldn't otherwise be able to use—the homeopathic remedies made from them contain all their energy but none of the poisonous constituents.

The homeopathic remedies referred to in this book are not accompanied by explanation. You'll need to look up the remedies yourself in a homeopathic materia medica or consult with a holistic veterinarian who uses homeopathy. See TheHerbalDog.com for suggestions.

Potency

Homeopathic remedies come in different potencies. The higher the number, the more potent the medicine; for example, a 30C remedy is more potent than a 12C remedy. Specifically, potency refers to dilution, and counterintuitively, the more dilute a remedy, the more potent its energetics. Most homeopathics come as small pellets contained in a vial. The medicine is on the outside of the pellets, so touch them as little as possible. Since they are energetic remedies, store them in a cool place away from electronics and wireless devices.

Dosing

As is the case for flower essences, dosing for homeopathy isn't dependent on the weight of your dog. I usually recommend two to four pellets as a dose, given at least twenty to thirty minutes away from food and water. Shake out the pellets into the vial's cap and then into the side of your dog's mouth. Hold their mouth closed for at least a few seconds. As soon as the pellets contact the mucosa of your dog's mouth, they will dissolve and be absorbed.

If your dog is finicky or you need to administer a remedy repeatedly for an acute situation, you may liquify a homeopathic dose. Making a liquid dose is easy. Place four pellets in a one-ounce amber glass bottle. Fill it with spring water or filtered water. Put on the cap and tamp the bottle against the heel of your hand for thirty seconds. Give a dropperful of the remedy per dose inside your dog's cheek. Dr. Dee Blanco recommends making a new remedy every three days.

For acute situations, if you're using remedies of 30C potency or less, give the dose every twenty minutes until you see a response. You may give up to five or six doses per day. With a higher potency, like a 200C, you can dose every thirty minutes for two or three doses or until you see a response. Stop the remedy when you see improvement. If symptoms reappear, dose again. Use a different remedy if you don't see positive results in two to three hours. Remedies don't cause any harsh side effects, so they are a safe choice for both acute and chronic illness.

. . . .

Tip! For further guidance on using homeopathic remedies Dr. Brendan Clarke, homeopathic and integrative veterinarian, suggests starting with the book *Dogs: Homeopathic Remedies* by George Macleod.

. . . .

Medicinal Mushrooms

In the past decade, medicinal mushrooms have become well known for their positive impact on health and longevity. They are beginning to play a much larger role in canine health and wellness as well. What I love about mushrooms is that they are easy to use and well tolerated by most dogs.

Tip! For nutritional purposes, add cooked mushrooms (all of the traditional culinary mushrooms are safe for dogs) or dried mushroom powder to your dog's meals. They offer a wealth of nutrients (vitamins and minerals), fiber, and prebiotics that feed your dog's microbiome. When consumed regularly, they improve immunity and overall organ health, which improves longevity!

Mushroom medicine has long been a part of traditional Western herbalism, Indigenous American medicine, and traditional Chinese medicine. Medicinally, mushrooms modulate the immune system, provide a rich base of antioxidants, and bring down systemic inflammation—which is key to disease prevention. Each species has its own unique mechanisms of action and effects on the immune system. (Due to lack of room, I couldn't cover all my mushroom friends in this book, but I have included some key fungi for you to explore in chapter 8.)

Mushrooms are the fruiting bodies of the fungi system, while their "roots" are mycelia. Each part is unique and contains varied constituents. As an herbalist, I use fruiting bodies, mycelia, or both depending on the case. Among other constituents, the fruiting bodies contain antibiotics, antioxidants, beta-glucans, ergosterols, fiber, glycoproteins, polysaccharides, and triterpenoids. Beta-glucans have been particularly well studied due to their ability to activate immune cells. Dogs have beta-glucan receptors in their intestines, so mushroom medicine is perfect for them!

Mushrooms have a hard coating, called chitin, that makes up their cell wall structure. This chitin needs to be broken down to extract the medicinal constituents. The two main solvents used for this purpose are alcohol and hot water. I usually extract mushrooms using both, a process that is referred to as a double extraction. Commercially, you can find hot-water-extracted mushroom powders and different types of extracts. I recommend both for my clients. For more information and sourcing recommendations, see TheHerbalDog.com.

Phytoembryonics

Phytoembryonic therapy is often referred to as gemmotherapy. People sometimes think this means therapy with precious gems, but this isn't about healing with crystals. The science of phytoembryonics centers around plant stem cells. They are found in the buds, tissues, embryonic seeds, barks, and rootlets of plants. Stem cells include everything needed for the total growth of the plant, including enzymes, minerals, hormones, genetic material, and other growth factors. Stem cell remedies help remove toxins by opening detoxification pathways.[18] This allows for better assimilation, organ function, and cellular health and can help prevent chronic disease.

There are two types of phytoembryonic remedies: mother tinctures and homeopathic dilutions. I refer to the homeopathic dilutions as gemmotherapy and the mother tinctures as phytoembryonic therapy.

Benefits of Phytoembryonic Therapy

Anti-inflammatory	Increases assimilation of nutrients
Autoimmune-friendly	Increases cellular oxygenation
Decreases destructive antigens, which hyperstimulate the immune system	Increases cellular voltage while balancing electrolytes*
Detoxifies autoimmune complexes, metabolic wastes, excessive mucus	Promotes lymphatic flow and immune modulation
Good source of amino acids, antioxidants, enzymes, trace minerals	Stimulates digestive enzyme production
Helps heal leaky gut	Supports healthy gut flora and digestive function
Helps maximize organ function	Supports liver function by reducing toxic load[19]

---

*Cellular voltage is the electromagnetic current in cells.

Measurements

The recipes and formulas for herbal remedies almost always need accurate measuring, but sometimes the units of measure need to be converted to whatever measure you are working with or have at hand. You can easily find conversion calculators online and in apps. I keep a book with a single page of the weights, measures, and conversions I use the most. This way, I've got everything I need before starting a recipe.

Volume and Weight

Some remedy components are measured by volume. Examples are liquids such as alcohol, infusions, tinctures, and oils like olive oil. Herbs can vary in size, shape, and density depending on drying and preparation methods, so you measure them by weight, not volume.

You can't measure weight unless you have a scale. Digital scales allow you to easily switch between ounces and grams without needing to do any conversion calculations.

It may be helpful to keep a record of volume-to-weight conversions for certain ingredients, such as beeswax. When used in salve recipes, beeswax is melted, and so recipes often call for it as a volume—for example, 1/4 cup beeswax. But beeswax is solid at room temperature, and to measure out 1/4 cup, you'd have to melt it first. If you knew beforehand that 1/4 cup of beeswax weighs approximately 58 grams, you could weigh out the appropriate amount at the start of the recipe.

Parts

The simpler's method, as it's called, is a traditional system of measuring ingredients in parts. Parts can be anything: teaspoons, pounds, milliliters, grams, cups. Recipes written in this way set up the ingredients as a ratio: 1 part this and 2 parts that, or a 1:2 ratio. This measurement method is versatile because you can use the ratio to make large or small amounts of medicine. Just make sure you stick to the same measurement for the part throughout the recipe.

·····
The Handful

The "handful" is a loose measurement found in many old herbals. As you can imagine, a handful can vary for obvious reasons. If you ever see a handful used as the unit of measure in a recipe, know that the recipe will use nontoxic herbs that can be loosely measured.

·······
The Drop

I often hear the question, what's a drop? The answer may seem simple, but it can get complicated, especially for those more scientifically minded folks. Difficulty arises when you are administering a significant number of drops. Viscosity matters. Water forms smaller droplets than alcohol. Twenty drops of one tincture may not equal twenty drops of another.

A general rule of thumb for a nonresinous extract is that the dropper in a one-ounce glass bottle will hold thirty drops, and the dropper in a two-ounce bottle will hold forty drops.

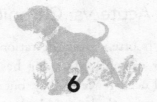

6

Planning Herbal Protocols

*Plants can either teach me what I do not know to do . . . or
give me what I need. . . . They are not only teachers, but also
Givers, who bestow knowledge to the tissue and mind, as well
as give me what my body lacks.*

JULIA GRAVES,
THE LANGUAGE OF PLANTS

When working with herbs, every protocol is a success. Why? If I choose
the incorrect herbs for a dog, the herbs speak loudly and dictate the
direction I should go. The purpose of any protocol is moving in the
right direction, even if that movement is miniscule. Observation is key.
Figuring out if an issue is acute or chronic and working with dosage
are ways to help hone your dog's herbal regimen. If you're not seeing
improvement, you might want to increase the dosage to see how that
amount interacts with your dog's body. Most of the herbs in this book
are nontoxic, meaning they have a high tolerance for error. If the increase
in dosage doesn't improve your dog's condition, discontinue the herb or
formula and try another. If your dog is tolerating an herb or formula and
you increase the dosage and they start showing adverse symptoms, go
back to the dosage where they were doing well.

Acute vs. Chronic

An acute health issue is often a manifestation of a deeper underlying chronic condition. For example, your dog has diarrhea a few times a month. The occasional occurrence is okay, but if they consistently have diarrhea throughout the month, I would look at diet, ear test their meals (see page 150), and look at the energetics of their food and supplements to determine the underlying cause(s).

One goal of holistic herbalism is to distinguish acute issues from chronic disease symptoms. Using herbs acutely is different from using them for chronic disease. Acute conditions need large amounts of herbs for short periods of time, while chronic conditions use smaller, continuous dosages or cycled/pulsed herbs.

First-aid episodes are almost always acute—symptoms manifesting from an outside source like a burn, a puncture, or eating something indiscriminate. Outside of first aid and the occasional turkey carcass consumption, symptoms like vomit, mucus, and diarrhea are the body's way of communicating what's happening inside.

Suppression occurs when you use remedies to force your dog's body to act a certain way. In acute situations, where symptoms can endanger the life or long-term health of your dog, suppression is warranted. With chronic illness, suppression should be avoided.

As a general principle, holistic herbalism aims to stimulate the body's self-healing mechanisms. Sometimes this isn't possible, or there isn't time for it in a moment of crisis, and some suppression must occur. If your dog has been having explosive diarrhea for two days, you need to do something to stop it, immediately, or they'll become dangerously dehydrated. Many acute solutions are stop-gap measures, allowing you more time to work with underlying issues. For example, an acute response to skin eruptions would help manage the discomfort and spread of symptoms, while at the same time you can work on supporting liver health, since the liver plays a role in recovery for almost all skin issues, and bolstering all the channels of elimination.

I emphasize individuality in everything I teach, from herbalism to feeding. What works well for one dog doesn't always work well for another. Examining the underlying cause of your dog's symptoms is critical to recognizing patterns. The bigger picture will then become clear. Why? Often, you'll be working with acute and chronic diseases simultaneously. You work with acute symptoms first and then chronic ones. Most acute issues should clear up within one day to two weeks.

> **Tip!** For acute situations, energetics aren't as important as they are with chronic conditions.

The Art of the Dose

Ahhh, dosage. It's one of the biggest issues when working with any herbal protocol or remedy. Theories on dosage strategy vary throughout history, geographical location, and field of study. As an herbalist, my view on dosage is just one of many. I determine dosage by looking at the dog as an individual, their tolerance and symptoms, and the energetics of the plants I'm working with.

You'll find more information about dosing for specific herbs, mushrooms, and other remedies in the monographs in chapter 8. Here, we'll go over the basics.

The Standard Dose

Depending on the manufacturer or the practitioner you're working with, the "standard dose" for any particular herb or remedy can vary, sometimes by a wide margin. Why do we see such variation? Herbal dosing schedules represent suggested doses for general use, not for specific energetic patterns, individual constitution, or disease profile. So, for example, most tincture labels advise you to give your dog a specific amount of tincture two or three times per day. But the effect of an herbal tincture varies from dog to dog, and that schedule isn't appropriate and won't be effective for all dogs. Dosage should instead be determined by the herbs(s) you're using, the needs and symptoms of your individual dog, and whether the illness is acute or chronic.

It can be hard to get out of the pharmacological mindset when considering dosage. Veterinary medicine and some holistic practitioners need uniform dosages. But for you, your dog's caregiver, rethink dosage and remember what you're trying to accomplish with herbs. The standard dose comes from a mechanical way of looking at things, not a holistic way.

I've included dosage ranges throughout this book. From a holistic perspective, for most chronic conditions you'd start with a low dosage and work your way up slowly.

Material Dosages

A holistic guideline called the Arndt-Schultz law says that low doses stimulate, medium doses regulate, and large doses suppress.[1] *Material dosage* is just another name for a large dosage. With tinctures, for example, a material dosage might be ten to thirty drops or more per dose (depending on the dog). Large dosages typically force the body to react, leading to digestive upset, side effects, and liver congestion. But sometimes you need high dosages to push the body—for example, if you are dealing with persistent diarrhea or vomiting, kennel cough, muscle spasms, urinary tract infections, abscesses, autoimmune disease, cancer, or respiratory distress. Large doses in such situations will help move toxins, fluids, and foreign materials.

The best way to give a large dose is to space it out over an hour, allowing your dog's body time to absorb and process the medicine. I learned this practice from herbalist Matthew Wood.[2] What I like about this method is that it gives you time to check your dog's reaction, since your dog can't readily tell you how a medicine feels. If your dog's stomach gets upset, decrease the dose to the tolerated amount for two days and then increase it by a quarter.

Dosing Guidelines

For general chronic conditions, I suggest giving remedies twice daily. You may need to give remedies three times daily for serious chronic conditions. When a dog has an immediate, acute issue, give them a tincture dose three to five times per day or every couple of hours, depending on the herb, until symptoms subside.

The dosing schedules in this book are generally drop dosages based on the weight of the dog, defined as follows.

Dog Sizes by Weight

Size	Weight	Example
Extra-small	10 pounds	Chihuahua or Maltese
Small	10–25 pounds	Pug or French Bulldog
Medium	22–55 pounds	Corgi or Spaniel
Large	55–100 pounds	Labrador or Golden Retriever
Extra-large	101+ pounds	Bernese Mountain Dog or St. Bernard

Tincture Dosages

When administering tinctures, I dilute them in a dropperful of water and squirt them into my dog's mouth. I start with drop dosages of gentle herbs for general chronic conditions. Drop dosing combines the energetic signature of the herb and the body's healing energy. For large doses, I divide the dosage into small increments and give them by mouth over the course of an hour. If my dog won't let me squirt the tincture into their mouth, I will apply the tincture to a treat.

General Tincture Dosing Schedule

Size of Dog	Dose
Extra-small	1 diluted drop–3 drops
Small	2–6 drops
Medium	4–8 drops
Large	6–10 drops
Extra-large	8–12 drops

Diluted drop dosage: diluted drops are for extra-small or sensitive dogs. To make a diluted drop, take 1 drop of the remedy and dilute in 1/2 ounce of water. Stir lightly for fifteen seconds and give one dropper of the mixed water.

Note: This schedule is for stimulating healing. Remember, some conditions warrant a more material (large) dose. Much like homeopathy, drop dosing depends primarily on finding the most relevant herb or herbal combination. The key is that you can always increase the dosage, but starting with a high dosage can be unforgiving.

Infusion and Decoction Dosages

Pour doses of an infusion or decoction over your dog's food or mix it into broth. As a general rule, decoction doses are half of infusion doses.

General Infusion Dosing Schedule

Size of Dog	Dose
Extra-small	⅛ cup
Small	¼ cup
Medium	½ cup
Large	¾–1 cup

General Decoction Dosing Schedule

Size of Dog	Dose
Extra-small	1 tablespoon
Small	⅛ cup
Medium	¼ cup
Large	6 tablespoons–½ cup
Extra-large	¾–1 cup

Dried Herb Dosages

The dosage of dried herbs depends on your individual dog and the herb or blend of herbs you're using. In commercial use, recommendations are based on weight. Please refer to the monographs in chapter 8 for detailed information on dosage. In general, for nontoxic herbs, Clark's rule can be used to determine a dried herb dosage for a dog if you know the dosage for a human adult. Take your dog's weight in pounds and divide it by the average weight in pounds of a human, which is 150 pounds. Take that number and multiply it by the milligrams of the adult dose. This will give you your dosage for your dog. For example, your dog weighs 70 pounds. You divide that by 150 and get approximately 0.47. Let's say the adult dosage of the herb you're considering is 500 mg. Multiply 0.47 by 500 and you get a 235 mg dosage for your dog.

Clark's rule, obviously, doesn't follow holistic principles. Your dog might need more or less.

Creating a Healing Protocol
for Chronic Conditions

Putting together a protocol can seem intimidating, but it doesn't have to be. It's all about preparing your dog's body for the regimen.

1. Help stabilize the nervous system. The nervous system is a huge part of any chronic condition. It needs a good healthy fat layer around each neuron for it to be responsive. Give herbs for nervous system support (see chapter 4) before beginning any other herbs to calm oversensitivity and chronic fight-or-flight responses. *Directions:* Give for 2 weeks, then move to step 2, while continuing to administer the herbs that support the nervous system.

2. Stimulate the lymphatics. You must get the lymph moving so it can transport toxins, clean the extracellular matrix (the fluid between the cells), and transport fat-soluble nutrition. Give lymphatic herbs (see chapter 4), and make sure your dog gets age-appropriate exercise and/or massage. *Directions:* Give for 2 weeks. Then move to step 3, while continuing with steps 1 and 2.

3. Gently support the liver system. Give herbs that support the liver and bile flow (see chapter 4) as a means of supporting detoxification. *Directions:* Give no more than three liver-supporting herbs or one formula for 2 weeks. Then move to step 4, while continuing with steps 1, 2, and 3.

4. Support digestion and enzyme production. If needed, add an herb that offers digestive support and promotes balanced enzyme production (see chapter 4). You may not need to do this depending on the herbs you choose in steps 2 through 4. *Directions:* If you add a digestive herb, use no more than one. Give for 2 weeks, then move on to step 5, while continuing with steps 1 through 4.

5. Add one or two herbs that address the general condition/imbalance of your dog. *Directions:* Work slowly up to the appropriate dosage for your dog, while continuing the herbs chosen in steps 1 through 4.

Slow and steady wins with preventing and healing chronic disease. Many people get impatient and start to go fast, but the key to success is to let the body get used to things, let symptoms clear, and then see if they start up again. Once you start step 4, give your protocol eight weeks to start seeing positive changes. Reassess at eight weeks to see if you need to stop one or more of the herbs, increase or decrease the dosage, or continue for another four weeks.

. . . .

Tip! Some of the herbs you choose for your protocol may have overlapping indications, which can reduce the total number of herbs you need to give to your dog. Make your herbal selections intentional; less is more. Look up each herb in chapter 8 to see its energetics and effect on the nervous system, lymphatics, liver, and gut.

. . . .

General Guidelines for Holistic Herbalism

Herbalism is a learning process. It works best when used according to energetics, individuality, and intention. When using herbs, remember to breathe and be patient with your dog and yourself. Herbalism takes time to learn, especially if you have never used plants as medicine. These pointers will help guide you in your journey.

Energetics and Intention

- Consider the energetics of your dog's core pattern. These energetics may differ from what you see happening in your dog right now, especially if your dog is dealing with an acute issue.
- Know an herb's intention. What are its cofactors and energetics?
- Have realistic expectations. Conditions of cold to deep cold need more time to heal due to the weakened vital force. Herbs are not quick like pharmaceuticals.
- What do you want the herb to do? Does that action match the herb's energetics and your dog's energetics?

Using Herbs

- Address acute conditions first, then chronic ones.
- Dosage depends on how serious or advanced your dog's condition is.

- If your dog is doing well at a certain dose, but when you increase the dose they show symptoms, go back down to the tolerated dose.
- When using herbs, keep the delivery system in mind. What form of delivery can you use for the herb you are considering? Does that work for your dog? Tinctures, glycerites, infusions, and decoctions are readily absorbed and work best for acute conditions. Dried herbs can be mixed into food or given in capsules.
- If possible, give tinctures diluted in a bit of water (for taste) and give in the mouth; give powders and infusions/decoctions in food.
- Your dog's tolerance can vary herb to herb. Keep a journal of sensitivities and progress.
- Herbs can cause what they heal—this can be a healing aggravation where the medicine temporarily causes the symptom it will heal or it can be a sign that the dosage is too high, the herbal choice is incorrect, or (in the case of strong herbs) your dog's constitution isn't ready. When your dog has a healing aggravation, the symptoms will go away in two or three days. If symptoms persist, look to an incorrect herb or an incorrect dosage. Stop the remedy, wait until symptoms clear, and reassess starting dosage or herb choice.
- Self-selection can be useful, though it is beyond the scope of this book. As noted earlier, I recommend the work of Caroline Ingraham; you can find her practice online. If you're familiar with the technique, you can offer fresh or powdered herbs, mushroom powders, infused oils, or infusions before feeding. Dogs can't self-select herbs to prevent illness or disease.

Timing

- It takes approximately three days for your dog's body to get used to a remedy. Any herbal or homeopathic remedy may aggravate symptoms. Wait seventy-two hours to see if your dog is okay with the remedy. Reduce the dosage or discontinue the remedy if irritation continues. For example, if your dog gets loose stool when they start using cleavers, this situation should correct itself after three days. If not, you would reduce the dosage or stop using cleavers. I've never encountered any life-threatening symptoms resulting from the use of herbs and homeopathics, but if they should occur, stop dosing immediately and bring your dog to your emergency vet.
- Start one herb or formula at a time and see how your dog reacts to it.

This way, you'll know what is working and what isn't working. Wait a full three to seven days between additions. Extra-sensitive dogs may need ten days or more.

- Timing for each herb or formula can vary and get complicated. Generally, give powdered herbs with food, infusions and decoctions with food, and tinctures before meals, preferably in the mouth. Remember, there are gray areas.
- Separate pharmaceuticals and herbs by three to four hours.
- Some dogs are reactive when given a tincture on an empty stomach. If that's the case for your dog, add tinctures to food or give them after your dog has eaten.
- You should see positive changes in a dog on an herbal regimen within six to eight weeks. If your dog is not moving in the right direction within this time period, reconsider dosages or remedy choices.
- Most herbs aren't meant for long-term use (meaning more than six months). The general goal is helping the body heal. The gray area is considering plant and dog individuality. If you think your dog is ready, slowly take them off the herb (one herb or formula at a time) and see how they do over a period of a few weeks to a month. During this time, don't make any other changes. If you see decline, put your dog back on the herb or formula.
- In my experience, healing takes three months to a year to fully balance out chronic disease. During this time, you'll need to see ongoing improvement.
- Short-term dosage schedules for acute situations can be given for between one and eight weeks. This exact dosage and timing depends on the herb and the condition.
- Long-term care employs nontoxic herbs. Pulse them by taking one day off weekly, one week off every six weeks, and a month off every six months. That said, with some herbs pulsing may not be possible; your dog will let you know. Note: pulsing schedules can vary.
- With any herbal regimen, it's important to know what works and what doesn't. So go slowly, giving your dog time to adjust to each herb.

Safety

- Every food, supplement, and remedy, including herbs, carries some risk. Be informed and do the best you can.

- Know the indications, cofactors, energetics, known side effects, and pharmaceutical interactions for any herb you're working with. The monographs in chapter 8 offer details on all these topics.
- If you see signs of an allergic response, like shaking or severe lethargy, discontinue the herb immediately and notify your veterinarian.
- Side effects can occur with any herb. The reasons might be that the herb is incorrect or energetically inappropriate, your dog cannot tolerate it or has a histamine intolerance, the dosage is too high, or the herb is of poor quality.
- Some herbs, such as chamomile, are safe even in large amounts, while others, such as goldenseal, need caution.
- Always use the Latin names to identify plants you're interested in. Common names can change from region to region.
- Many herbs will increase urination; this is normal. If incontinence occurs, decrease the dosage.
- Less is more most of the time, and when dosages seem small, they're small for a reason. Doubling the dosage of a remedy won't double its effectiveness, and the high dosage may burden your dog's body and cause unwanted and uncomfortable reactions. The goal is to give the least amount of a remedy that will provide the desired benefit.
- Standardized herbal extracts lack a plant's synergistic constituents and create more side effects than their whole-plant counterparts. Signs of toxicity or sensitivity include excessive chewing, diarrhea, drooling, loss of appetite, shaking, restlessness, vomiting, and hair loss.
- Nutritive herbs, like fruits and greens, are mild and safe for long-term use. An example of this would be nettles.
- Limit more medicinal herbs to two to three weeks of use because certain constituents (such as alkaloids) can affect organs like the liver. Examples include Oregon grape root and oregano.
- Giving your dog too many herbs and supplements all at the same time is known as "kitchen sinking," and it confuses your dog's ecosystem. This practice has good intentions but often makes matters worse. If you see a list of ten herbs for arthritis, don't give your dog all ten herbs at once, hoping one will work. Instead, look at each herb in the list as an individual. Figure out which herbs match your dog. It may be one or a combination of herbs from the list, but not all.

- If your dog isn't getting better despite your best efforts, bring them to your holistic vet for testing.
- Many herbs can speed up or hinder the metabolism of pharmaceuticals. Be aware of possible negative interactions. Most concerning herb-drug interactions involve blood thinners, tranquilizers, antidepressants, and thyroid medications.
- Discontinue most herbs one week before surgery unless otherwise instructed by your veterinarian.
- Avoid using herbs with diabetic, pregnant, or lactating dogs unless supervised by a holistic vet.

Working with Extra-Sensitive Dogs

Sensitive dogs or dogs experiencing chronic deep-seated illness need extra care. Less is more with most dogs, and a sensitive dog's constitution is usually easily overwhelmed. One of the most important things to note about working with a sensitive dog is to add only one thing at a time. Don't rush. If an herb consistently doesn't work with your dog, move on to a different one after following the guidelines below.

Pace of change: Once you've introduced an energetically appropriate herb to your sensitive dog, don't change anything until your dog is showing zero signs of sensitivity to the remedy and things are moving forward. This may take weeks, depending on your dog's ecosystem and how it's progressing. Remember to breathe and be patient.

Tincture/Glycerite Dosing: Start your dog, no matter what their size, with 1 drop of a remedy in 1 ounce of liquid. Give one dropperful per dose. If your dog doesn't show any reaction to the remedy, you can increase the number of droppers of the diluted mixture until you get to three. Then slowly transition to 1 drop of the pure remedy mixed with 1 to 2 ml of water. Stop the remedy if your dog shows any reactions to it and let the symptoms clear. Continue to add drops to the dose until you have reached the limits of your dog's tolerance or the recommended dosage.

Remember that your dog may need less than the recommended dosage. Note: Reactivity symptoms include itchiness, scratching, vomiting, diarrhea, loose stool, and lethargy.

Dried Herb Dosing: Start with one-eighth of the recommended dose of an energetically appropriate herb and like above, discontinue if your dog shows a reaction to it. Let the reaction clear then start again.

Infusion/Decoction Dosing: Water-based herbal medicine is a gentle way to introduce your dog to plant medicine. Start with one-quarter the recommended dose, following the same guidelines for reactivity outlined above.

7

Herbal Applications

Welcome! This chapter covers common canine conditions and how to work with them. Each section gives you an explanation of the condition, its common energetic patterns, causes of the condition, and effective dietary and herbal strategies. Keep in mind the following:

- This material is comprehensive but not exhaustive.
- Some conditions don't have obvious dietary, herb, mushroom, phyto-embryonic, essential oil, or homeopathic solutions, so you won't see all these categories listed among the healing strategies for each of them.
- Warm and cool energetics are included—but remember, most herbs are appropriate for acute use (less than two weeks) and occasional use in balanced, healthy dogs.
- Dosages for almost all of the suggested herbs, mushrooms, and phyto-embryonics can be found in the monographs in chapter 8.
- Essential oils are listed for self-selection only.
- For guidance on using homeopathic remedies, you'll need to consult with a homeopathic vet or look up the remedies in a good veterinary homeopathy book (see page 126).

Acid Reflux

Common energetic pattern: damp heat

Acid reflux is an uncomfortable, involuntary symptom of a larger issue. It occurs when your dog's stomach contents (or sometimes the intestines) flow in the wrong direction, causing discomfort. Some signs in dogs involve vomiting bile, burping, lip smacking (nausea), restlessness, and anxiety with walking around or pacing.

The immediate response for most people is to give an acid reducer or an antacid. While these medicines can give temporary relief, they can also cause a cascade of food allergies by decreasing stomach acid, which is vital to digestion and immune function.[1] Most acid reflux is caused not by too much stomach acid but by low stomach acid or stomach acid in the wrong place.

Causes of Acid Reflux

Acid reducer	Gut inflammation
Anesthesia	Hiatal hernias
Antacid	Histamine intolerance
Citric acid	Leaky gut
Digestive insufficiency	Low vagal tone
Energetically inappropriate	Obesity
foods	Pancreatitis
Esophagitis	Stress
Fermented foods (too much)	Ulcer
Food sensitivities	

Helpful Herbs and Supplements

Herbs can help shift gut function and give your dog temporary or permanent relief, depending on the issue causing the reflux. Review the list of possible causes of reflux above and address as appropriate. Especially pay attention to the energetics of the foods you're feeding; working with your dog's diet is a good way to begin to address reflux.

Herbs for warm dogs: aloe vera, artichoke, burdock root, chamomile, goldenseal, gotu kola, lemon balm, licorice root, marshmallow root, milky oat seed, Oregon grape root, slippery elm bark, yellow dock root

Herbs for cool dogs: ashwagandha, ginger, licorice root, meadowsweet, slippery elm bark

Mushrooms: lion's mane, reishi, tremella, turkey tail

Phytoembryonics: cowberry, fig

Essential oils for self-selection: fennel, ginger, lime, peppermint, rosemary, spearmint

Homeopathic remedies: Arsenicum album, Carbo vegetabilis, Iris versicolor, Lycopodium, Nux vomica, Phosphorus
Supplements: apple cider vinegar, betaine HCL, digestive enzymes
Foods: apple, carrot, liver, organic oats, raw goat milk, raw cow milk, spinach, sweet potato

Allergies and Sensitivities

True allergies produce anaphylaxis. If this is the case for your dog, work with your vet and contact a homeopathic veterinarian to work out a plan for long-term care and healing. Most "allergies" are sensitivities.[2] As veterinarian Peter Dobias observes, "If we consider that almost 80 percent of immune system function resides in the gut, there's no surprise that heavily processed foods, poor quality ingredients, drugs and vaccines, toxic substances, and food preservatives can get the immune system into overdrive and make it overreact."[3]

Many sensitivities are triggered by the presence of undigested proteins in the small intestines, which cause inflammation and can lead to leaky gut, where the gut lining thins, becomes permeable, and allows "leaks" into the bloodstream. This causes extreme sensitivity to normal foods. (We'll talk specifically about leaky gut later in this chapter.)

Many sensitivities arise from insufficient stomach acid. Strong stomach acids are integral for the breakdown of proteins into amino acids. When proteins don't get broken down properly, they're marked for termination by the immune system and then the liver. Overloading the immune system leads to many issues, including acid reflux, depleted microflora, food sensitivities, hot spots, itchiness, poor assimilation and elimination, liver congestion, yeast overgrowth, and leaky gut. If it's not dealt with, you can end up with a dog who can't eat any proteins without reacting.

Stomach Acid and Digestive Enzyme Antagonists	
Acid reducers	Chlorine
Antacids	Dewormers
Antibiotics	Dryness
Antihistamines	Flea and tick medicines
Bromide	Fluoride

Glyphosate	Pesticides
Heavy metals	Pharmaceuticals
Kibble	Poor diet
Leaky gut	Steroids
NSAIDs	Sympathetic excess
Overcooked food	Vaccines

Liver and Lymphatics

It's important to support the liver and lymphatic system for dogs with allergies/sensitivities because congestion in either system can have a negative impact on both the immune system and the digestive system. A slowdown in liver function will back up the portal vein and cause a cascade of excessive histamine and blood toxins as well as difficulties with nutrient assimilation and waste elimination. Lymphatic congestion can make overall congestion worse. Stimulating lymph circulation helps improve all organ function as well as cellular nutrition.

Seasonal Allergies

Many dogs who suffer from allergies throughout the spring and summer deal with the release of histamine. Upon contact with an allergen, mast cells release histamine and cause the typical allergic reactions like backward sneezing and itchiness. (These reactions happen continually, rather than seasonally, when a dog has a mast cell tumor.) Remember, histamine is a normal part of how the body works. For more on seasonal allergies, or what I like to call *reactions* or *intolerances*, see also the Histamine Intolerance section of this chapter, page 195.

Histamine

As discussed in chapter 4, histamine isn't an enemy. It's essential for bodily functions like appetite regulation and brain, immune, muscle, and nerve function. It's also intricately linked with digestion and stomach acid levels. Allergic-type reactions are often treated with over-the-counter antihistamines, but these medications can themselves cause allergies and sensitivities. Their side effects include nausea, diarrhea, dizziness, weakness, loss of appetite, stomach pain, rapid heart rate, hives, and painful urination.[4]

In contrast, natural antihistamines help repair and work with your dog's natural histamine cycle. You can add herbal antihistamines to your dog's protocol, or try supplementing with quercetin, which naturally helps regulate histamine.

Natural antihistamines: chaga mushroom, cordyceps mushroom, ginger, green tea (decaffeinated), maritime pine bark, nettle, reishi mushroom, spirulina, turmeric

Natural sources of quercetin: apples, black currants, blueberries, broccoli, kale, rose hips

• •

Tip! For a powerful antihistamine combination, mix equal parts of nettle, maritime pine bark, and chaga mushroom powder. Give 1/8 teaspoon for every 10 pounds of your dog's weight, twice daily in food.

• •

If you think your dog has issues with histamine, avoid bone broth, fermented foods, and any leftover foods, which are all high in histamine. You can work these back into your dog's diet when their symptoms have calmed down and you've done work to support their liver.

Digestive Enzyme Supplements

Digestive enzymes can help dogs with food sensitivities and allergies by helping them thoroughly break down proteins and in turn avoid a triggered immune response from partially broken down proteins.

When looking at supplementing digestive enzymes in your dog's diet, it may take some trial and error to find the right one. Options include pancreatic enzymes (amylase, protease, and lipase), papain, and betaine HCL. Once you find one that works well for your dog, continue to supplement with it until any sensitivities clear. Continue giving enzymes if you feed your dog kibble or cooked food.

. . . .

Tip! In my experience, warm dogs should avoid enzymes with bromelain. Extra-sensitive dogs need slow, gentle support for building tolerance and may do best with homeopathic-based enzymes.

. . . .

Protocol: Basic Elimination Diet

The goal of this elimination diet is to bring down inflammation, increase stomach acid, and support liver function, assimilation, and elimination. I've seen this protocol work miracles.

While you have your dog on this diet, be patient. If you feel bad about having to put your dog on this diet, don't vocalize that. For example, "Oh, poor Fluffy can't have his favorite carrots because he is on a special diet. I feel so bad for him." Don't do this to yourself or your dog. Vibration is everything. Be confident, and let your dog know they will feel better soon.

1. **Temporarily simplify your dog's diet.** Feed your dog a simple diet consisting of meat, bone, and organ for 6 to 12 weeks. This can be muscle meat with organ and calcium powder or, if you are an experienced raw feeder, give fresh bone and organ. Feed the equivalent of 2 to 4 percent of your dog's body weight to start. If your dog loses weight, increase their portion by 0.5 percent of their body weight until their weight stabilizes. Work to find an energetically appropriate protein that your dog can tolerate. Commercially, there are meat, bone, and organ grinds out there that you can purchase for simplicity.

   Note: If you normally feed your dog kibble but want to try this elimination diet, cook your dog's protein and add in organ and bone powders. If you are only willing to feed kibble, look for a limited ingredient option. See TheHerbalDog.com for suggestions.

2. **Use targeted supplements to support the digestive system.** In addition to this simplified diet, supplement with an oil that is rich in essential fatty acids—unless you suspect yeast (candida) involvement, in which case hold off until the yeast is under control. To feed the microbiome, supplement with chlorella, moringa, spirulina, or phytoplankton (pick one). Add fulvic acid for trace minerals. Include

digestive enzymes with all meals, avoiding bromelain for warm to hot dogs.

3. **Use ear testing to identify potential inflammation responses.** Ear testing is a quick way to see if you are feeding your dog anything that causes a highly inflammatory reaction. First, feel your dog's ears for temperature and make a note of it. (For example, my dog's ears are usually slightly warm; she's a warm dog.) Feed the item in question, wait 30 to 45 minutes, and then recheck your dog's ears. A drastic change in temperature indicates an immediate inflammatory response—that is, an immune cascade response. Check every ingredient you are giving your dog in this simplified diet. When testing dried or fresh herbs, put them in some type of food that you know your dog doesn't have an ear-based response to.

4. **Supplement with *Saccharomyces boulardii*.** Supplementation with this beneficial probiotic yeast reduces inflammation, boosts digestive enzyme production, and helps beneficial bacteria colonize, support, and repair the gut mucosal layer. Use it for 6 to 8 weeks. During this time, avoid ferments, bone broth, and probiotics. Start low and slow for extra-sensitive dogs; slowly work up to the full dose. If *Saccharomyces boulardii* consistently upsets your dog's system, try colostrum or sodium butyrate.

5. **Make sure your dog is getting enough B-complex vitamins.** You can use a supplement, but be sure it is non-synthetic and includes folate (avoid folic acid when possible).[5]

6. **Support the nervous and lymphatic systems.** Add lymphatic stimulants and nervous system supports to your dog's regimen; see chapter 4 for suggestions. Make sure your dog gets at least 30 minutes of daily age-appropriate exercise or interactive play.

7. **Support the liver.** Add gentle support for the liver to your dog's regimen for 6 to 8 weeks; see chapter 4 for details.

8. **Start to add foods back into your dog's regimen.** When you feel your dog is stable, slowly add foods back into their regimen. Test the ears with every new addition, discontinue anything that your dog reacts to, and make a note of it. This includes the supplement suggestions above.

Helpful Herbs and Supplements

Herbs for warm dogs: burdock root, chamomile, cleavers, dandelion, echinacea, eyebright, marshmallow root, nettle, rose hips, skullcap, slippery elm, yarrow, yellow dock

Herbs for cool dogs: astragalus, calendula, ginger, green tea (decaffeinated), licorice root, nettle, rosemary, slippery elm, turmeric

Mushrooms: cordyceps, lion's mane, reishi, turkey tail

Phytoembryonic: black currant, horsetail, mountain pine

Essential oils for self-selection: eucalyptus, German chamomile, helichrysum, lavender, peppermint, ravensara, sandalwood

Homeopathic remedies: Arsenicum album, Euphrasia officinalis, Histaminum, Natrum muriaticum, Rhus toxicodendron, Staphysagria, Sulphur

Supplements: chlorella, colostrum, digestive enzymes, N-acetylcysteine (NAC), phytoplankton, prebiotics, probiotics, propolis, quercetin, spirulina, vitamin C

Foods: apple, blueberries, broccoli, eggs, kale, kelp, leafy greens, moringa, organ meats, raw cow milk, raw goat milk

Anal Gland Conditions

Common energetic pattern: dampness, relaxation

Your dog's anal glands are anatomically like sacs, emptying a mix of toxins and lubricating fluid through a small narrow duct near the anal sphincter under the tail to the left and right of the anus. Oily and pungent smelling, anal gland fluid softens stool and releases when your dog defecates. Anal glands back up when they don't naturally express. Since the anal duct is narrow, it isn't good at passing any solid or semi-solid substance. If allowed to fester, the sacs will become inflamed and then infected, sometimes causing an abscess.

The belief that expressing a dog's anal glands will keep fluid from building up is a fallacy. This practice makes the anal sacs lose tone and their natural ability to empty. The anal sac stays at least half full most of the time. With my own dogs, I look at their anal glands every couple of weeks to note if anything looks swollen, especially if I see one of my dogs licking the area.

When anal glands produce a bit of a smell, it doesn't necessarily mean there is a problem. Many people think that when their dog is dragging their bottom across the floor, they must rush their dog to the vet to have the glands expressed, but this isn't the case. Dogs will do this occasionally to help stimulate movement in a stagnant gland.

When the anal glands aren't expressing properly, they can swell and leak along with being irritated and inflamed. When severe inflammation develops, they can stay open, which is when you get leakage and straining of the anus. Most of the time, the issue is not the anal glands themselves but the consistency of the stool. For example, thin stools can cause anal glands to get backed up, as can chronic diarrhea. Dogs can develop an impaction or blocked gland when the glands get too plugged.

Causes of Anal Gland Conditions

Docked tails	Lack of exercise
Expressed anal glands	Low-residue diets
Fleas and tapeworms	Muscle and spine injuries
Food sensitivities	Obesity
Kibble*	Tumors

Poulticing for Impacted Anal Glands
Anal gland impaction isn't life-threatening; home care can be used before resorting to antibiotics or emergency veterinary care. Yes, you'll need to do some hands-on work, but in most cases, impaction can be worked out at home.

Calendula is one of the best herbs for most anal gland issues except for abscesses. For general use, prepare a strong infusion of dried calendula flowers, steeping them in hot water for twenty minutes. Then take out the calendula flowers and wrap them in muslin, making a poultice. Soak the poultice in the warm infusion and apply to your dog's bottom. I reheat the infusion as needed. If you don't have any calendula flowers, you can use calendula tincture diluted one-to-one with warm water.

Sometimes this is all you need to loosen a backed-up anal gland. If you need something stronger, try the following.

---

*Kibble strains the digestive system and dries out the tissues robbing the gastrointestinal system of moisture.

✒ Anti-inflammatory Poultice

Nettles help decrease inflammation, soothe tissues, increase circulation, and cleanse the area, while plantain, a mild antibacterial, helps draw out any infection. Oregon grape root is a cooling antibacterial and anti-inflammatory.

8 ounces water
1 tablespoon dried nettles
1 tablespoon plantain (fresh if you have it)
½ teaspoon Oregon grape root
Muslin, for wrapping the poultice

Heat the water until it is almost boiling. Pour the hot water over the herbs, cover, and let steep for 20 minutes. Remove the herbs and wrap them in muslin. Dip the poultice into the warm infusion and apply it to your dog's bottom. Do this for 20 minutes, on and off, repeating two or three times. You'll notice the glands loosening, and you can then try to gently apply pressure, squeezing outward. If a gland doesn't expel the fluid easily, do another round of compresses until it softens.

When a backed-up or impacted anal gland releases, you might sometimes see blood flowing out of the duct. If this is the case, after most of the flow has stopped, do one more round of the poultice. This time, add 1 teaspoon of dried white yarrow or 1 ml of white yarrow tincture to the tea just before you dip your poultice in it. Apply the poultice for 20 minutes, then gently apply pressure in an attempt to drain any remaining any fluid.

Preventive Dietary Strategies

Dietary choices can help prevent gland problems in the first place.[6] For raw food feeders, feeding raw meaty bones (10% or less of total diet) can help with healthy anal gland excretion. Ensure that your dog gets quality pre- and probiotics with their food and freshly ground seasonal veggies to bulk up their stool.

Organic olive oil is a good addition if your dog's stool tends to be a bit dry, especially during the summer months. The ever-popular pure pumpkin can also help firm up stools. For either olive oil or pumpkin puree, give the following doses daily.

Olive Oil/Pumpkin Puree Dosing Schedule

Size of Dog	Dose
Extra-small dogs	½ teaspoon
Small dogs	1 teaspoon
Medium dogs	2 teaspoons
Large dogs	1 tablespoon
Extra-large dogs	2 tablespoons

Helpful Herbs and Supplements

Herbs: aloe, angelica, calendula, chickweed, marshmallow root, milk this-tle seed, nettle, slippery elm, yarrow, yellow dock

Mushroom: turkey tail

Phytoembryonic: fig

Essential oils for self-selection: calendula, geranium, helichrysum

Homeopathic remedies: Arsenicum album, Calcarea sulphurica, Hepar sulphuris, Mercurius solubilis, Myristica

Supplements: larch arabinogalactan, L-glutamine, MCT oil, probiotics

Foods: apple (cooked), apricot (dried), beets, celery, flaxseed (freshly ground), olive oil, plantain seed, prune, pumpkin

Antibiotics Recovery

Antibiotics (ciprofloxacin and metronidazole) saved my life but altered my microbiome. I took cipro and metronidazole for eight weeks. Later, testing showed that these two antibiotics had killed off more than 30 percent of my gut bacteria. I developed food sensitivities and eczema. Within a year, I developed hypothyroidism. This is a case of "I wish I knew then what I know now." That experience helped me better understand food sensitivities, leaky gut, and autoimmune disease and, eventually, heal myself and help my animal clients do the same.

Flagyl (the brand name for metronidazole) is the standard of care for canine idiopathic (unknown) diarrhea.[7] One of the side effects of Flagyl is that it kills fusobacteria, which help the gut digest proteins. A decrease in protein digestion can lead to food sensitivities. This activity can trigger inflammatory pathways responsible for skin disorders and liver disharmony.[8]

Another example of the impact of antibiotics is my little Finnbar. He was seventeen but looked ten, and he was healthy for his age. I brought him in to the vet to get one tooth extracted because it was bothering him. The vet pulled fourteen teeth—without consulting me first. He gave Finnbar clindamycin (another antibiotic) and Flagyl, as well as NSAIDs and, of course, anesthesia. The vet called me when everything was over, telling me the wonderful things he did for the "health" of my pug. I was furious. The doctor had simply decided that his teeth looked bad and that Finnbar would be better off without them. This is a decision he and I should have made together, and I could have helped Finnbar through it and done a cleaning. The doctor said, "It was just easier to pull them." He obviously didn't know much about pug teeth.

Sadly, Finnbar's health quickly declined after the antibiotic treatment, and he died within a year, five months from his eighteenth birthday. I see many geriatric dogs quickly decline after they are given antibiotics. Good gut health is often all old dogs have to keep themselves together! Don't give antibiotics to an old dog unless their life is threatened. It takes time to reverse gut microbiome damage; in Finn's case, we ran out of it.

Old dogs aren't the only ones susceptible to the ill effects of antibiotics. I try to avoid giving any puppies antibiotics unless their life is threatened. In adult dogs, I will exhaust other options before using antibiotics. Avoid using "preventive antibiotics" if you can. The overuse of antibiotics is leading the way for antibiotic resistance and chronic disease.[9]

How Antibiotics Damage the Body

Everything is connected in the dog-as-ecosystem, and your dog's microbiome has far-reaching actions throughout the body. Your dog's systems of assimilation and elimination are dependent on these microbes. They help break down food, nourish your dog's brain, support the nervous and lymphatic systems, and manufacture vitamins and nutrients for systemic health.[10] Your dog literally cannot live without them.

Antibiotics destroy bacteria, and most are indiscriminate, killing off the beneficial bacteria of the microbiome just as readily as the pathogenic ones. Microbes—whether pathogenic or beneficial—produce toxic by-products when they die off, so antibiotics leave behind a mess of toxic waste, congesting the liver, hyperstimulating the immune system, and raising oxidation levels. Antibiotics open up the body to a slew of yeast, fungi, and pathogenic bacteria.[11] It takes years to recover from long-term antibiotic use. Without support to foster recovery, the body will need two years to balance out after just one round of antibiotics.[12]

Effects of Antibiotics

Aggression	Mitochondrial damage
Anal gland conditions	Nausea
Anxiety	Panic
Biofilm formation	Personality changes
Bloody stool	Poor appetite
Candida overgrowth	Tooth discoloration (especially
Cognitive decline	with doxycycline)
Diarrhea	Urinary tract infections
Enzyme insufficiency	Vomiting
Leaky gut	

Preventive Antibiotics

Many times, vets will prescribe antibiotics preventively, hoping to ward off infection. I think this is the wrong choice. Take, for example, pancreatitis. Antibiotics degrade pancreatic function and kill off beneficial bacteria, making gut function worse while weakening the immune system.[13] The die-off from the bacteria can flood the body with metabolic wastes, increasing liver and systemic toxins. For a dog with pancreatitis, the liver is already dealing with necrotic tissue from premature pancreatic enzymes release.

Protocol: Antibiotics Recovery Regimen

This plan is designed to address recovery after antibiotic use. The recommended supplements can also be used concurrently with antibiotics administration to prevent or minimize some of the negative effects. Probiotics should be given at least three hours after the antibiotics.

If you are considering a fecal transplant as a form of probiotic aid to recovery, prepare the gut with steps 1 through 3 before your dog undergoes the procedure or takes any fecal pills.

See the relevant monographs in chapter 8 for dosage recommendations for the herbs suggested here.

For Long-Term Antibiotic Damage

Dogs that have suffered damage from long-term antibiotic use need to go slow, starting with one-quarter (or less) of the recommended dosage for any of the herbs or supplements and slowly increasing over a period of weeks. Add remedies to the regimen one at a time. Don't give more than four herbal remedies at a time.

Goals for Recovery

1. Support the nervous system.
2. Support the lymphatic system.
3. Restore glycocalyx and IgA levels.
4. Add fulvic acid.
5. Give prebiotics.
6. Give probiotics.

Step 1: Support the Nervous System

Supporting the nervous system is an important part of healing any chronic condition, and it's especially important for antibiotic recovery because a big part of your dog's nervous system lies in the gut. Give fig phytoembryonic (if available) combined with skullcap for 8-12 weeks (if your dog is tolerant of each). After 2 weeks continue to step 2.

Step 2: Support the Lymphatic System

You want your dog to have strong lymphatic function during this process. Use cleavers for a warm dog or calendula for a cool dog. If you are unsure, choose calendula. Follow steps 1 and 2 concurrently for 2 weeks before continuing to step 3. Keep your dog on the cleavers or calendula for a total of 8–12 weeks.

Step 3: Restore Glycocalyx and IgA Levels

As discussed in chapter 4, glycocalyx is the protective coating that lines the gut's epithelial cells so that beneficial bacteria can adhere to the gut lining. The production of the antibody IgA is dependent on glycocalyx levels. Antibodies help the immune system fight infection, toxins, pathogenic bacteria, and viruses. Together, low glycocalyx levels and IgA production put dogs at risk for pathogenic overgrowth. Additionally, without proper IgA and glycocalyx levels, any probiotics you give your dog, including fecal transplants, will go right out with your dog's poop. You must prepare the gut first.

One of the best ways to increase glycocalyx and IgA production is by supplementing the gut with *Saccharomyces boulardii,* which is resistant to antibiotics and helps beneficial bacteria colonize, support, and repair the gut's mucosal layer while increasing glycocalyx and IgA production. Start supplementation with *S. boulardii* slowly, working up to the recommended dosage, which is a billion or more organisms per dose. When you get to the full dosage, continue for 4 to 6 weeks. After 3 weeks of following steps 1 through 3 concurrently, you can proceed to step 4.

Some dogs can't tolerate this much *S. boulardii.* Grass-fed colostrum is an alternative; it can improve IgA and glycocalyx levels, but most hot dogs can't tolerate it. Symptoms of intolerance can include excessive scratching, acid reflux, flatulence, and hot ears. If your dog can't use *S. boulardii* or colostrum, use a plantain leaf tincture or glycerite for 6 to 8 weeks instead.

Caution: *Saccharomyces boulardii* helps rid the body of heavy metals and can cause temporary lethargy. To facilitate its work, you can use it with a binder like zeolite.

Zeolite Spray

Use nano-sized zeolite to help bind toxins and heavy metals and get them out of the body. Look for purified clinoptilolite zeolite for dogs. Alternatives to zeolite include bentonite clay, cracked-wall chlorella, fulvic acid, pectin, and activated coconut charcoal.

Step 4: Add Fulvic Acid

Fulvic acid is high in trace minerals, antioxidants, and electrolytes. It increases assimilation and acts as a prebiotic.

Start fulvic acid supplementation slowly and work your way up to rec-ommended dosage. Now you are doing steps 1 to 4 concurrently; after three weeks continue to step 5. Keep your dog on fulvic acid for 12 weeks

Step 5: Give Prebiotics

Your dog's microbiome needs food, just like plants need soil. Without healthy soil, you can't grow anything. Most prebiotics are made of insoluble and soluble fiber that pass through the stomach mostly undigested, pass into the colon, and nourish the bacteria there.

Besides providing a food source for hopeful probiotics, the main importance of prebiotics is their production of short-chain fatty acids (SCFAs). When fiber is consumed, SCFAs produce beneficial compounds like acetate, butyrate, and propionate that help protect your dog's intestinal barrier and decrease inflammation.[14] Incorporate prebiotics into your regimen for 2 weeks, then continue to step 6.

Cooked mushrooms or dried mushroom powder are my favorite prebiotics due to their soluble and insoluble fiber content, which feeds the microbiome and helps the colon function properly.

I also recommend cooked organic apples; I give my dogs 1 teaspoon per 30 pounds of body weight. Cooked apples are high in pectin, which can help heal the gut lining.

Prebiotics: apples, bananas, burdock root, chlorella, collagen in bone broth, dandelion root, elecampane, fermented vegetables, Jerusalem artichokes, mushrooms, raw honey, raw milk, rose hips, sea vegetables, sweet potatoes

Step 6: Give Probiotics

Probiotics repopulate the microbiome, which is important when it's been decimated by antibiotics. Give your dog probiotics concurrently with prebiotics for 6–8 months, rotating different strains for variety. If you can, test your dog's microbiome first to assess which species might be best.

Consider giving your dog probiotics along with the antibiotics. This practice decreases the side effects of the antibiotics and results in decreased commensal bacteria damage. Remember to give the probiotics at least 3 hours after the antibiotics.

Raw cow milk, goat milk, and kefir can be beneficial sources of probiotics. Both are slightly warming, so avoid them with dogs that have difficulty staying cool or excessive dampness. Give 1 ounce of milk or kefir for every 20 pounds of body weight.

Probiotics can also be found in fermented vegetables. A dog needs only a small amount, starting at 1 teaspoon per 25 pounds of body weight. Fermented vegetables are rich in lactobacillus bacterium. They are more warming than goat milk, so limit their use with warm dogs. (Before feeding anything fermented to a warm to hot dog, do an ear test to check for an inflammatory reaction; see page 150.)

Green tripe is a good source of probiotics as it's rich in commensal bacteria and digestive enzymes. Feed 1 tablespoon for every 20 pounds of body weight.

I frequently recommend *Weizmannia coagulans* (previously known as and still marketed as *Bacillus coagulans* and before that *Lactobacillus sporogenes*), a spore-form probiotic, for antibiotics recovery. Sporebiotics have an increased chance of surviving the stomach and don't open until they feel comfortable, usually in the small or large intestine.[15]

. . . .

Tip! Dogs need sulfur in their diets for a healthy skin, coat, and musculoskeletal system as well as efficient food metabolism. It's also an integral part of cell reproduction. Sulfur is absorbed in the intestines, and antibiotics can create a sulfur deficiency when they destroy intestinal bacteria. Feeding probiotics together with sulfur, such as MSM (methylsulfonylmethane), can be helpful.

. . . .

Tip! Dogs with small intestinal bacterial overgrowth (SIBO) must avoid probiotics like bifidobacteria, lactobacilli, and fructobacilli, as well as prebiotic inulin. Your vet can test your dog for SIBO through breath hydrogen testing.

. . . .

Additional Herbal Supports

Milk thistle seed can support the liver with detoxification. Give either tinctured or dried milk thistle during and after antibiotic use. For long-term antibiotic damage, give milk thistle seed for the duration of the protocol.

Flower essences provide vibrational assistance, helping to balance your dog's mental and emotional state during recovery. Combine equal parts of crab apple, echinacea, and self-heal flower essence. Give one to six drops of the mixture twice daily for a month during or after antibiotic use.

🌿 Formula for Antibiotics-Related Diarrhea

If antibiotics cause your dog to have diarrhea,
add this blend to their regimen.

15 ml blackberry leaf tincture
13 ml plantain tincture
2 ml black walnut tincture

Combine the tinctures in a 30 ml bottle with a dropper top. Give the blend three times daily, diluted in warm water, until symptoms clear, following the dosing schedule below.

Dosing Schedule

Size of Dog	Dose
Extra-small	3 drops
Small	6 drops
Medium	10 drops
Large	15 drops
Extra-large	20–25 drops

Helpful Herbs and Supplements

Herbs for warm dogs: burdock root, cleavers, dandelion root, licorice root, milk thistle seed, olive leaf, plantain, rose hips, skullcap

Herbs for cool dogs: calendula, elecampane, licorice root, milk thistle seed, olive leaf, rosemary

Mushrooms: chaga, maitake, reishi, turkey tail

Phytoembryonics: beech, cowberry, fig, olive, walnut, willow

Flower essences: black walnut, crab apple, echinacea, self-heal

Homeopathic remedies: Arnica, Calendula officinalis, Thiosinaminum 12C

Supplements: chlorella, collagen, digestive enzymes, inulin, larch arabinogalactan, *Saccharomyces boulardii,* fulvic acid, humic acid, sodium butyrate, spirulina, zeolite

Foods: colostrum, fermented raw dairy, fermented vegetables, raw dairy, variety of tolerated vegetables

. . . .

Tip! Antibiotics can interfere with vitamin A absorption. Long-term antibiotic usage can cause vitamin K deficiency. Vitamin A and K levels can be checked by your veterinarian.

. . . .

Arthritis and Chronic Musculoskeletal Pain

Common energetic patterns: dryness, damp heat

Arthritis is a blanket term for musculoskeletal inflammation arising from different causes, including diet, environment, genetics, gut health, lymphatic congestion, and a hyperstimulated or depleted immune system.

Your dog's musculoskeletal (muscular-skeletal) system comprises cartilage, bone and marrow, joints, and muscular tissue. Voluntary and involuntary muscles work together with nerves to initiate movement, which produces heat and helps circulate blood. The body's bones protect vital organs, create red blood cells, and store vitamins and minerals such as calcium and phosphorus.

Consider kidney and liver function if your dog is prone to musculoskeletal problems. The buildup of toxins and stagnant elimination pathways can lead to the development of chronic ailments like arthritis, systemic inflammation, and spinal degeneration. Strategies might involve different types of herbs used internally and externally. Anti-inflammatory herbs can help reduce swelling and support the joints and muscle tissue. Cleansing and lymphatic herbs help eliminate built-up toxins in the muscle tissue. Herbal diuretics help support kidney function by facilitating the removal of wastes and relieving stagnation. Many times, relaxing herbs can assist with releasing trauma, tension, and stress.

Poor nutrient absorption in the intestinal tract can lead to chronic muscle and bone conditions like arthritis. Make sure your dog's diet supports healthy gut function.

The Role of Fluids

Your dog's musculoskeletal system and joints depend on fluids. Synovial fluids help protect cartilage and keep bones from bone-on-bone contact.

Inflammation causes damage to the entire system, fluids, and cartilage. Chronic inflammation causes heat, which causes dryness, which puts pressure on ligaments, muscles, tendons, and connective tissues. Arthritis can be a sign of dryness, especially in the kidneys.

Soft tissues and joints need fluids for flexibility and decreased heat. Without moisture, your dog's body can't cool, producing excess heat and protein-based waste. This dryness can be experienced as painful joints and tight ligaments.

Pain

Arthritic and musculoskeletal pain, obvious or hidden, can be dealt with at home with some trial and error. Testing different remedies and finding the right remedy or combination of remedies can make a world of difference for your dog.

Pain Cofactors

Abnormal posturing	Excessive licking
Aversion to normal routine	Groaning (sound of the kidney)
Aversion to touch	
Aversion to walking	Hiding
Arched back	Inability to jump
Changes in behavior	Lethargy
Crying out	Limping
Decreased appetite	Restless positioning

Helpful Herbs and Supplements

Herbs: alfalfa, angelica, ashwagandha, burdock root, cayenne, dandelion flower, ginger, goldenseal, gotu kola, gravel root, licorice root, marshmallow root, mullein root, nettle leaf and seed, rose hips, Solomon's seal, St. John's wort, teasel, turmeric, yarrow

Mushrooms: cordyceps, reishi, tremella

Phytoembryonics: black currant, bramble, mountain pine, willow

Essential oils for self-selection: balsam, copaiba, fir, myrrh

Flower essences: beech, gentian, marshmallow, rock water

Homeopathic remedies: Aconitum, Arnica, Baptisia, Belladonna, Calcarea phosphorica, Calendula officinalis, Chamomilla, Echinacea,

Hamamelis virginiana, Hypericum, Ledum, Nux vomica, Rhus toxico-dendron, Ruta graveolens, Symphytum officinale, Staphysagria

Supplements: biotin, bone broth, bromelain, chondroitin, full-spectrum CBD oil, green-lipped mussel, hyaluronic acid, magnesium, MSM (sulfur), PEA, propolis, silica, trace minerals, vitamins A, C, D, E, K, and B-complex

---

Nightshades

Monitor your dog's reactions to nightshades (plants in the Solanaceae family). In certain dogs, this family of herbs and vegetables can increase inflammation in the digestive and musculoskeletal systems. Look for symptoms like joint pain, acid reflux, gastrointestinal distress, and lip licking. Most dogs are fine with small amounts of nightshades. Dogs with autoimmune and leaky gut are more susceptible to irritation. Nightshades include ashwagandha (which tends to cause just mild reactions), cayenne, eggplant, goji berries, peppers, potatoes, and tomatoes. Consider feeding these foods only during their harvest season.

Bladder and Urinary Tract Conditions

Your dog's bladder and urinary tract can cause myriad issues but the main conditions that most dogs deal with are urinary tract infections, incontinence, and bladder stones and gravel. It's important to remember that, looking at these conditions holistically, they are symptoms of a larger imbalance. They are warning signs, in different degrees, that your dog's ecosystem needs support and balancing.

Urinary Tract Infections

Urinary tract infections (UTIs) often result from kibble diets, energetically inappropriate diets, dog diapers or pads, humping of toys, stress, and/or toxic overload. When a urinary tract infection occurs, you must do more than get rid of the infection . . . your dog's body is telling you that elimination has decreased and toxicity is up. When toxicity increases, you'll get increased inflammation. So toxicity must be addressed!

The conventional answer to UTIs is antibiotics; as detailed earlier in this chapter, antibiotics destroy not just the infection but also the ever important gut microbiome. If you don't take further action to repopulate the microbiome and address the root cause of the infection, you can bet that the infection will return within a few months.

If you think your dog is developing a UTI, it must be addressed; if ignored, it may turn into a kidney infection. Look at your dog's energetics and patterns for guidance. Visit your veterinarian for diagnostics, especially if your dog has chronic infections, to rule out something more serious like diabetes, stones, or tumors. Most UTIs are symptomatic of a larger issue.

Be sure to balance out the renal system after the infection disappears; see the discussion of the renal system in chapter 4.

☙ Formula for Urinary/Bladder Infection in Cool Dogs

> 10 ml calendula tincture
> 8 ml parsley tincture
> 5 ml echinacea tincture
> 4 ml olive leaf tincture
> 3 ml uva-ursi tincture

Combine the tinctures in a 30 ml bottle with a dropper top. Give the blend three times daily, diluted in warm water, in the side of the mouth or dripped on a small treat, following the dosing schedule below. Give the formula for 10 days.

Once symptoms clear, prepare another batch of the same blend, but without the echinacea and uva-ursi. Give this blend three times daily, diluted in warm water, for another 10 days, following the dosing schedule below.

Dosing Schedule

Size of Dog	Dose
Extra-small	3 drops
Small	8 drops
Medium	15 drops
Large	20 drops
Extra-large dog	25–30 drops

❧ Formula for Urinary/Bladder Infection for Warm Dogs

10 ml plantain glycerite
8 ml marshmallow root glycerite
4 ml cleavers glycerite
3 ml echinacea tincture
3 ml uva-ursi tincture
2 ml yarrow tincture

Combine the glycerites and tinctures in a 30 ml bottle with a dropper top. Give the blend three times daily, diluted in warm water, in the side of the mouth or dripped on a small treat, following the dosing schedule below. Give the formula for 10 days.

Once symptoms clear, prepare another batch of the same blend, but without the echinacea and uva-ursi. Give this blend three times daily, diluted in warm water, for another 10 days, following the dosing schedule below.

Dosing Schedule

Size of Dog	Dose
Extra-small	3 drops
Small	8 drops
Medium	15 drops
Large	20 drops
Extra-large	25–30 drops

Helpful Herbs and Supplements

Note: Keep in mind, a urinary tract infection can be chronic but can be tended to as an acute situation to provide relief. Feel free to use any of the herbs listed below for less than two weeks, especially in a formula.*

Herbs for warm dogs: chamomile, cleavers, couch grass, dandelion root and leaf, echinacea, goldenseal, lemon balm, marshmallow root, nettle, Oregon grape root, plantain, rose hips, usnea, uva-ursi, yarrow

---

*This guidance applies to most acute situations. See chapter 6 for more information on acute versus chronic.

Herbs for cool dogs: ginger, goldenrod, goldenseal, gravel root, green tea (decaffeinated), juniper berry, nettle, olive, parsley, rose hips, turmeric

Mushrooms: poria, reishi, tremella

Phytoembryonics: cowberry, heather, horsetail, olive

Essential oils for self-selection: cinnamon, coriander seed, eucalyptus, rosemary

Flower essences: bladderwort, crab apple, impatiens

Homeopathic remedies: Apis mellifica, Berberis vulgaris, Cantharis, Equisetum hyemale, Nux vomica, Pulsatilla

Supplements: bone broth, cranberries, D-mannose, glandulars, omega-3 fatty acids, magnesium, PEA, vitamins B$_6$, C, D, E, and K

Urinary Incontinence

Incontinence can be frustrating and its causes varied. It ranges from urine dribbling to full-blown emptying of the bladder. When working with an incontinent dog, I generally focus first on the kidneys and urinary system. Determining whether a dog's incontinence is hormone-related is an important step. (Did the incontinence occur after a spay or neuter? Are there issues with your female dog's cycle? Issues with cortisol?)

Causes of Incontinence

Abnormal growths/blockages	Nervous system conditions
Emotional/nervous conditions	Pharmaceutical side effects
Enlarged prostate	Physical abnormalities
Hormonal conditions	Stress
Inflammation	Too much of an herb or
Involuntary muscle	supplement (diuretic)
contractions	Urinary/bladder conditions
Low estrogen from spaying	Urinary/bladder stones
Musculoskeletal conditions	Vaccination

Hands-on methodologies that can help end canine incontinence include age-appropriate exercise, acupressure, acupuncture, and chiropractic.

Helpful Herbs and Supplements

Herbs for warm dogs: chamomile, corn silk, dandelion, licorice root, mullein root, nettle, plantain, red clover, uva ursi (used acutely)

Herbs for cool dogs: angelica, juniper berry, licorice root, mullein root, nettle

Herbs for hormonal incontinence: dandelion, chaste tree, raspberry

Mushrooms: poria, reishi

Phytoembryonics: bramble, cowberry, heather, horsetail

Essential oils for self-selection: basil, clary sage, copaiba, cypress, geranium, juniper, lavender, thyme, ylang-ylang

Flower essences: crab apple, Easter lily (flower essence is not toxic), oak

Homeopathic remedies: Causticum, Belladonna, Equisetum hyemale, Ferrum phosphoricum, Kreosotum, Lycopodium

Foods: apple, asparagus, berries, coconut, pumpkin seed, baked sweet potato, watermelon seed

Bladder Gravel and Stones

Lack of moisture can lead to gravel and stones in the bladder and kidneys. Make sure your dog is drinking enough water. Avoid giving your dog hard water, as it can lead to stone and gravel formation. Kibble can cause bladder gravel and kidney stones, as it's low in moisture and tends to be drying. If your dog suffers from gravel or stones, feed them a fresh food diet and focus on herbal infusions and tinctures/glycerites.

Symptoms of Bladder Gravel and Stones

Bloody urine	Off-smelling urine
Leaking urine	Straining to pee
Lethargy	Urinating in the house
Licking of genitals	Vomiting
Low appetite	

❧ Gravel and Stone Formula

Use this acute gravel and bladder stone formula if you think your dog has a buildup of sediment in their bladder or they've been diagnosed with stones. You can also give this formula for 1 week per month to dogs who are prone to bladder stones while you work to balance their constitution.

4 parts marshmallow root glycerite
4 parts nettle leaf tincture
3 parts cleavers leaf and flower tincture
2 parts blackberry leaf tincture
2 parts gravel root tincture
2 parts plantain leaf tincture
2 parts uva-ursi leaf tincture
1 part yarrow flower and leaf tincture

Combine the glycerites and tinctures in an amber glass bottle with a dropper top and shake well.

Give 3 drops for every 10 pounds of your dog's body weight three times daily until symptoms clear or for a maximum of one month.

Caution: Do not use this blend for dogs with kidney or liver disease or for dogs that are pregnant.

Helpful Herbs and Supplements

Note: although stones are a symptom of a chronic problem, you can begin balancing your dog's system by using an acute blend of herbs, despite your dog's energetics, for a period of two weeks or less and then move to a more energetically appropriate formula.

Herbs for warm dogs: burdock seed, celery seed, cleavers, couch grass, dandelion, juniper berry, lemon balm, licorice, marshmallow root, milk thistle seed,

Herbs for cool dogs: ginger, gravel root, juniper berry, licorice, meadowsweet, milk thistle seed, parsley, turmeric

Herbs for calcium oxalate stones: celery seed, cowberry (phytoembryonic), marshmallow root

Mushroom: tremella

Phytoembryonics: bramble, cowberry, heather

Essential oils for self-selection: fennel, grapefruit, helichrysum, lemon, lemongrass, orange

Flower essences: crab apple, fireweed, goldenrod, marshmallow, mimulus, rock water, oak, vine, violet

Homeopathic remedies: Belladonna, Berberis vulgaris, Calcarea carbonica, Cantharis, Lycopodium

Candida Overgrowth

Common energetic pattern: cool to cold, dampness

Yeasts, and specifically the species *Candida albicans,* are a normal part of the gastrointestinal microbiome. They and other microorganisms in the microbiome, such as bacteria, keep each other in check through competition for food. When factors lead to an imbalance in bacterial colonies, however, that system of checks and balances can fail and candida populations can grow quickly. When allowed to proliferate, these yeasts act like mushrooms, creating a mycelium-like structure that allows them to work in tandem as a larger organism, and they begin a hostile takeover of your dog's gastrointestinal tract.

The mucosal lining in your dog's intestinal lining is normally tight and helps control bacteria, viruses, and yeasts like candida from getting through and going into the bloodstream. The interesting fact about candida is that it helps your dog absorb nutrients—but only when it's balanced. Candida overgrowth can damage the intestinal lining, leading to a host of issues with digestion, elimination, leaky gut, and more.

> *For dogs with a major yeast infestation, all of that dead yeast has an impact. Toxins from dead candida become too much to handle all at once. The cells of this shocking enemy create toxic chemicals that kill beneficial bacteria, bacteria that are paramount to the health of the immune system. . . . Its waste produces toxic alcohols, acetone and hydrogen sulphide, which are known to be nerve poisons. And if that's not bad enough, these single-cell organisms can change form into multi-celled or mycelial [fungi] that have pileous (hairy) root-like projections. These penetrate the intestine causing gut trauma or leaky gut syndrome, decreasing the body's ability to absorb vitamins, minerals, amino acids, and fatty acids. This leads to nutritional deficiencies, autoimmune disease, malabsorption, allergies, cancer, arthritis, and more.*
>
> JULIE ANNE LEE,
> "SKIN DISEASE IN DOGS: WHAT TO DO
> WHEN YEAST ATTACKS," A BLOG POST ON
> THE ADORED BEAST APOTHECARY WEBSITE

Signs of Yeast Overgrowth

Allergies

Bad breath

Black skin

Bloating and abdominal pain

Butt itchiness

Chronic diarrhea

Chronic constipation

Chronic itchiness

Chronic kidney and bladder
  infections

Ear discharge

Essential fatty acid intolerance

Feet chewing

Food sensitivities

Fungal infections on the skin

Hair loss (especially on the tail
  or upper back)

Joint swelling

Mouth lesions

Mucus in the stools

Odor of corn chips or gym socks

Redness between toes

Sensitivity to humidity

Sinus infections

Causes of Candida Overgrowth

Antibiotics

Chemotherapy

Diabetes

Environmental toxins
  (like glyphosate or mercury)

Pharmaceuticals

Processed diet

Stress

Sympathetic excess

Vaccines

Breaking Down Biofilm

Biofilm is a slimy matrix that bacteria and yeasts, like candida, create to protect themselves in the gastrointestinal tract. Biofilm formation is a normal function of the organisms in the microbiome, and in a healthy system, it's kept in check by the immune system. With the right stimulus, however, biofilm can run amok.

As an example, when bacteria and yeast are threatened by antibiotics and antifungal medications, they can accelerate their production of biofilm. When the use of steroids shuts off the immune system, it opens the door for pathogens. Without the immune system to keep biofilm in check, they expand.

Biofilm works so well as a protective coating that it can make it challenging to overcome candida overgrowth and other yeast and bacterial issues. The signs that biofilm might be at play inside your dog's gastrointestinal tract include poor or no response to protocols for healing leaky gut or yeast overgrowth.

Successful biofilm care includes supporting the immune system, breaking down biofilm, normalizing and balancing gut bacteria, and cleaning up the by-products of yeast and bacteria die-offs through the elimination channels. Many herbs and fungi have the dual properties of helping to minimize and break up biofilm while also balancing microbe populations. Examples include dandelion, olive leaf extract, lion's mane mushroom (fruiting body and mycelium), oregano, reishi mushroom, rosemary, shitake mushroom, teasel, and turmeric. You can also give your dog digestive enzymes (including cellulase) between meals and before bed; they help break down biofilm.[16]

Eliminating Heavy Metals

Heavy metals hide in your dog's supplements, kibble, vaccines, pharmaceuticals, household environment, and water. Heavy metals increase oxidation and free radical production, taxing liver detoxification and contributing to systemic stress. Too many heavy metals in your dog's tissues contribute to low immune function, cognitive decline, and yeast overgrowth!

Candida attaches itself to mercury and other heavy metals. Remedies that rid the body of heavy metals deprive candida of attachment sites, allowing it to be more easily flushed from the body. Supplementing biotin can help with removing heavy metals, especially mercury (and yeasts). Use it in conjunction with chlorella and clay water (see below), which help bind the metals and remove them throughout the colon. Give 5 mg of biotin for every 10 pounds of your dog's body weight.

MSM (a bioavailable form of sulfur) is another option. It cleanses the body of heavy metals. The starting dose is 50 mg of MSM for every 10 pounds of your dog's body weight, given once daily.

✤ Clay Water

Clay water is simple to make and so beneficial when trying to remove heavy metals from your dog. Bentonite clay has a molecular negative ion surface area that expands and binds to positive ions, which include heavy metals and air pollutants.

> 1 teaspoon bentonite clay
> 4 ounces purified water

Combine the clay and water. Mix with a wooden spoon until the clay is dissolved. Let sit for at least 1 hour; letting it sit overnight will make it even more effective as the water will have more time to mix with the clay.

Stir the clay water before administering. Give 1/8 teaspoon for every 10 pounds of your dog's body weight. Wait at least 2 hours before feeding your dog.

Supporting Glycocalyx and IgA

Like antibiotics, yeasts deplete IgA and glycocalyx in the digestive tract. Supplement with *Saccharomyces boulardii* to help increase levels of both, which will support a healthy microbiome balance that suppresses yeast overgrowth. See the discussion of the digestive system in chapter 4 for more details.

Colostrum is sometimes used as an alternative for dogs that don't tolerate *S. boulardii*. However, don't use colostrum when your dog is dealing with yeast overgrowth, as it can aggravate the condition.

The Anti-yeast Diet

Sugar is candida fuel. When a dog is dealing with candida overgrowth, all sugars, even natural ones, must be eliminated. Feed your dog meat, organs, bone, and nothing else except supplements and herbs. (There may be exceptions if your dog has underlying health issues like kidney disease, chronic pancreatitis, or diabetes; in these cases, consult with your vet.) See the protocol for the basic elimination diet on page 149. Stick to protein, fats, and greens and eliminate dairy (milk sugar) and other foods with any type of sugar until you clear the yeast. Then you can add in more vegetables, broths, and raw dairy. Make sure to add foods one at a time and test ears for immune response. Give your dog at least three to five days to get used to each new food. Make a note in your journal of your dog's reactions.

Going slow is key to conquering candida overgrowth. How slow? Extremely slow. Your dog should be well and symptom-free for at least two months before you add any foods with naturally occurring sugars to their diet. When you are ready to reintroduce foods, add a new energetically appropriate food item each week while monitoring your dog's reaction.

Support for the Cleanse

Yeast isn't a benign substance, whether living or dead. When yeasts die, they give off toxins and increase your dog's toxic load. If you treat yeast overgrowth too fast, your dog can experience symptoms from the volume of yeast die-off. Signs that you're cleansing your dog too fast include diarrhea, hot spots, severe itchiness, lethargy, thinning hair and hair loss, and discharge from the eyes, ears, skin, and anus.

Dealing with candida or candida-based leaky gut is *always* slow-and-steady-wins-the-race. Repair doesn't happen overnight. Too much, too soon, causes excessive yeast die-off. The slow goal is to rebalance candida populations while avoiding excessive die-off.

If you see signs that your dog is experiencing an excessive yeast die-off, slow your protocol and begin a regimen of clay water (page 172), chlorella, and mountain pine phytoembryonic (if available). When yeasts die they release toxins and heavy metals that can make your dog feel sick. Clay, chlorella, and mountain pine buds can help alleviate your dog's toxic burden, binding to the metals and removing them from the body through the stool and urine. Zeolite can be a good alternative to chlorella if you need it.

Always support the liver when working with anything gastrointestinal-related; this includes yeast overgrowth. See chapter 4 for details.

Exercise is also a key factor in recovery. Breathing fresh air helps oxygenate cells, which decreases inflammation and supports a healthy immune system. Movement also helps stimulate the lymphatic system, which is imperative when eliminating toxins.

Helpful Herbs and Supplements

Herbs for warm dogs: chamomile, echinacea leaf and flower, goldenseal, licorice root, marshmallow root, milk thistle seed, mullein, Oregon grape root, rose, usnea

Herbs for cool dogs: calendula, ginger, licorice root, milk thistle seed, oregano, olive leaf, pau d'arco, turmeric

Mushrooms: lion's mane

Phytoembryonics: beech, olive, walnut, willow

Essential oils: bergamot, copaiba, cypress, eucalyptus radiata, geranium, helichrysum, lavender, lemongrass, myrrh

Flower essence: chestnut bud, crab apple, oat, scleranthus, willow

Homeopathic remedies: Baptisia, Berberis vulgaris, Bryonia, Calendula officinalis, Candida albicans nosode, Hydrangea arborescens, Viscum album

Supplements: activated charcoal, apple cider vinegar, bifidobacterium, chlorella, digestive enzymes, fermented foods, humic/fulvic acid, MCT oil, monolaurin, N-acetylcysteine (NAC), *Saccharomyces boulardii,* spirulina, zeolite

· ·

Tip! Omega-3 fatty acids are among the strongest candida killers. They both help remove heavy metals from the body and fortify the immune system. They can cause die-off symptoms, including dizziness, uneven gait, stomach distension, and lethargy. When a dog reacts negatively to essential fatty acid supplementation, it can indicate a yeast infection.

· ·

🌿 Anti-yeast Rinse and Soak

This rinse eliminates itchiness and odor from a candida infection. Prepare the thyme as a cold infusion, using apple cider vinegar instead of water and letting it steep overnight. Thyme works as an antifungal and helps relieve itchiness. Chamomile also relieves itchiness when used as a rinse; prepare it as a cold overnight infusion if you decide to use it. You could add 2 to 3 ounces of patchouli infusion, if you like; patchouli kills yeast and makes tissues inhospitable to pathogenic fungi.

2 ounces coconut water
1 ounce thyme-infused apple cider vinegar
6 ounces cold chamomile infusion (optional)

Combine all the ingredients and shake to mix. Use as a rinse daily to help relieve active symptoms. Just squeeze the rinse into your dog's fur and work it through the coat with your hands. Don't rinse it out.

Constipation

Common energetic pattern: coolness and dryness with tension

When your dog has constipation, it can feel like a panic situation. Constipation happens in the large intestine. As digestive wastes move through the colon, large amounts of bacteria break down waste, water is absorbed, and waste mixes with bile to form your dog's stool. When wastes fail to pass through the colon fast enough, too much water is removed, leaving your dog's stool dry, hard, and difficult to expel. This process leads to an overabundance of feces in the colon as wastes build up, stretching the colon lining.

What causes constipation? The answer isn't as easy as it would seem. When I look at a dog with constipation, I first determine whether the issue stems from dryness in the colon, excessive heat in the digestive tract, or stagnancy throughout the dog's ecosystem. Dogs shouldn't go more than forty-eight hours without a bowel movement, so it's important to quickly figure out what is happening and how to deal with it.

Evaluating Potential Causes

First, let's explore constipation as it relates to energetics and diet. When dogs that are energetically warm to hot eat energetically warm foods like lamb, venison, or salmon, they can easily develop constipation because their digestive tract is hot and quickly dries up circulating fluids. On the other hand, when cool dogs are fed an overabundance of cooling foods like pork, duck, sweet potatoes, and chlorella, contractions in the intestines can occur and cause constipation or diarrhea. Other diet-related problems include lack of water, insufficient fiber intake, or, in some cases, too much fiber, like the overfeeding of pumpkin. Too many bones in the diet can cause constipation. A kibble diet, grain, or excessive flour-based treats can also cause constipation; these foods turns to sugar and lead to stagnation in the large intestine, especially when water consumption is insufficient.

Another factor in constipation is weight. Obese dogs usually have slower waste mobility through the large intestine. Stress can be another factor; dogs who don't get enough exercise or who exercise excessively without rest periods can be very stressed, which can lead to either constipation or diarrhea.

When diet, water, and stress have been ruled out as a cause, look for physical manifestations of difficulty like anal gland infections, spinal weakness, arthritis, or muscle and back injuries. Pharmaceuticals, including anesthesia, painkillers, nausea medicines, and vaccinations, can cause constipation, as can iron-rich supplements. Benadryl and other antihistamines can cause severe constipation.

Sometimes there can be a more dire cause for constipation, an inedible object that's been swallowed or a tumor that obstructs passage through the bowel. Most foreign obstructions work themselves out within forty-eight hours. Still, if they persist and your dog loses their appetite, starts to vomit, becomes lethargic, and develops a hard distended stomach, they must be seen by a veterinarian.

Laxative Strategies

An easy first step in addressing constipation is to lubricate the gastrointestinal tract. Gentle laxatives should be your first choice. Mild laxatives such as marshmallow root and tremella mushroom coat the insides of the colon and create a slippery environment, helping move stool along the colon so it can be excreted.

Support for the liver is also imperative because constipation traps toxins inside your dog's body causing a heavier toxin burden for the liver. Herbal bitters such as artichoke, burdock root, and milk thistle can help support detoxification and release bile, which helps increase digestive enzymes in the small intestine; this in turn helps relieve constipation. See chapter 4 for details on how to support the liver.

Helpful Herbs and Supplements

Herbs for warm dogs: burdock, chamomile, cleavers, couch grass, chickweed, dandelion, licorice, marshmallow root, Oregon grape root, passionflower, plantain, slippery elm, violet, wood betony, yellow dock

Herbs for cool dogs: angelica, fennel, licorice, olive, passionflower, slippery elm, wood betony

Herbs for constipation resulting from pharmaceuticals: burdock root, marshmallow root, milk thistle seed, Oregon grape root, slippery elm

Herb for constipation alternating with diarrhea: yellow dock root

Mushroom: tremella

Essential oils for self-selection: chamomile, fennel, ginger, lemon, orange, peppermint, sweet basil

Phytoembryonics: bramble, cowberry, fig, mountain elm, olive, walnut

Flower Essences: angelica, aspen, beech, bottlebrush, crab apple, lilac, self-heal

Foods: apple, berries, broccoli, carrots, celery, chard, chia, freshly ground flax seed, green beans, kale, kelp, lettuce, moringa, mushrooms, pumpkin, spinach

Coughing

Coughing can have many causes, but whatever the case, you need to determine the energetics of the cough. Is it dry or moist? The answer will guide you.

Causes of Cough

Aspiration pneumonia	Heartworm
Collapsed trachea	Kennel cough
Flu	Pneumonia
Heart disease	

Kennel Cough

Kennel cough is scary to experience. It sounds awful; it can be dry or wet, and sometimes it makes dogs hack and gag. Know that kennel cough usually runs its course in three to five days. During this time, focus on making your dog comfortable and work toward boosting immune function. Kennel cough affects the mucosa of the upper respiratory system. Once dogs are exposed to it, it takes five to ten days for symptoms to occur. Healthy dogs don't normally get kennel cough. I see this affliction as a red flag for immune health. Full healing usually takes four to five weeks.

Note: If your dog comes down with kennel cough but has another health condition or is immune-compromised, you may need veterinary assistance.

. . . .

Tip! Celestial Seasonings Sleepytime Tea stops coughing for up to four hours. Give as an infusion or use it as the base of a cough syrup.

. . . .

❧ Canine Cough Syrup

Prepare a strong infusion or decoction of an appropriate herb from the lists that follow. Mix together equal parts of this infusion or decoction and honey (preferably manuka or buckwheat). If you like, add 1–2 ml of an appropriate tincture or glycerite (again, choose from the list of herbs on the facing page).

The dose is 1/2 teaspoon for dogs under 10 pounds, 3/4 teaspoon for dogs between 10 and 25 pounds, and 1 teaspoon per 25 pounds of body weight for bigger dogs. Give this dose up to three times per day.

🌿 Kennel Cough Formula for a Cool Dog

15 ml astragalus root tincture
10 ml echinacea tincture
10 ml licorice root tincture
3 ml angelica tincture
2 ml New England aster tincture

Combine the tinctures in a 30 ml amber glass bottle with a dropper top and shake well. Give 2 drops for every 10 pounds of your dog's body weight, twice daily.

Note: For both formulas, you can use glycerites in place of the tinctures except for New England aster and angelica; they must be in tincture form. If you use glycerites, double or triple the dosage.

🌿 Kennel Cough Formula for a Warm Dog

10 ml marshmallow root glycerite or decoction
10 ml mullein tincture
5 ml echinacea tincture
3 ml licorice root tincture or glycerite
2 ml New England aster tincture

Combine all the tinctures or glycerites in a 30 ml amber glass bottle with a dropper top and shake well. Give 2 drops for every 10 pounds of your dog's body weight, twice daily.

Helpful Natural Remedies

Herbs for dry coughs: burdock root, chamomile, licorice root, marshmallow root, mullein, plantain, red clover, rose petals, Solomon's seal, usnea

Herbs for wet coughs: astragalus, calendula, elecampane, ginger, goldenseal, olive leaf, plantain, rose hips, usnea

Herbs for spasmodic coughs: angelica, bee balm, chamomile, elecampane, licorice, mullein, passionflower, red clover, skullcap

Herbs for immune support: angelica, astragalus, chamomile, echinacea, ginger, goldenseal, licorice root, marshmallow root, mullein, olive leaf, Oregon grape root, plantain, rose hips, skullcap, thyme, turmeric, usnea

Mushrooms: chaga, cordyceps, reishi, tremella (dry cough)

Essential oils for self-selection: cardamom, chamomile, eucalyptus, ginger, lavender, lemon, orange

Flower essences: crab apple, fireweed, oat, olive, nasturtium, Rescue Remedy, white chestnut

Homeopathic remedies for dry coughs: Bryonia, Causticum, Phosphorus, Rumex, Spongia, Sticta pulmonaria

Homeopathic remedies for wet coughs: Ammoniacum gum, Antimonium tartaricum, Hepar sulphuris, Lycopodium, Pulsatilla

Homeopathic remedies for spasmodic coughs: Coccus cacti, Corallium rubrum, Drosera, Hyoscyamus niger, Ignatia

Supplements: full-spectrum CBD oil, manuka honey, propolis, raw buckwheat honey, trace minerals, vitamins C, E

Diarrhea

Diarrhea is a common occurrence in dogs, and it's caused by food passing too quickly through the intestines and not going through the proper assimilation process. Diarrhea can take many forms. For instance, an increase in stool, no matter its consistency or size, can be classified as diarrhea. Diarrhea can be watery, bloody, or loose stool. It doesn't necessarily have to be the smelly, explosive type of stool that makes us gag. It is simply poop that interferes with your dog's regular evacuation routine.

Diarrhea is often temporary, resulting from an unknown gastrointestinal event that goes away quickly. It's essential to look for cofactors. Diarrhea accompanied by abdominal swelling, fever, gas, mucus, pus, and in extreme cases vomiting can be a sign of something more serious.

Diarrhea is the body's way of ridding itself of toxins. Allowing your dog time to expel those pathogens is integral to clearing up diarrhea. Where things get tricky is finding that fine line between a healthy bodily expression and dehydration from rapid water and electrolyte loss. Most diarrhea causes a depletion of water, sodium, and potassium; replenishing these substances is vital to your dog's recovery. Encourage your dog to drink plenty of water or broth during this time.

Sometimes it's helpful to have your dog fast during diarrhea and focus on fluid intake. Many dogs will do this naturally, but if you have one of those breeds that will eat no matter what, try giving them just small amounts of bone broth or electrolyte fluid. Most diarrhea resolves itself in one to three days. If the event lasts longer and is accompanied by pus or extreme pain, go to the vet immediately. If your dog is vomiting and having diarrhea, this is a reason for ruling out something more extreme.

Dehydration

From a whole-body perspective, diarrhea is a manifestation of gastrointestinal imbalance. Fluids build up in the intestines and cause rapid evacuation of stool—for example, runny, watery, and explosive diarrhea. When this occurs, especially in chronic diarrhea, the malabsorption of nutrients and chronic dehydration can occur. Therefore, preventing dehydration is a must. Fluid loss happens quickly. Look for signs including dull, sunken eyes; dry, thickly coated gums; and lethargy and weakness. Possible dehydration warrants the use of an electrolyte solution. If your dog won't drink, use a syringe to *slowly* give them fluids until you can get them to the veterinarian.

Easy electrolyte solutions include raw goat milk, raw cow milk, and coconut water mixed with a little salt. Here is an easy electrolyte solution recipe for dogs over six months of age. For puppies, use salted coconut water (eliminating the honey and vinegar from the recipe below).

☙ Canine Electrolyte Formula

1 cup water, coconut water, or bone broth
2 teaspoons raw honey
½ teaspoon apple cider vinegar
⅛ teaspoon Himalayan salt

Warm the water enough to melt the honey, add the other ingredients, and stir. Give by the teaspoon or tablespoon two or three times daily, as needed, following the dosing schedule below.

Dosing Schedule

Size of Dog	Dose
Extra-small	⅛ cup
Small	¼ cup
Medium	½ cup
Large	I cup
Extra-large	I½ cups

Caution: Do not give Pedialyte to dogs with Addison's disease as it interferes with their potassium and sodium balance. In general, use caution when using commercial products for humans; they can contain artificial sweeteners that are toxic to dogs—such as xylitol.

Acute vs. Chronic Diarrhea

There are two types of diarrhea: acute and chronic. Acute diarrhea is more common and usually resolves itself. However, acute diarrhea can happen on consecutive days. I've found acute diarrhea to be associated with antibiotic usage, bacterial infections, coccidia, dairy products, food sensitivities, food poisoning, food volume, inflammation in the intestines, and ingestion of foreign or inappropriate objects. For puppies, conditions like parvo and distemper can cause rapid diarrhea. See your vet immediately when puppies have excessive diarrhea.

Chronic diarrhea happens over a long, drawn-out period, such as loose stools occurring on one or two days a week for months. Chronic loose stools are usually caused by a digestive issue like a bacterial infection. Since chronic diarrhea is not as overt as the acute variety, it can often be overlooked—or it can manifest as an explosive runny stool when you least expect it. Diarrhea that happens for more than two consecutive days always needs attention. Antibiotic usage, bacterial infections, cancer, chronic stress, giardiasis, kidney imbalance, leaky gut, liver imbalance, pancreas imbalance, thyroid imbalance, and viral infections can all have a diarrhea component.

Acute Diarrhea Formula

This formula helps stop general diarrhea. It works quickly.

15 ml calendula tincture
10 ml blackberry leaf tincture
5 ml yarrow tincture

Combine all the tinctures in an amber glass bottle with a dropper top. Give three times daily, following the dosing schedule below, or until symptoms clear. Don't give for more than 3 days.

Dosing Schedule

Size of Dog	Dose
Extra-small	2–3 drops
Small	6 drops
Medium	10 drops
Large	15 drops
Extra-large	20–25 drops

Hot vs. Cold Diarrhea

You can analyze the color and consistency of your dog's stool to help you choose the best herbal protocol. If stools are dark and have a foul odor, your dog usually has heat in their digestive system. Diarrhea in this case may be accompanied by anal burning and itchiness. You'll want to use cooling herbs. (Remember, despite your dog's energetics, address the acute situation first and then the energetics of the acute condition.)

When dogs are kibble-fed, heat-induced diarrhea is usually caused by rancid ingredients. If your dog's intestines make loud noises followed by smelly loose stools, you're looking at undigested food.

Diarrhea that is characterized by copious amounts of water and a mild smell is usually a cold condition. If weakness and lethargy are present, look to a pathogen. Small amounts of blood or mucus are usually characteristic of pathogenic bacteria (unbalanced gut flora) and inflammation.

Bloody Diarrhea

Bright red blood in the large intestine or the stool usually indicates inflammation and isn't a cause for panic. Yes, it's good to go to the vet and ensure that the blood is only inflammation, but *don't* give "preventive" antibiotics to clear up any unknowns unless it's your last resort. Antibiotics will only worsen your dog's gut balance and cause long-term damage to their microbiome. The standard of care for most diarrhea is Flagyl, which, as discussed earlier in this chapter, can activate inflammation genes and cause a cascade of gut issues, including leaky gut, SIBO, and yeast overgrowth.[17]

🌾 Bloody Diarrhea Formula

*As noted earlier, for dogs, bloody diarrhea isn't something to worry
too much about, especially if you're sure your dog hasn't eaten a
cooked bone or something sharp. The most common cause is bacteria or
inflammation. The goal is to calm the intestines and stop the bleeding.
Yarrow helps stop the bleeding, while calendula soothes tissues and
calms the intestines. Oregon grape root is antibacterial.*

3 parts calendula tincture
1 part Oregon grape root tincture
1 part yarrow tincture

Combine all the tinctures in an amber glass bottle with a dropper top. Give
twice daily, following the dosing schedule below, for no more than 5 days.

Dosing Schedule

Size of Dog	Dose
Extra-small	1 or 2 drops
Small	2 or 3 drops
Medium	4–6 drops
Large	8–10 drops
Extra-large	10–12 drops

Diarrhea Caused by Giardiasis

For puppies and adult dogs, giardia, a protozoal parasite, can cause rapid
onset of diarrhea. Usually dogs get giardia from drinking out of streams
and other outdoor water sources. Giardiasis diarrhea is characterized
by uncontrollable, liquid diarrhea that persists for a week or more.
Always test for giardia and rule out chronic diarrhea or a severely strain-
dominant microbiome where there is too much of one microorganism.

🌾 Formula for Giardiasis Diarrhea

3 parts echinacea tincture
1 part goldenseal tincture

Combine the tinctures in an amber glass bottle with a dropper top.
Give three times daily, following the dosing schedule below, for 7 days.
Between meals and before bed, give small amounts of digestive enzymes
(including cellulase). Take a 10-day break from the tincture blend, while

continuing with the enzymes, and then do another 7-day round of the tincture blend.

Dosing Schedule

Size of Dog	Dose
Extra-small	3–4 drops
Small	8 drops
Medium	16 drops
Large	20–25 drops
Extra-large	30 drops

Helpful Herbs and Supplements

Herbs for acute diarrhea: agrimony, blackberry leaf and root, calendula, echinacea, goldenseal, Oregon grape root, slippery elm, usnea, yarrow, yellow dock root

Herbs for chronic diarrhea: agrimony, blackberry leaf, calendula, slippery elm, yellow dock root

Essential oils: chamomile, eucalyptus, helichrysum, lavender, peppermint

Homeopathic remedies: Aconitum napellus, Arnica montana, Arsenicum albulm, Baptisia tinctoria, Carbo vegetabilis, Chamomilla, Chincho officinalis, Juglans regia, Lycopodium clavatum

Supplements: colostrum, digestive enzymes, fiber, gelatin, probiotics, pumpkin

🌿 Formula for Diarrhea Caused by Ingestion of Cat Feces

It is very common for dogs to indulge in cat feces. However, those delicious cat turds are teeming with bacteria and cause many cases of diarrhea. Use blackberry leaf tincture mixed with Oregon Grape root or echinacea/goldenseal combination when diarrhea, specifically from cat poo, is present.

> 3 parts blackberry leaf tincture
> 1 part Oregon grape root tincture, usnea tincture, or a 1:1 blend of echinacea and goldenseal tinctures

Combine the tinctures in an amber glass bottle with a dropper top. Give the blend twice daily, diluted in warm water, in the side of the mouth or dripped on a small treat, following the dosing schedule below.

Dosing Schedule

Size of Dog	Dose
Extra-small	2 drops
Small	4 drops
Medium	8 drops
Large	12 drops
Extra-large	15 drops

◥ Diarrhea Clean-Up Formula

Cleaning up your dog's digestive tract and normalizing tissue after a dog has diarrhea is vitally important. Calendula, marshmallow root, and plantain will help clean up the intestinal tract and calm tissue inflammation. Crab apple flower essence helps cleanse and balance your dog's system and emotional state during sickness, while oak flower essence helps with any physical weakness or debilitating conditions.

> 10 drops marshmallow root tincture
> 10 drops plantain tincture
> 5 drops calendula tincture
> 2 drops crab apple or oak flower essence
> 2 ounces filtered water

Combine the tinctures, flower essence, and water. Administer twice daily, following the dosing schedule below, for 3 to 4 days.

Dosing Schedule

Size of Dog	Dose
Extra-small	1 teaspoon
Small	2 teaspoons
Medium	1 tablespoon
Large	2 tablespoons
Extra-large	3 tablespoons

Ear Infections

Common energetic pattern: dampness

Ear infections can be many things, but with chronic ear infections, look to the gut, kidneys, and lymphatics. Support and nourish these three systems and watch your dog's ear infections disappear.

With an acute ear infection, it's often best to visit your veterinarian so you know what you are dealing with—whether there's a foreign object involved, where in the ear the infection is located, and so on.

Inside the ear canal, most of the time a buildup of bacteria and yeast cause ear infections. Diet, kidney weakness, and the shape of the ear can play a contributory role. Dogs who swim can be prone to ear infections.

. . . .

Tip! When dogs chronically itch the side of their faces, it can indicate an ear infection.

. . . .

Contributors to Ear Infections

Autoimmune disease	Kidney weakness
Digestive insufficiency	Liver congestion
Food sensitivities	Lymphatic congestion
Hyperactive immune system	Vaccines
Hypothyroid	Water in the ear
Irregular ear shape	(from swimming)

Working with Ear Infections
Focus first on relieving the inflammation, pain, and swelling, then work on clearing up the infection. For chronic ear infections, focus on kidney weakness. It's important to act quickly to keep the infection from becoming severe. Visit your vet if you don't see relief with any of these protocols within three days.

Most important, make your dog as comfortable as possible. Administer full-spectrum CBD oil directly on your dog's gums or chamomile tincture/glycerite to help relax your dog's nervous system.

Clean the ears and then address the infection with an ear oil. The herbal formulations you use for the cleaner and oil will depend on whether the infection is caused by bacteria or yeast. Here's how to tell the difference:

- Bacterial infection: yellow and green discharge
- Yeast infection: brown discharge with a stinky, vinegary smell.

Ear Cleaners

When your dog is prone to ear infections, herbal ear cleaners can help keep inflammation and infections from occurring by decreasing the buildup of bacteria and yeast inside the ear canal. Mixing natural anti-inflammatory, antiseptic, and soothing herbs can decrease your dog's discomfort level and their urge to incessantly scratch their ears.

Note: Store the cleaners in a dark, cool area or refrigerate. Let warm to room temperature before using. They will keep for approximately thirty days.

⁂ Bacterial Ear Infection Cleaner

Clean the ear with this cleaner and then apply oil formula below.

> 15 ml aloe vera juice
> 15 ml distilled witch hazel
> 8 ml meadowsweet tincture
> 8 ml St. John's wort tincture
> 8 ml usnea tincture
> 6 ml rosemary tincture

Combine all the ingredients in a 60 ml amber glass bottle with a dropper top and shake well. Apply to your dog's ears twice daily, before the ear oil, and let your dog shake out the liquid before applying ear oil.

⁂ Yeast Ear Infection Cleaner

Clean the ear with this cleaner and then apply oil formula below.

> 15 ml green tea (decaffeinated)
> 10 ml apple cider vinegar
> 10 ml olive phytoembryonic
> 8 ml St. John's wort tincture
> 6 ml meadowsweet tincture
> 6 ml mullein flower tincture
> 5 ml calendula tincture

Combine all the ingredients in a 60 ml amber glass bottle with a dropper top and shake well. Apply to your dog's ears twice daily, before the ear oil, and let your dog shake out the liquid before applying ear oil.

Ear Oils

Ear oils are a good way to help clear infections and soothe your dog's ears. These recipes are made with infused oils, *not* essential oils.

Note: Store the ear oils in a dark, cool place. They should keep for a few months. You can add a few drops of vitamin E oil for longer storage.

🌿 Ear Oil for Bacterial Infection

    10 ml pumpkin seed oil
    6 ml echinacea flower and leaf infused oil
    5 ml mullein flower infused oil
    5 ml plantain flower infused oil
    2 ml rosemary infused oil
    1 ml garlic infused oil

Combine all the ingredients in a 30 ml amber glass bottle with a dropper top and shake well. Apply to your dog's ears twice daily, after cleaning them, and let your dog shake out the liquid before applying ear oil.

🌿 Ear Oil for Yeast Infection

    10 ml MCT oil
    5 ml calendula infused oil
    5 ml mullein flower infused oil
    5 ml plantain infused oil
    5 ml St. John's wort infused oil

Combine all the ingredients in a 30 ml amber glass bottle with a dropper top and shake well. Apply to your dog's ears twice daily, after cleaning them, and let your dog shake out the liquid before applying ear oil.

🌿 Ear Mite Oil Drops

Similar to an ear infection, ear mites can cause some of the same symptoms as an ear infection, including pain, discharge, itching, and inflammation. Two main differences between ear mites and ear infection is that ear mites come from other dogs and your dog will have a dirt-like discharge and possibly sores inside the ear canal.

    10 ml aloe vera juice
    8 ml distilled witch hazel
    5 ml echinacea root tincture
    5 ml Oregon grape root tincture
    1 ml garlic tincture

Combine all the ingredients in a 30 ml amber glass bottle with dropper top and shake well. Apply to your dog's ears twice daily, after cleaning them, and let your dog shake out the liquid before applying ear oil.

Helpful Herbs and Supplements

Herbs for warm dogs: chamomile, cleavers, echinacea, goldenseal, nettle leaf and seed, Oregon grape root

Herbs for cool dogs: astragalus, bee balm, calendula, nettle leaf and seed, olive, parsley, rosemary

Herbs for yeasty ear infections: calendula, chamomile, echinacea, mullein flower, pau d'arco, plantain, St. John's wort

Herbs for bacterial ear infections: echinacea, mullein flower, olive leaf, plantain, St. John's wort

Phytoembryonics for yeast ear infections: beech, black currant, heather, olive

Essential oils for self-selection: bergamot, chamomile, lavender, niaouli, oregano, patchouli, petitgrain, tea tree, yarrow

Homeopathic remedies: Aconite, Apis mellifica, Arnica, Capsicum annum, Causticum, Cinchona officinalis, Conium maculatum, Dulcamara, Kali sulphuricum cell salt

Supplements: digestive enzymes, full-spectrum CBD oil, omega-3 fatty acids, probiotics, *Saccharomyces boulardii*, vitamin E

Grief

This discussion of grief addresses you, the reader, and your animals. If one of you is grieving, so is the other. Grief is a mother, a teacher, and sometimes a friend holding us tight as we mourn those we've lost. It can be a weight that takes hold of you or your dogs if left unnoticed. Telling others that we are grieving and being vulnerable is hard for many people, as they feel ashamed of their feelings or the difficulties they're having with the loss of a loved one. As a culture, humans—with or without social media—concentrate on "looking good," putting on a good face, and acting like everything is fine. "Oh, I'm fine, I'm ok, don't worry about me." How many times have we said this despite feeling like a gaping wound? Our dogs feel the same and partake in many of the same coping mechanisms, feeding off our energies and being strong for us.

Sometimes the mere mention of grief can clear a room or make others feel uncomfortable. Many people find it confrontational, especially in cultures where looking good is the focus of social interaction. Some folks cannot deal with their own grief, and the sorrow they are dealing with or carrying around, so hearing about other people's grief is too much. Yet grief is not the enemy or something to be embarrassed or ashamed of; it's part of you. If someone is uncomfortable with your grief, it's more about them than you. We can't expect to move forward without looking at the present, what is happening now, or how we relate our past to our future. We must unite (with good boundaries) and hold space for people.

When grieving, it's important to know that people deal with loss in different ways, express it in different ways, and experience the cycle of grief in different ways. Grief affects us both mentally and physically through loss, heartache, stress, tension, passion, gratitude, missing, longing, emptiness, illness, and, surprisingly, love. And grief is not limited to the loss of a loved one. Physical and emotional grief can occur with any type of loss, including anticipated loss, or when circumstances affect your sense of belonging or security.

As we heal ourselves, we heal the web of life, our pets, and ourselves. Everything is connected. Grief works on a system of opposites; grief's opposite is acceptance and love. We wouldn't know what joy and love are without sorrow and grief. Life and death, yin and yang, up and down—the world is built upon a system of opposites so we can experience the knowing of each. Without one, we wouldn't have the other. Without love, we wouldn't be able to experience grief. So, in essence, grief is love.

Losing a loved one never has a right time. However, having a plan for support, if possible, may benefit you and your dog in a time of need. Our plant allies are here to help us build a bridge to the other side and hold space as we go through the loss process. Acceptance is a part of the healing process, but some of us, including our furry companions, might not know what is needed or how to move through the grief. Our plant allies offer transformation and understanding of the unknown.

Dogs grieve for many reasons. They can react to our emotions, experiencing what is known as secondhand grief. They may also feel grief after trauma, loss of a partner or housemate, and other unknowable factors, seen or unseen by their guardians. The issue is that the grief our dogs feel often goes unnoticed. What makes this worrisome is that the emotional can manifest in the physical because everything is connected.

Signs Your Dog Might Be Grieving	
Constipation	Nervous pooping
Excessive fear	Personality changes
Grinding of teeth	Restlessness
Lethargy	Tail tucking
Loss of appetite	Twitching
Lung weakness	Whining or the sudden
Nervousness	inability to be alone

Behavior Management

When your dog is grieving, whatever the reason, provide lots of fresh air and exercise. Stick to a routine to relieve stress. If your dog likes to play, spend at least fifteen minutes multiple times per day engaging in play or attempted play. Try to balance, support, and give your dog personal space without reinforcing the grieving behavior. However, if your dog is clingy, be available, but be careful not to reinforce the grieving behavior.

Helpful Herbs and Supplements

Plants can open cellular energy, transform stagnant emotions, and support emotional and physical healing. From a holistic herbalist's perspective, four forms of herbal medicine help transform grief: herbal tinctures, essential oils, flower essences, and homeopathic medicine.

Herbs for warm dogs: cleavers, hawthorn leaf and flower, mullein leaf and flower, passionflower, rose petal, skullcap, violet

Herbs for cool dogs: bee balm, calendula, hawthorn berry, nettle, St. John's wort

Phytoembryonics: beech, fig

Essential oils for self-selection: bergamot, myrrh, neroli, rose, sweet marjoram

Flower essences: agrimony, baby blue eyes, bleeding heart, boneset, bougainvillea, comfrey, echinacea, gorse, mullein, olive, passionflower, pine, star of Bethlehem, water violet

Homeopathic remedies: Aconitum, Arsenicum album, Calcarea phosphorica cell salt, Ignatia, Natrum muriaticum cell salt, Phosphoricum acidum, Pulsatilla

Growths and Warts

Dog warts can be confusing. They vary in color (pink, black, brown, or gray) and texture, making them look scary. When you see a small lump, how do you tell if it's a wart? What should you do?

My advice? Breathe. Your dog looks to you for reassurance; focus on being calm. From a holistic perspective, warts on the skin are a warning sign that the body, and especially the liver, isn't functioning as well as it should. Most warts are viral in nature, but others have unknown causes, and some have a genetic component. Warts are common near and inside a dog's mouth, hairy toes, eyes, and armpits. Almost all warts are noninvasive, but some can cause pain and quickly multiply.

It's good to have your holistic veterinarian look at any warts you find on your dog to ensure they look normal. Your vet can quickly tell you if your dog has warts or what is known as papillomatosis. Papillomas are more prevalent in younger dogs with immature immune systems and look like a small head of cauliflower.

Often mistaken as warts, skin tags are more prevalent in older dogs, which is the opposite of canine warts. Skin tags are fibrous growths and are more apt to appear on the chest, neck, and legs. They can be any shape and usually hang or have flexible appendages.

Transmission and Susceptibility

Warts take a long time to develop, sometimes over months, making it hard to trace the origin of the infection. A viral contagion causes most warts and is most likely to infect dogs with low vitamin D levels, young dogs, those with compromised immune systems, or those having had surgery. Some breeds, like my favorite, pugs, are more prone to getting warts.[18] Spaniels, Weimaraners, and Vizslas are more susceptible to papillomatosis.[19]

Wart viruses (yes, there is more than one type) aren't transmitted from dogs to humans; however, the virus can be transmitted to dogs from toys, bedding, and other dogs. With papillomas, wash bedding, toys, or anything your dog touches, as they can spread quickly from dog to dog. During an active episode, keep your dog out of dog parks, daycare, and boarding facilities.

Conventional Wart Treatment

Warts can be scary in this age of cancer. Your vet is most likely good at recognizing warts and can ease your mind. While most warts don't cause any issues and go away on their own, some can bleed, itch, or become infected. Eye and mouth warts might obstruct vision or make eating difficult. The standard of practice is freezing them off, which is a painless outpatient procedure. In some cases surgical intervention might be needed.

Holistic Wart Care

Prevention is one of the best ways to deal with warts. Supporting your dog's immune system can go a long way in keeping your dog from getting warts, even if they're young.

To get rid of warts, look at improving immune and organ health. Ensure that your dog eats a balanced diet with adequate antioxidants, trace minerals, and live enzymes. In addition to general immune and system support, there are internal and external options using herbs and homeopathy, but patience is needed. Wart removal takes time. Give a remedy eight to ten weeks before discontinuing (unless there are complications) and trying another.

Healing Strategies: Immune Focus

Age-appropriate exercise	Increased fiber-rich foods
Decreased stress (for you too!)	Kidney support
Energetically appropriate food	Liver support
Filtered water (no plastic water bottles!)	Lymphatic stimulation
Fresh-food diet with enzymes	Microbiome support with pre- and probiotics
Fresh outdoor air	Minimal vaccination and
Increased antioxidant-rich foods	prescription drugs

Helpful Herbs and Supplements:
Internal Use
Herbs for warm dogs: cleavers, echinacea, milk thistle seed, red clover
Herbs for cool dogs: calendula, milk thistle seed
Mushrooms: chaga, reishi, turkey tail (all in higher dosages than is normally recommended)
Phytoembryonics: black currant, dog rose, maritime pine, olive, willow
Flower essence: crab apple
Homeopathic remedies: Antimonium crudum, Dulcamara, Graphites, Kali bichromiucum, Natrum sulphuricum, Nitricum acidum, Phosphorus, Phytolacca decandra, Psorinum, Saponaria officinalis, Sulphur, Thuja occidentalis
Supplements: chlorella, full-spectrum CBD oil, phytoplankton, spirulina

External Strategies
With time, warts can be eliminated with consistent application of black currant phytoembryonic, black walnut tincture, dandelion phytoembryonic, dog rose phytoembryonic, or oak phytoembryonic.

The stem sap of calendula and dandelion are also excellent topicals for reducing or eliminating warts. Break off a stem of calendula or dandelion as close to the ground as possible. Gently squeeze the sticky, milky sap from the stem onto the wart. Apply twice daily until the wart is gone. It should take approximately two weeks. (Note: Dandelion sap may be initially irritating, but the irritation stimulates the immune system, which fights warts within.)

Histamine Intolerance

Histamine is often misunderstood, especially regarding leaky gut. Dogs who can't effectively metabolize histamine can display leaky gut symptoms. Unfortunately, treating histamine intolerance the same way you treat leaky gut makes things worse. Histamine works with acid in the stomach. As your dog ingests food, any pathogens are targeted with a histamine response. Histamine helps break down your dog's food. In the stomach lining, histamine stimulates gastric acid, which helps digest vitamins, minerals, and proteins.[20]

The enzymes HNMT (histamine N-methyltransferase) and DAO (diamine oxidase) break down histamine so it doesn't build up in the body. HNMT deals with intracellular (inside the cells) histamine, and DAO deals with extracellular (outside the cells) histamine, meaning the histamine found in the matrix (interstitial fluid) around cells and organs.[21]

The goal is for histamine to be metabolized and excreted by the body. HNMT metabolizes most of your dog's histamine using methylation, which depends on vitamins B_6 and B_{12}, calcium, copper, and folate. If your dog does not consume or absorb adequate B_{12} and consumes too much folic acid (a synthetic form of folate), their histamine methylation cycle can be disrupted and histamine can accumulate, causing issues.[22]

The body ensures that DAO is doing its job because histamine and DAO are released simultaneously in the small intestine. Unfortunately, DAO production can dwindle for several reasons, including antibacterials, antihistamines, aspirin, dewormers, leaky gut, NSAIDs, poor diet, SIBO, steroids, and vaccines. (In humans, too much alcohol can cause the decline of DAO.)

Low DAO levels can pressure the liver because food isn't being broken down as it should and the liver isn't metabolizing histamine. When proteins, fats, and starch aren't broken down, they can enter the blood, and your dog's body sees them as foreign, which causes sensitivities and allergies. DAO depends on copper, B vitamins, and vitamin C as precursors to histamine metabolism.

High Histamine Cofactors

Alcohol	Hypertension
Allergies	Hyperthyroidism
Anxiety	Itchiness and scratching
Chronic skin conditions	Leaky gut
Difficulty breathing	Nausea
Fatigue	Poor body temperature
Food sensitivities*	regulation
Hives	Sinus congestion
High heart rate	Sun intolerance

*Note that a dog can have food allergies and food sensitivities without having histamine intolerance.

DAO Antagonists

Antacids	Pathogenic bacteria
Antiarrhythmics	Pharmaceutical immune
Antidepressants	modulators
Antihistamines	SIBO
Aspirin	Stress
Copper deficiency	Vetprofen (an NSAID)
Genetic factors	Vitamin B6 deficiency
Inflammation	Vitamin C deficiency
Leaky gut	

Lyme disease and its coinfections, too, can cause high histamine levels and immune overload.[23]

The Microbiome-Histamine Connection

Your dog's microbiome can give off large amounts of histamine. Most dogs with an imbalance of histamine have an overgrowth of pathogenic bacteria in their guts. What does this have to do with histamine? Microbiome health can affect DAO activity, and healthy levels of DAO are integral in managing histamine. Imbalanced microflora and high histamine cause higher inflammation levels.

The answer to good gut health is good, energetically appropriate foods, normal levels of stomach acid, proper levels of DAO, and healthy vagus nerve function. Working toward this involves live enzymes, prebiotics, and probiotics. Unfortunately, some probiotics produce histamine. This is okay for a dog without histamine issues but not for those with high histamine levels (or for those with diseases like mast cell cancer).

Histamine-Producing Microbes

Citrobacter spp.	*Lactobacillus delbrueckii* ssp.
Enterobacter spp.	*bulgaricus* (aka *L. bulgaricus*)
Enterococcus faecalis	*Lactococcus lactis* (aka *Lactobacillus lactis*)
Escherichia coli	*Limosilactobacillus reuteri*
Lacticaseibacillus casei	(aka *Lactobacillus reuteri*)
(aka *Lactobacillus casei*)	*Salmonella typhimurium*

Low-Histamine Bacteria

Bifidobacterium spp.
Lacticaseibacillus paracasei (aka *Lactobacillus paracasei*)
Lacticaseibacillus rhamnosus (aka *Lactobacillus rhamnosus*)
Lactiplantibacillus plantarum (aka *Lactobacillus plantarum*)
Lactobacillus gasseri
Ligilactobacillus salivarius (aka *Lactobacillus salivarius*)

As discussed earlier in this chapter, in regard to allergies, many factors, including histamine, cause food sensitivities, in which a dog's immune system targets specific foods for termination, seeing them as a threat to the dog-as-ecosystem. No fun. Food sensitivities are usually symptoms of leaky gut, nutrient deficiencies, or a breakdown of the enzymes responsible for working nicely with histamine.

When the body targets a thing like broccoli as a harmful invader, you know the gut is in trouble and needs balancing. I use broccoli as an example because of a sweet pug I knew named Innis, who would have been euthanized over her "allergies." She had been to numerous vets and dermatologists. Innis was so itchy that she would scratch her skin bloody. Her health improved with a fresh food diet, but her skin issues didn't clear until we finally identified the culprit as broccoli, her favorite treat, and removed it from her diet. It took more than a year of therapeutic work before she was able to eat her favorite snack again, but she got there.

An immune attack isn't fun. The heat, scratching, biting, . . . the list goes on. But over-the-counter antihistamines are hard on the liver, causing congestion. Research has shown that regular use of antihistamines can actually cause an increase in histamine levels due to the negative effect on stomach acid and DAO production.

Signs of Too Much Histamine

Car sickness	Heightened anxiety
Congestion	Hives
Constipation	Hot skin
Diarrhea	Low blood pressure
Farting	Rapid heartbeat
Gas	Rashes

Rubbing belly on carpet   Sneezing

Runny nose   Vomiting

Scratching   Weak muscle tone

As high histamine levels can be caused by undigested food, many of the above symptoms will occur after your dog eats.

Avoiding Histamines

High levels of histamine and the breakdown of DAO can lead to histamine intolerance. Things get tricky when a histamine-intolerant dog is exposed to histamine-producing microbes and high-histamine foods, such as ferments and bone broth. In these situations, histamine's effects accumulate, resulting in the dog having constant symptoms.[24]

Foods that contribute to high histamine levels include both foods that are themselves high in histamine and foods that block DAO production, thus preventing the breakdown of histamine. They should be removed from your dog's diet while the dog is healing from the effects of high histamine.

Foods that contribute to high histamine levels: anchovies, artificial dyes and preservatives, avocados, bananas, beans, bone broth, cashews, citrus, cow milk (pasteurized/homogenized), cured meats, dried fruit, eggplant, ferments*, gluten, goat milk (pasteurized/homogenized), green tea (can block DAO production), kefir, kibble and processed treats, kiwi, leftover foods, mackerel, papaya, peanuts, pecans, pork, sardines, shellfish, soy, spinach, strawberries, tomatoes, tuna, vinegar, walnuts

Food that is not freshly prepared, whether it's a prepared meal stored in the fridge or leftovers from an earlier meal, can be an issue. Food starts to ferment via bacteria as it sits in the refrigerator or out on the counter. The longer it sits, the higher its histamine content. Freezing leftovers or prepped meals is your best option, as freezing stops the decay process. Figure out how long it takes for your dog's food to get from frozen to room temperature once you take it out of the freezer. Take it out, set a timer, and then serve once it's reached room temperature.

---

*Ferments are beneficial for the gut, especially in an energetically cool dog, but not for dogs with histamine intolerance because the fermentation process creates histamines.

An Antihistamine Diet

A controlled, naturally antihistaminic diet can rest your dog's digestive and immune systems and reduce inflammation. Many histamine-friendly foods are high in quercetin, an antioxidant that reduces inflammation, allergic-type sensitivities, and negative heart response to inflammation and naturally helps the body with histamine by calming and stabilizing the cells that release histamine.

While focusing on natural antihistamines in the diet (see the foods list below), also supplement with vitamin C. This vitamin is a histamine intolerance superhero. It helps with histamine overload by increasing antioxidant efficiency and DAO production and slows histamine release in immune cells.

Helpful Herbs and Supplements

Herbs for warm dogs: chamomile, cilantro, echinacea, elderberries, lemon balm, licorice root, milk thistle seed, milky oats, nettle, peppermint, slippery elm, yarrow

Herbs for cool dogs: dill, elecampane, fennel, ginger, holy basil, licorice root, milk thistle seed, moringa, nettle, parsley, slippery elm, thyme, turmeric

Mushrooms: chaga, reishi, turkey tail

Phytoembryonics: beech, black currant, mountain pine, nettle bud

Essential oils for self-selection: eucalyptus (*E. radiata*), ginger, helichrysum, holy basil, lavender, manuka, myrrh, peppermint, ravensara, Roman chamomile, rosemary, sweet fennel, sweet marjoram, tarragon, thyme, vetiver

Flower essences: agrimony, beech, centaury, golden yarrow, heather, impatiens, Joshua tree, nettle, oak, Rescue Remedy, vervain, walnut

Homeopathy: Histiminum, Ledum, Urtica urens

Supplements: black cumin oil, bromelain, DAO, methylated B vitamins, pantothenic acid, quercetin, taurine, trace minerals, vitamin B_6, vitamin C

Foods: apples, beef, blueberries, broccoli, brown rice, Brussel sprouts, cabbage, celery, chicken, coconut, cranberries, flax seed (freshly ground), kale, organic oats, olive oil, plums, squash, turkey, watercress

Tip! It's important to filter your dog's water of all chlorine because chlorine compounds histamine reactions.[25] Dogs who swim in chlorinated water or drink chlorinated water can have more anxiety, sensitivities, and histamine reactions. To mitigate the effect of chlorine, filter your dog's water. If your dog swims in chlorinated water, give your dog vitamin C and the amino acid taurine the day before, day of, and day after they swim.

Hot Spots

Common energetic pattern: damp heat

Most hot spots stem from chronic imbalances within the body, especially liver imbalances, food sensitivities, or muscular skeletal pain and tightness. Flea and other bug bites can cause hot spots, too, but this is less often the case. Hot spots that appear suddenly are a sign that the body is eliminating toxins through the skin or an environmental allergen has overwhelmed the immune system. The most common places you'll see hot spots is on the side of your dog's face, the neck, the hind end, and the top of the tail.

Energetically, hot spots are damp and bring heat and inflammation to the skin. Most hot spots result from too much heat being produced in the body. They're prolific, quickly kicking out hair and spreading into a sticky, painful, itchy mess.

The conventional approach to treating hot spots is a path of suppression. But suppressing symptoms doesn't address the underlying cause of the hot spot and can put your dog into a cycle of sickness. Natural at-home protocols are usually effective. A trip to the vet is warranted if you can't control the spread of the hot spot and it gets large and painful. This happens most often with dogs that are immune-compromised or have severe thyroid disease.

The natural approach to resolving a hot spot is two-fold: First address internal systems, building support for the immune system and the organs of elimination like the digestive tract, lymphatic system, liver, and kidneys. Then turn your attention to topical applications for the hot spot itself.

Internal Protocol

Internal protocols focus on the liver, kidneys, lymphatic system, and digestive system, specifically the microbiome. Chapter 4 offers details on how to support all of these systems. At the same time, make sure that you are feeding your dog energetically appropriate foods and treats.

The next step: apply topicals. If your dog is in pain and won't tolerate your efforts, give them calming herbal tinctures. These include California poppy, chamomile lemon balm, passionflower, skullcap, and St. John's wort. You'll need a material dose to relieve pain, which is typically fifteen to twenty drops for every twenty pounds of your dog's body weight. Or you could simplify and give 30 ml of tincture for every twenty pounds of weight. You can also use full-spectrum CBD oil (rub it on your dog's gums), but it takes longer to work.

Topical Options

After you secure your dog and help calm them, you'll have access to the hot spot. For almost all hot spots, you'll want to gently trim the hair around the lesion. Flush with a mild, soothing, antibacterial rinse (see the recipe on the facing page). Spray or flush the hot spot with this solution three or four times per day for the first one to two days. If your dog is extra sensitive, drizzle the solution on the hot spot with a dropper. Let the hot spot air-dry and keep your dog from licking it.

When the hot spot dries out and starts to heal, apply a calendula salve to support the healing process (see the oil recipe on the facing page and the salve instructions on page 204). I like to use a calendula salve mixed with echinacea, catnip, or yellow dock infused oil. Yellow dock helps quell the itch and reduce heat; echinacea and catnip have a cooling and detoxifying effect. Apply the salve twice daily until the hot spot heals.

If the hot spot is too sensitive for a salve, dab it with St. John's wort infused oil, on its own or mixed with calendula infused oil, twice daily until it heals. Both herbs help relieve inflammation and heat. You can make these oils and preserve them with vitamin E oil so you have them on hand or purchase them commercially. The calendula infused oil recipe provided on the facing page can easily be adapted to make other varieties of infused oil such as the echinacea, catnip, yellow dock, and St. John's wort oils suggested here for hot spot relief.

🌿 Hot Spot Rinse

8 ounces boiled and cooled filtered water
15 drops echinacea tincture
10 drops crab apple flower essence
10 drops self-heal tincture
8 drops usnea tincture
Pinch of Himalayan salt

Combine all the ingredients and shake to mix. Spritz or flush a hot spot with this solution three or four times daily for 1 or 2 days.

🌿 Calendula and Goldenseal Hot Spot Spray

Use this calendula and goldenseal spray for painful, dry, or healing hot spots. It's ideal when your dog won't let you touch their hot spot. Don't add to any hot spot that has pus, as this spray will seal in infection.

1 cup filtered water
15 drops calendula tincture
15 drops goldenseal tincture

Combine all the ingredients in a bottle with a spritzer top and shake well. Mist the hot spot with this solution three or four times a day.

🌿 Calendula Infused Oil

You can use this simple recipe to slowly infuse most dried herbs into oil. Make sure the herbs are cut small to expose more surface area. Herbs must be completely dry to avoid mold.

4 ounces dried calendula flowers or petals
1 cup organic sunflower oil (or enough to cover the flowers)
1 tablespoon non-GMO vitamin E oil

Combine ingredients in a crock pot that has a warm setting and a glass top. Cover and let warm, stirring a few times daily, for 48–72 hours. Temperature must remain under 110°F. Wipe away any condensation that forms on the glass lid and don't use the oil until you have zero condensation showing up over a 12-hour period. Strain with cheese cloth or a fine metal strainer and add vitamin E oil. Pour liquid into a glass jar and seal, placing natural waxed paper under the lid. Label and store in a dark place. This oil can be used to make the salve below. Or it can be mixed with St. John's wort oil and dabbed onto a particularly sensitive hot spot twice daily until it heals.

🌿 Calendula Salve

This salve supports the healing process as a hot spot begins to dry out and heal.

1 ounce beeswax
4 ounces calendula infused oil

Melt the wax with a double boiler by taking a saucepan with an inch or two of water and placing the beeswax in a heat-resistant glass bowl nestled in the pan so that it fits snugly without touching the water. Simmer water in the saucepan until the wax in the bowl melts. Measure 1 ounce of the melted wax and mix it with warm calendula oil. To test the consistency, take a small sample and refrigerate it for 15 minutes. You don't want it too hard. Add more oil if needed. When you have a good consistency, pour the mixture into glass containers and let cool. Apply calendula salve to hot spot twice daily until it heals.

Bentonite Clay Paste

Bentonite clay is another topical remedy to try. It disinfects hot spots and quells itchiness and scratching. To use it, mix bentonite clay powder and water together to make a paste, and gently apply a thin layer to the area of the hot spot. Let the paste sit until dry. With a warm damp cloth, pat the area until the clay dissolves. This will take some patience but helps a hot spot heal quickly.

Some hot spots lack moisture and remain dry, with limited bacteria growth. For these, you can apply a simple calendula salve or infused oil to heal tissues and calm the itch.

If your dog's hot spots keep returning, muscle tension, injury, and pain could be the cause. These situations are most common for hot spots over the spine. Look for tension in the area under the hot spot, moving downward or slightly to the left or right of the area. With this type of hot spot, you might see several hot spots over a short period of time. In most cases, there will be excessive licking; chiropractic adjustments, acupuncture, or acupressure may help. They can clear stagnant energy and bring much-needed circulation to the area.

· ·

Tip! If your dog's hotspot is bright red and hot, you can give homeopathic belladonna 30c two or three times per day. If redness and heat decrease, discontinue.

· ·

Itchiness and Scratching

Dogs are covered in hair, and so scratching occasionally throughout the day is normal. If your dog is losing fur due to scratching, preoccupied with scratching, or damaging their skin by scratching, it's important to find them some relief. Itchiness and scratching can have many underlying causes. You must rule out fleas, as well as detergents (especially the popular commercial ones, like the kind that comes in an orange container), dryer sheets, laundry scent boosters, carpet powders, floor cleaners, and any other products your dog regularly comes in contact with. I can't count the number of times I have seen dogs with excessive itchiness have a sensitivity to products in the above list.

Itchiness, scratching, biting, and gnawing are all reactions to skin afflictions. These types of issues can make us desperate to find quick solutions for our pet, but most of the time, when fleas and flea allergy have been ruled out, itching and scratching are due to underlying causes like low immune function, liver congestion, emotional imbalance, or microbiome imbalance, especially candida overgrowth. When looking at herbs and supplements for itching, focus on immune and liver support, antibiotic recovery, and yeast or leaky gut herbs. Remember to always support your dog's nervous and lymphatic systems while you are trying to quell the itch.

Causes of Itching

Airborne irritants	Digestive enzyme insufficiency
Constipation	Ear infections (head and face scratching)
Contact sensitivities	
Dampness	Food sensitivities
Damp heat	Lack of B-vitamins
Depleted skin oils from too much bathing	Leaky gut
	Imbalanced microbiome
Depleted nervous system	

Sometimes, having strategies for calming your dog's itching and scratching can go a long way while you work on the inside. Here are a few tried and true methods.

Rinses for Itchiness

Herbs that are good for itch-relieving rinses include calendula, chamomile, chickweed, cleavers, dandelion root, echinacea, lavender, plantain, yarrow, and yellow dock. (See chapter 5 for instructions on making and using rinses.)

☙ Rinse for Dry, Scaly Skin with Heat

Heat describes the energetics of this condition. Yarrow is specific for hot, dry skin. St. John's wort is an anti-inflammatory and specific for redness and heat, and goldenrod is specific for scaly dry skin. Prepare the St. John's wort as a cold infusion, using apple cider vinegar instead of water and letting it steep overnight. You can use dried or fresh herbs to make the infusions here.

6 ounces goldenrod infusion
2 ounces yarrow infusion or 15 drops yarrow tincture
1 ounce St. John's wort–infused apple cider vinegar or infusion

☙ Rinse for Itchy, Irritated Skin with Heat

Lavender infusion is specifically for itchy, dry skin, with an emphasis on the itch. The apple cider vinegar can be plain or infused with any itch-relieving herb (and if your dog is sensitive to vinegar, replace it with more infusion). Chickweed relieves itching; when it doesn't work, use yellow dock root. Both will cool the skin and relieve the itch.

6 ounces chickweed infusion or dried yellow dock root decoction
2 ounces lavender infusion
1 ounce apple cider vinegar

☙ Rinse for Inflamed, Red, Itchy Skin

Plantain relieves inflammation, draws heat out of the skin, and quells the itch. Yarrow will help bring down the redness and heat.

8 ounces fresh or dried plantain infusion
1 ounce apple cider vinegar
1 ml yarrow tincture

Leaky Gut

Common energetic patterns: cold, damp stagnation and damp relaxation

The gut, as discussed throughout this book, is the gastrointestinal tract and its microbiome. Leaky gut happens when carbs, fats, proteins, and inflammatory pathogens (bacteria, viruses, yeast) cross the epithelial lining of the gut and leak into the bloodstream. This instrusion activates your dog's immune system, which launches an attack, causing an immune cascade.

A healthy gut lining is thin but tight. It lets nutrients (amino acids, fatty acids, glucose, minerals, vitamins) pass, but not undigested food molecules or pathogens. Your dog's microbiome helps keep this lining intact and tight. This is one reason a high level of commensal (healthy) gut bacteria is important.

Causes of Leaky Gut

Antibiotics	Histamine
Antihistamines	Processed foods
Candida overgrowth	Stress
Energetically inappropriate diet	Sympathetic excess
Enzyme insufficiency	Vaccines
Flea and tick medications	

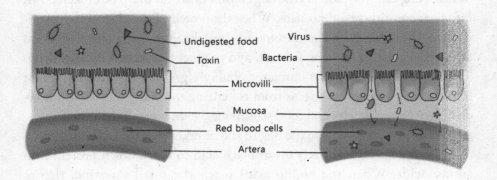

Healthy gut   Leaky gut

Symptoms of Leaky Gut

Anxiety	Food sensitivities
Arthritis	Gastric ulcers
Asthma	Insulin resistance
Autoimmune disease	Irritable bowel syndrome (IBS)
Chronic constipation or diarrhea	Joint pain
Chronic heart disease	Kidney disease
Cognitive decline	Lethargy
Dementia	Nutritional deficiencies
Dermatitis	Obesity (can't lose weight)
Diabetes	Seasonal allergies
Disrupted sleep patterns	SIBO
Dry skin conditions	Thyroid disorders

Testing

Levels of the protein zonulin can be elevated when leaky gut is present, especially in dogs with histamine issues and SIBO.[26] You can test for increased levels of zonulin, but the research isn't clear on its reliability as a predictor of leaky gut.

Antibodies, Enzymes, and Proteins

When a dog eats, the proteins the dog consumes are meant to be broken down into their constituent amino acids. When the proteins instead cross the gastro-intestinal lining and slip into the bloodstream, the immune system reads them as intruders, marks them as a threat, and produces antibodies against them. These antibodies, known as immunoglobulins (IgA), are designed to prevent infections by keeping pathogens from colonizing the body. In this case, however, they cause allergies and food sensitivities. Even though the immune system means well, it can make the dog ill and at odds with the environment.

When dogs eat, they rely on stomach acid to break down protein into amino acids. When the amino acids reach the small intestine, they're absorbed into the gut lining for systemic distribution. If your dog doesn't have enough stomach acid (an enzyme deficiency), these proteins don't get broken down enough, and your dog's body sounds the alarm. This is what I call a "high allergen" issue. Once the immune system has marked a type of protein as an intruder that should be terminated, it will keep responding in the same way every time it encounters that protein. Your dog ends up not being able to eat that type of protein without having the immune system leap into action. This type of overstimulation reduces energy and cellular voltage and deactivates the vagus nerve.

The Lymphatic Connection

When working with leaky gut, always include support for the lymphatic system. The gut contains lymphoid tissues called Peyer's patches that help your dog's body keep pathogens in check and the gut lining tight. Peyer's patches need lymph stimulation or else they can't assimilate fats or filter pathogens as they should, leading to leaky gut. Your dog needs a healthy lymphatic system for a tight gut lining.

Leaky Gut and Seasonal Allergies

When the gut barrier becomes leaky and allows unapproved passage, it can influence your dog's lungs, making them more susceptible to seasonal allergies. Lung mucosa normally can keep allergens and histamines in check, but when your dog's immune system and gut are challenged, that hyperstimulated defensiveness can pour over into the liver and lung systems. This along with liver congestion causes reactions to everyday airborne particles like pollen.

Strategies for Leaky Gut

Healing leaky gut requires you to address inflammation, rebalance the immune response, and support a healthy microbiome. Make sure your dog is getting adequate vitamins (preferably from herbs and food), with healthy levels of vitamins A, B, C, D, E, and K. If you are adding multiple remedies or supplements to your dog's regimen, add them one at a time, giving your dog a few weeks to adjust before adding the next one. This is especially important if you have an ultra-sensitive dog.

Helpful Herbs and Supplements

Herbs for warm dogs: aloe vera, burdock root, gotu kola, licorice root, marshmallow root, plantain, slippery elm, yarrow

Herbs for cool dogs: astragalus, calendula, licorice root, nettle, St. John's wort, slippery elm, turmeric, wood betony

Mushrooms: cordyceps, poria, reishi, tremella, turkey tail

Phytoembryonics: fig, mountain elm, mountain pine

Essential oils for self-selection: fennel, ginger, lavender, lime, oregano, peppermint, thyme

Flower essences: agrimony, aloe vera, beech, borage, buttercup, comfrey, crab apple, rock rose, self-heal, yarrow

Homeopathic remedies: Arnica, Calendula officinalis, Colocynthis, Magnesia carbonica, Magnesia muriaticum, Nux vomica, Silicea, Thiosinaminum

Supplements: betaine hydrochloride, butyric acid, colostrum, digestive enzymes, fiber, full-spectrum CBD oil, humic and fulvic acids, larch arabinogalactans, L-glutamine, magnesium, omega-3 fatty acids, probiotics (soil-based), quercetin, *Saccharomyces boulardii,* trace minerals (including zinc), vitamin B-complex, vitamin D, vitamin E

Lipomas

Common energetic pattern: damp stagnation

Lipomas are benign tumors of fatty cells, hormones, and toxins. They're usually found below the skin in your dog's fatty layer. However, sometimes lipomas can be found in the intramuscular tissue, where they can cause pain and restrict movement. If your dog's lipomas are large and don't respond to herbal strategies, they might need to be surgically removed (if possible). Most lipomas form in the chest, armpit, torso, neck, and legs. They feel rubbery and move slightly when you press down on them. They are not cancerous, though checking your dog's lumps and bumps to see if they change shape or bleed is always a good idea. *Note:* When you find a lipoma on your dog, bring it to your veterinarian's attention to confirm that you're dealing with a lipoma instead of another type of tumor.

Surgery is one of the only options you're given when you go to the vet. Surgery is needed if it's a life-and-death concern. But lipomas like to multiply after surgery, as the procedure congests the liver, lymphatics, and immune system and doesn't address the root cause. Enter holistic herbalism.

Warning Signal

I can't count the times I've heard people say that lipomas are just part of a dog getting older. This is a fallacy. Lipomas are a warning sign that something more serious is happening inside your dog. The liver and other elimination systems are not functioning correctly. The liver is congested. The body is trying to protect itself from circulating toxins by forming a fatty tumor. Whenever you're working with lipomas, look at toxic load. How is the liver within the dog-as-ecosystem?

Lipoma Causes

Genetics can contribute to lipoma formations, but this is a predisposition, not an absolute. Dogs with lipomas have damp stagnation. Look at anything that taxes the liver: diet, water quality, medications, household cleaners, grooming supplies, stress, surgery, and more.

Diet

Kibble contributes to liver stagnation, dampness, kidney dryness, poor digestion, and overall systemic toxicity due to its processed ingredients, poor-quality proteins, lack of enzymes, and unhealthy oils.[27] If you feed kibble, make sure it is a baked style or air-dried. Work toward feeding a minimally processed diet of energetically appropriate fats, greens, and proteins. If you're feeding cooked food, remember that cooking destroys enzymes, and add digestive enzymes to your dog's regimen to help your dog assimilate the food.

Since lipomas are a sign of dampness, avoid dampening foods, including dairy, eggs, honey, mussels, pork, and spinach. Instead, focus on more drying foods like apple, celery, chamomile, chlorella, ginger, kelp, parsley, pumpkin, roasted (not boiled) sweet potatoes, and seaweed. Don't overfeed; it congests the liver and contributes to lipoma formation.[28] While working with lipomas, feeding your dog once daily can speed up the process so their organs can rest and repair while they focus on detoxification.

Raw feeders are often baffled and shocked when their dogs get lipomas. "How can my dog have a lipoma? They're raw-fed!" Unfortunately, we can't protect our pets from all toxins. Even the cleanest diets have toxins, and we all live in a toxic environment. Pollution is real until we all decide to protect our planet's resources, including its air, water, and soil.

Water

Clean water is another factor in reducing toxic load. Ensure your dog is not ingesting chlorine or fluoride, as they disrupt the endocrine system and wreak havoc on the liver.[29] Even if your dog is drinking well water, filter it. Invest in a water filtration system. Even a simple countertop filter is better than tap or bottled water. Water bottled in plastic is filled with endocrine disrupters and microplastics.[30] Soda companies own most of the bottled water sold in the United States; more than half of all bottled water comes from tap water.[31]

Cleaners

Cleaners and detergents are a powerful source of household toxins. Work to replace all your name-brand cleaners with nontoxic, all-natural formulas. You must read labels; don't believe what the front of the bottle tells you. Check out the Environmental Working Group website for guidance. Don't forget laundry detergents, dryer sheets, and laundry scent boosters, which are considerable contributors to liver congestion.[32] As a rule of thumb, avoid any laundry detergent sold in plastic bottles. Instead, use a natural soap brand, soap nuts, or ionic washer balls.

Pharmaceuticals

Look carefully at your dog's medications. Many pharmaceuticals can contribute to lipoma formation, including antibiotics, heartworm medications, flea and tick medications, levothyroxine, steroids, NSAIDs, and gabapentin.[33] Don't overvaccinate. Here in the United States, the only vaccine required by law for dogs is rabies.

Tick Disease

Tick-borne diseases can cause lipomas. If your dog has multiple lipomas, have the dog undergo a C6 antibody test for Lyme and its coinfections.[34] If the test comes back positive, use a Lyme and coinfections homeopathic nosode formula and work with a holistic practitioner to address the tick-borne disease.

Environmental Toxins and Air Quality

Consider the use of pesticides (including lawn chemicals), herbicides, and fungicides in your home and neighborhood. Wash your produce and invest in air purifiers throughout your home.

Glyphosate, the active ingredient in the pesticide Roundup, is of particular concern. Glyphosate levels in dogs can be twice as high as in humans, and it is known to harm the microbiome, decrease vitamin absorption, and interfere with a dog's ability to manufacture fatty acids.[35] A dog's immune system, gut health, liver, and kidneys can all be negatively affected by glyphosate exposure. Though science has only started to explore the adverse effects of glyphosate exposure, they know it can accumulate inside the kidneys. Some options for mitigating the effects of glyphosate include humic and fulvic acid, kelp, chlorella, modified citrus pectin, the amino acid glycine, and high fiber foods.[36]

Stress and the Nervous System

Stress can cause stagnation in the liver and gastrointestinal system. As mentioned in chapter 4, when your dog is in fight or flight (sympathetic excess) either from your stress or stimulus specific to them, they have limited access to their digestive fire, including liver function. Excess stress and low vagal tone can put extra pressure on the liver. It is important to include nervous system support as a part of your overall lipoma protocol.

Lipoma Strategies

With lipomas, you'll want to focus on three things: keeping new lipomas from forming, making sure current lipomas don't get any larger, and slowly shrinking current lipomas. To do this, you'll focus on your dog's internal ecosystem through lymphatics, energetics, and liver support (including elimination) and work from the outside in by applying reducers to your dog's lipomas and getting energy moving.

Support Lymphatics

The lymphatic system actively supports the digestive, endocrine, immune, liver, and renal systems. Unfortunately, the lymphatic system doesn't have a pump, so when dogs are given detoxifying herbs, the toxins that are released end up stuck in circulation if lymph is stagnant. Help prevent stagnation by using either calendula (warming) or cleavers (cooling). Both herbs are safe for long-term use. Another strategy is to get your dog moving with age-appropriate exercise, which is key for proper lymphatic drainage.

Balance Energetics

Liver congestion and detoxification are two reasons even raw-fed dogs get lipomas. Another reason is that dogs are fed foods that are energetically off for their ecosystem—for example, a warm to hot dog eating lamb, which is warming. Consistently mismatched energetics in the diet can lead to inflammation and stagnation. Feed your dog energetically appropriate foods to prevent and relieve inflammation and stagnation; see appendix 5 for information on the energetics of various foods.

Stimulate Circulation

Circulation moves fluids, nourishes all parts of the body, and supports elimination. Working with blood and lymphatic circulation is essential when helping the body address toxins and support toxin release. Most lymphatic herbs support these functions.

Prevent Growth with Liver Support

Keeping lipomas from multiplying or getting larger is a secondary goal. Turkey tail mushroom is my go-to for this. It supports the liver and helps prevent tumor formation. I use material dosages of the hot-water-extracted powder, given twice daily, using the following schedule.

Dosing Schedule

Size of Dog	Dose
Extra-small	⅛ teaspoon
Small	¼ teaspoon
Medium	½ teaspoon
Large	¾ teaspoon
Extra-large	1–2 teaspoons

Note: If a lipoma has grown in size after four weeks of taking turkey tail, you may need to increase the dosage by one-quarter.

Lipoma Reducers

Some herbs can be effective in reducing the size of lipomas. Use one that is energetically appropriate for your dog, and apply to lipoma(s) two or three times daily.

Reducer for warm dogs: Mix burdock, red clover, and self-heal tinctures in equal parts.

Reducer for cool dogs: Mix angelica tincture, calendula tincture, and apple cider vinegar in equal parts.

Salve reducer: Cooling chickweed and violet salve

Move Stagnation

Stagnation throughout the body needs stimulation. Exercise, fresh air, chiropractic adjustments, acupuncture, acupressure, and massage push through stagnation and stimulate energy.

Expectations

Lipomas don't form overnight and will not disappear overnight. Though some will start to shrink in just a couple of weeks, it's common for them to take four to six weeks before showing signs of progress, so patience and consistency are essential. Don't give up.

Finding an herbal combination that works for your dog may take trial and error. If you don't notice any shrinkage of the lipoma at all after the first four weeks, use a different remedy or assess dosage.

Helpful Herbs and Supplements

Herbs for warm dogs: artichoke, burdock root, chickweed, cleavers, dandelion root, echinacea, milk thistle seed, red clover, rose hips, self-heal, violet

Herbs for cool dogs: angelica, ashwagandha, calendula, milk thistle seed, olive leaf, turmeric

Mushrooms: maitake, poria, reishi, turkey tail

Essential oils for self-selection: copaiba, grapefruit, helichrysum, lemon, myrrh, peppermint

Flower essence: crab apple

Homeopathic remedies: Baryta carbonica, Calcarea carbonica, Phytolacca decandra, Silicea, Sulphur, Thuja occidentalis, Uricum acidum

Supplements: apple cider vinegar (for cool dogs), full-spectrum CBD oil, fulvic acid, MCT oil, N-acetylcysteine, probiotics (soil-based), sargassum seaweed, superoxide dismutase, trace minerals, vitamin A, vitamin C, vitamin D,* vitamin E

Foods: baked beet root, baked sweet potato

---

*First test your dog's vitamin D levels to see if supplementation is necessary.

Nausea, Vomiting, and Poor Appetite

Common energetic pattern: heat and dampness

Regurgitation is the ejection of undigested food, mainly from inside the esophagus, coming up through the mouth and out. Regurgitation is mostly a normal process when dogs swallow a large amount of food. The expelled contents are usually stuck together, covered in mucus, and almost entirely undigested. Even though it's gross, it's perfectly normal for dogs to eat their regurgitated food, usually tearing it up into small pieces to fit into the esophagus.*

Vomiting, on the other hand, comes from the stomach and the upper intestines. It usually has a unique color, texture, and smell quite distinct from those of regurgitated food. Though occasional vomiting is normal and usually benign, sometimes vomiting can mean something serious. When a dog that never vomits suddenly starts to heave, you should take notice, especially if it turns into dry heaving.

Causes of Vomiting

Acute vomiting is usually caused by something your dog ingested, a food allergy or sensitivity, a reaction to a drug, a parasite, stress, or an organ malfunction.

Poisoning

Poisoning symptoms are vomiting, diarrhea, loss of muscular control, swellings, convulsions, and rashes. It's especially apparent when your dog displays more than one of these symptoms. If you suspect poisoning, contact your emergency vet straight away. Don't induce vomiting unless you're sure of what your dog has ingested. In some cases, making your dog vomit can make matters worse. Some examples of poisonous substances for dogs are pesticides, cleaners, antifreeze, arsenic, over-the-counter medications, xylitol, chocolate, and certain household plants. If you suspect poisoning, administer four times the standard dose of milk thistle seed (see the monograph in chapter 8) as a diluted tincture in the mouth, and then give activated charcoal at 3 to 5 grams for every 10 pounds of your dog's weight.

---

*Chronic regurgitation, where your dog can't keep any food down for more than a few seconds, isn't common, and I recommend seeing a veterinarian immediately if this occurs.

Giardia

Giardia is a parasite that can induce vomiting and cause diarrhea. Dogs can pick it up from contaminated water, food, and soil. If you suspect giardiasis (infection by giardia), have your dog's stool tested before starting the following protocol:

First 10 days: Give *Saccharomyces boulardii* and a 1:1 blend of echinacea and goldenseal tinctures twice daily for ten days, using the following dosing schedule. Give digestive enzymes and CoQ10 between meals.

Next 7 days: Discontinue the echinacea and goldenseal. Continue the *S. boulardii* and digestive enzymes.

Final 10 days: Repeat the protocol from the first 10 days.

Dosing Schedule for 1:1 Echinacea-Goldenseal Blend

Size of Dog	Dose
Extra-small	2-3 drops
Small	8 drops
Medium	15 drops
Large	20 drops
Extra-large	30 drops

Obstruction

When it comes to obstruction, I think of the quintessential golden retriever eating socks. When items stay in the stomach for too long and can't pass through the digestive system, they cause continued irritation until your dog vomits them up. For example, even though it isn't common, dogs can have obstructions from items like small toys and underwear, which they may vomit up weeks after consuming them. If you suspect that your dog has swallowed a small object that could cause an obstruction, give copious amounts of slippery elm. Mix slippery elm with enough warm water to make a gruel. Syringe into your dog's mouth four to six times per day. This protocol helps lubricate the gastrointestinal tract and coat the object in mucilage, so that it can slip out your dog's back end.

Keep an eye out for dry heaving or unproductive vomiting, lack of stool production, blood in the stool, and panting or shaking. If these symptoms occur, your dog may have a serious obstruction. See your vet immediately.

Morning Vomiting

On occasion, your dog may vomit bile and foam. This happens when stomach acid collects on an empty stomach. Officially called bilious vomiting syndrome, it usually happens in the mornings, though it's not a common condition. I've found that offering dogs a small meal or snack before bed resolves the situation.

Gastric Vomiting

A diagnosis of acute gastritis means the "stomach is inflamed and we can't figure out why," and it is associated with acute vomiting. Gastritis is usually caused by something your dog ingested that the body considers a toxin and wants expelled as soon as possible.

Vet-Warranted Symptoms

Aside from the symptoms mentioned above, consult with your vet if your dog displays any of the following symptoms:

- Bloody vomit
- Chronic water regurgitation
- Constipated for more than three or four days
- Lethargy (combined with other symptoms)
- Nonstop vomiting
- Refusal to eat or drink for more than a day
- Won't urinate

Dehydration from Vomiting

If you have a puppy or an older dog that is vomiting, watch carefully for signs of dehydration. Weakness, dull eyes, and dry gums are all signs that fluids need to be replaced. You may need to bring your dog to the vet for intravenous fluids if they can't keep things down.

Post-Vomiting Care

When vomiting occurs, most people are concerned that their dog will become hungry and keep offering them small meals and waiting to see if their dog will vomit again. This is a mistake. After an episode of vomiting, resting the digestive tract is essential. I recommend withholding food for at least six hours or until the following day. This allows the digestive organs time to rest.

When you're ready to feed your dog again, it's important to give warm or room temperature meals (not cold) due to the spleen's weakened condition. Begin with a small amount of broth every hour or so.* If your dog can't keep broth down, stop, wait five to six hours, and try again. Once your dog has been able to keep down broth for twelve to twenty-four hours, you can reintroduce solid food. Begin with small amounts of lightly steamed non-fatty protein and more broth. If all goes well, give your dog a smaller-than-usual portion of their regular diet, and take it from there.

If you feel like you don't know what you are doing or you're worried about your dog, take the dog to your vet.

Strategies for Nausea and Vomiting

There are many herbs can that soothe an upset stomach, relieve nausea, and support your dog's digestive system.

I love using flower essences for dogs with any type of upset stomach, especially related to nausea, vomiting, or low appetite. Here is a good formula for helping a dog keep fluids down: Mix equal parts crab apple, olive, star of Bethlehem, and walnut essences. Give 2 drops every four hours, either internally or sprayed or dripped on your dog's ears and muzzle, avoiding its eyes.

Lack of Appetite

Lack of appetite or disinterest in food can be a sign of nausea, bacterial infection, viral infection, urinary tract infection, injury, cardiac abnormality, stress, or advanced age. It's essential to consult with your vet about possible medical causes for loss of appetite especially if your dog refuses to eat for more than a couple of days. Common medical causes

---

*Avoid human broths containing onion and garlic.

include anemia, bladder infection, gastrointestinal upset, and respiratory duress. Also consider obstruction, pancreatitis, and parasites.

Possible Causes for Loss of Appetite

Anemia	Liver disease
Bad tooth	Obstruction
Bladder infection	Pancreatitis
Cancer	Parasites
Dehydration	Respiratory duress
Gastrointestinal upset	Side effects of an herb
Kidney disease	Side effects of a pharmaceutical

It's important to identify the cause of a dog's lack of appetite, and then, if it's appropriate for your dog's condition—such as, for example, if the underlying cause is a nonmedical issue like stress, fear, anxiety, or your dog's lack of interest in what they have determined unpalatable food—herbs can play a role in stimulating appetite.

. . . .

Tip! Low doses (1 to 3 mg) of full-spectrum CBD oil can effectively stimulate a dog's appetite.

. . . .

Here are two recipes based on energetics to help with your dog's appetite. If you don't know your dog's energetics, pick the cool dog formula.

❧ Appetite Stimulant for Warm Dogs

Dandelion, burdock root, and wood betony cool heat in the liver and digestive tract, and chamomile calms the nerves in the stomach.

    1 ounce cooled chamomile infusion
    6 drops burdock root tincture
    5 drops dandelion root tincture
    5 drops wood betony tincture

Mix all the ingredients in an amber glass bottle with a dropper top. Administer two or three times daily following the dosing schedule on facing page.

❧ Appetite Stimulant for Cool Dogs

This combination is bitter and will activate digestive secretions, helping to increase appetite. Make a fresh batch daily.

1 ounce ginger infusion
5 drops chamomile tincture

Mix the ingredients in an amber glass bottle with a dropper top. Administer two or three times daily, following the dosing schedule below.

Dosing Schedule

Size of Dog	Dose
Extra-small	½ teaspoon
Small	1 teaspoon
Medium	1½ teaspoons
Large	2 teaspoons
Extra-large	1 tablespoon

Helpful Herbs and Supplements

Herbs for warm dogs: catnip, chamomile, lemon balm, milk thistle, peppermint

Herbs for cool dogs: bee balm, calendula, fennel, ginger, meadowsweet, milk thistle, parsley, turmeric

Mushrooms: reishi

Essential oils: fennel, ginger, lavender, lemon, peppermint, orange

Phytoembryonics: fig

Flower essences: crab apple, olive, mimulus, star of Bethlehem, violet, walnut

Homeopathic remedies: Chamomilla, Iodium, Ipecacuanha, Nux vomica, Pulsatilla, Sepia, Zingiber

Supplements: B₆

Paw Problems

Dog paws consist of connective tissue, tendons, ligaments, and skin. The pads themselves consist of thick fibrous tissue with a sublayer of fat that helps absorb shock and steady their gait.

Dogs can suffer from many paw afflictions, some chronic and others acute. Chronic maladies can arise from allergies, food sensitivities, autoimmune disease, certain types of yeast, and interdigital cysts. Acute issues revolve around injuries: nail tears, cuts, scrapes, and various types of burns and wounds. Chemicals like pesticides, industrial salt, and other highly absorbable chemicals can cause burns on the pads. In wintry conditions, ice can wear your dog's paws raw and cause dryness and cracking.

Most of the time, you can tell when there is something wrong with your dog's paws. They'll either refuse to stand on all fours, hold the affected paw in the air, or limp. However, some dogs just don't show any symptoms when they have paw troubles. I try to make a habit of looking at my dog's feet several times weekly to check for problems.

Herbal soaks, sprays, and salves can go a long way in resolving most acute paw-related issues. One of my favorite remedies for paws is the mushroom poria. It's anti-inflammatory and works well for various types of paw inflammations. A bonus is that it helps support and modulate the immune system.

Tip! You can use powdered chaga mushroom extract and bentonite clay pastes (page 204) to help with interdigital cysts. Clay and chaga are drawing, dry up moisture, decrease inflammation, and help decrease any pathogenic bacteria.

Embedded Objects

Embedded objects like grass seeds or foxtails are acute issues that must be dealt with quickly. A single dose of homeopathic Silicea 30C is a good place to start. Then use a plantain poultice, which can draw out the object enough that you can remove it. If this fails, soak your dog's paw in a warm solution of Epsom salts or bentonite clay.

Dry Paws

Salves are excellent medicine for dry paws. Emollient herbs like dandelion, plantain, and chamomile infused in oil (olive, apricot kernel, or almond) and mixed with beeswax or vegan wax can turn pad dryness around in a few days. Chronic dryness can signify an imbalanced kidney, so a salve may be only palliative, easing symptoms. With kidney issues, you'll see redness between the toes, heat, and usually musculoskeletal weakness, especially in the hind end. The kidneys can get dry when the body doesn't contain enough moisture and fluids.

Bleeding Paws and Torn Nails

Paw wounds can be dealt with the same as skin wounds. Rinse the wound with clean water or the herbal flush remedy below. Inspect it for foreign objects. If it's bleeding, pour powdered white yarrow into the wound and gently apply pressure until the bleeding stops. Wrap the paw afterward if needed. If the wound is deep, you may need to administer calming herbs (see the discussion of the nervous system in chapter 4) before providing care.

. . . .

Tip! Yarrow powder can help heal even the deepest cuts. Pour it straight on the wound.

. . . .

🌿 Wound-Cleansing Paw Flush

This is my go-to strategy for an acute paw injury. If a wound is still bleeding after being flushed, apply yarrow powder and gentle pressure until the bleeding stops.

6 ounces warm distilled or filtered water
1 teaspoon Himalayan salt
6 drops crab apple flower essence

Combine all the ingredients in a sanitized application bottle and shake until the salt dissolves. Flush the wound with this solution twice daily until it heals.

For a torn nail: Soak the affected toe in this solution for at least 5 minutes twice daily until it heals.

If the origin of the puncture is unknown: Add 20 drops of echinacea tincture, 10 drops of usnea or Oregon grape root tincture, and 15 drops of plantain tincture to the solution. This will help disinfect the wound as well as draw out infection.

You can run into problems with paw wounds because you must wrap them most of the day, and dogs sweat through their paws. This type of moisture and lack of air can cause bacteria to proliferate. Make sure to change the dressing at least once daily and give the paw time to air out whenever possible.

Paw Wash

Apple cider vinegar soaks are beneficial for cleansing and balancing the pH of your dog's feet. Use a 50:50 solution of vinegar and distilled or filtered water. If you are washing off chemicals your dog may have come in contact with, like rock salt, refresh the solution every five minutes, pouring the spent solution into a rock or gravel substrate outdoors instead of down the sink or toilet. This way, it can be filtered by the earth instead of ending up in the water supply. After you're finished, pat your dog's feet dry. Do not rub.

. . . .

Tip! You can use herb-infused vinegar for foot soaks and washes, too. Bee balm, calendula, nettle, plantain, and self-heal are all good choices for soothing, healing soaks. Rosemary-infused vinegar is a great solution for cleansing your dog's feet, as it's antibacterial and improves circulation.

. . . .

Yeasty Paws

To combat yeasty paws, soak your dog's paws with the anti-yeast solution below and then apply the salve recipe that follows. This protocol is very effective for getting rid of yeast infections on the paws and skin. Don't forget that yeast infections on the skin come from within. Remember to support the immune system and work with your dog's internal terrain, as you would with any healing regimen.

🌿 Yeasty Paws Soak

8 ounces apple cider vinegar
8 ounces cooled pau d'arco decoction
2 ml bee balm tincture
2 ml calendula tincture

Combine all the ingredients. Soak the affected paws in this solution for 10 minutes twice daily for 5 days. Store any leftover solution in the refrigerator, where it will keep for more than a week.

❧ Yeasty Paws Salve

2 parts olive oil
1 part tamanu oil
1 part black cumin seed oil
Beeswax or vegan wax, as needed

Combine the oils in a pan over low heat. Add a bit of wax and stir until it melts. Then check for consistency by removing a small sample and chilling it in the refrigerator until it cools. If it is not thick enough, add more wax and then test the consistency again. When the salve has achieved your desired consistency, pour it into a heatproof container of your choice and let the mixture cool.

Stings and Bug Bites

Stings from wasps, hornets, and bees can be unsettling and emotionally and physically painful. Most stings create some inflammation from the toxins injected into the skin.

If your dog does get stung in the face or throat, administer homeopathic Apis mellifica 200C every 25 minutes for three doses. When you see improvement, stop. You can dose again if your dog's symptoms start to worsen. If after the second dose you don't see an improvement, switch to Belladonna 30C.

My main remedy for stings is bentonite clay. I always bring some premoistened clay in a small container with me wherever I go in the summer. All you do is mix bentonite or green clay with enough water to make a paste. Apply the paste to the sting and leave it on until it dries and cracks. Wash off the clay and repeat twice. I've seen this method work quickly to relieve pain and inflammation from all types of stings and spider bites.

Another quick and easy way to address stings in summertime is a fresh plantain poultice. Just chew up some broad-leafed plantain and apply the moist wad of plant material to the sting. Plantain helps relieve the pain and soothe the inflammation while it works to pull out the toxins.

ᩘ Bug Bite Skin Spray

Clay is my go-to for all types of insect bites; it draws out stingers and venom. Plantain and bee balm help calm the irritation of a bug bite and dissipate heat while lavender soothes the skin.

1 tablespoon bentonite or green clay
1 ml plantain tincture
1 ml bee balm tincture
16 ounces filtered water or fresh lavender infusion

Combine all the ingredients in a spritzer bottle. Apply as needed.

Surgery Preparation and Recovery

This section presents my protocol for helping a dog prepare for and recover from any kind of surgery. The more invasive the surgery, the longer it will take to heal. Being prepared is the most important part of recovery.

Before the Surgery: Preparation

Step 1: In the weeks leading up to the surgery, feed your dog a nutrient-rich diet, including greens. Add infusions of nutritive herbs like alfalfa, nettle, and shiitake and turkey tail mushrooms. Include double doses of omega-3 fatty acids and trace minerals. If appropriate, give small amounts of fermented veggies a few times daily, along with bone broth, N-acetylcysteine, milk thistle seed, and *Saccharomyces boulardii*. One week prior to surgery, mist your dog daily with flower essences of white, pink, and golden yarrow along with arnica and echinacea (available commercially as Yarrow Special Formula), or add this blend to your dog's food. Throughout this time period, make sure your dog gets age-appropriate exercise, if possible.

Step 2: Five days before the surgery, discontinue all herbs and supplements except for N-acetylcysteine and *S. boulardii*. Add a daily dose of homeopathic Arnica 30C to the regimen.

Step 3: On the day before the surgery, give Rescue Remedy three times throughout the day. Give yourself a few sprays, too, if you're anxious. I know I'm a wreck when my pets have surgery.

Step 4: On the morning of the surgery, give your dog (and yourself) a final dose of Rescue Remedy. Give your dog homeopathic Hypericum 30C to help calm their nerves.

After the Surgery: Recovery

Post-surgery, your dog can suffer from the usual side effects of the procedure and anesthesia, including chills, cognitive confusion, constipation, depletion of the immune system, discomfort, dry mouth, incontinence, itchiness, lameness, nausea, musculoskeletal pain, unsteadiness, and, over time, weight gain or loss. Your dog's cells have lots of work to do. When connective tissue, muscles, and tendons are cut, healing is essential.

. . . .

Tip! Low phosphate levels are common after surgery. Nettle infusion can be an effective supplement to restore phosphorus levels in dogs, as can meat.

. . . .

Phase One: Inflammation

The heat, swelling, and redness that occur immediately after surgery will last for approximately seven days.[37] After that, the body has an exceptional ability to heal, and remember, it's always attempting to balance itself out. You can help your dog get through this inflammation stage in the following ways.

Step 1: Continue homeopathic Arnica and Hypericum on the day of surgery and for seven days afterward. As you did before the surgery, mist your dog daily with flower essences of white, pink, and golden yarrow along with arnica and echinacea, or add this blend to any liquids or food you are feeding your dog. Give nutritive liquids and bone broth until your dog can resume a regular diet. You can add milky oats, chamomile, or lion's mane mushroom to the broth to support your dog's nervous system during this time. You can add nettles, marshmallow root, or broccoli sprout infusion for nutrition.

Step 2: Manage pain; see the discussion of arthritis and pain earlier in this chapter for suggestions. Give your dog mountain pine gemmotherapy, a potent anti-inflammatory, three to five times per day.

Phase Two: Repair

Beginning a few days after surgery and for up to six months, depending on your dog and the severity of the surgery, the body starts producing new blood vessels and collagen and goes about repairing vascular tissue. It's essential to give your dog's body what it needs for this phase.

Resume a nutrient-rich, enzyme-rich, energetically appropriate diet. Many people panic after their dogs have surgery, worried about the toll surgery has taken on their dog's body. It's all about having a plan. After surgery, dogs need a building diet and *gentle* detoxification. Too much detoxing can tax your dog's vital force and cause further depletion. Note: After surgery, dogs can experience poor appetite, constipation, and diarrhea.

Below is a list of herbs you can add to your dog's regimen based on energetics and need. Notice that many categories overlap in the herbs they contain. For example, calendula supports circulation as well as your dog's heart and lymphatic system. Don't overdo it. Make sure to look at the energetics of everything (unless using acutely) to help you decrease the amount of herbs you're working with.

Nutritives: alfalfa sprouts, bone broths, gotu kola, marshmallow root, milk thistle seed, milky oats, mullein, mushroom broth, mushrooms, nettle, parsley, raw cow milk, raw goat milk, violet

Circulation support: calendula, cleavers, hawthorn, lion's mane mushroom, maitake mushroom, milk thistle seed, red clover, reishi mushroom, rosemary, turmeric, wood betony, yarrow

Heart support: alfalfa, artichoke, astragalus, calendula, cordyceps mushroom, dandelion, gotu kola, hawthorn, lemon balm, maitake mushroom, milk thistle seed, reishi mushroom

Connective tissue support: chickweed, echinacea, gotu kola, gravel root, mullein root and leaf, nettles, rose, tremella mushroom

Lymphatic support: calendula, chickweed, cleavers, milk thistle seed, red root, turmeric, violet

Supplements to support the digestive system: digestive enzymes, humic and fulvic acids, prebiotics, probiotics

Helpful oils to heal the skin: Full-spectrum CBD oil and oils infused with St. John's wort, plantain, comfrey leaf, and/or yarrow oil can help heal your dog's skin and scars and relieve pain, especially St. John's wort oil.

Phase Three: Remodeling

Remodeling is the process by which your dog's body repairs itself and works to rebuild its tissues so that they are as close to the original as possible. The goal of this phase (and phase two) is repairing and minimizing scar tissue. This involves supporting the musculoskeletal system directly and through kidney interaction while supporting healthy nerve and organ function, especially elimination, because there is a proliferation of metabolic wastes during this time. Keep focusing on your dog's lymphatics, nutrition, and gut health, and use herbs and supplements that minimize scar tissue. Give liver support herbs (see chapter 4 for examples) to help with metabolic wastes from scar tissue breakdown.

Herbs for warm dogs: short-term calendula (two to three weeks), echinacea, gotu kola

Herbs for cool dogs: calendula, short-term echinacea (two to three weeks), rosemary, turmeric combined with bromelain

Mushrooms: chaga, cordyceps, lion's mane, maitake, poria, tremella, turkey tail

Phytoembryonics: bramble, hazel, Judas tree, lemon tree, mistletoe

Homeopathic remedies: Calcarea fluorica, Graphites, Thiosinaminum

Supplements: digestive enzymes

Vaccine Preparation and Recovery

My philosophy on vaccines is less is more. I'm not against vaccination, but I do consider the risks versus the benefits for my dog. The only vaccine that's required by law here in the United States is rabies; all others are optional. As a general rule, I do not recommend vaccinations for dogs with seizures, autoimmune diseases, or cancer. In these cases, you can work with your veterinarian to obtain a certificate of exemption.

In my practice, I've developed protocols to help prepare a dog's body for vaccination and prevent damage from the vast amount of inert ingredients, including foreign proteins. Vaccination can be considered an acute situation, so the protocols are designed for an acute response, and most dogs can use them regardless of their particular energetics.

The primary goals of protocols for vaccine support are to bring down inflammation, support the digestive system, help remove heavy metals, and balance the nervous system. We'll run through the specific herbs and homeopathics first and then summarize the pre- and post-vaccination schedule.

Note: You might want to see how your dog responds to the remedies weeks before you vaccinate them—particularly if your dog is sensitive or chronically ill—in order to gauge their response to the suggested dosage or remedy. If your dog doesn't tolerate a specific remedy, adjust the dosage or skip it altogether.

You should introduce remedies three to five days apart from each other. Once you know your dog will tolerate a newly introduced remedy, you can mix it together with the other ones your dog is already taking. Mix all the liquid remedies in a shot glass, add some warm water, and syringe them into the side of your dog's mouth, followed by a yummy treat.

Helpful Herbs and Homeopathics

Birch bud phytoembryonic. Choose birch if your dog has had reactions to prior vaccines or is sensitive to pharmaceuticals. But check with your vet before using birch, and be cautious about using it with prescription medications. Birch buds help clear pharmaceuticals from the body through the liver. Go slow with birch, as it can cause a strong detoxification response. You may have to offer your dog as little as 1 diluted drop, depending on how your dog reacts. Give twice daily for six weeks post-vaccination. Cut back on or discontinue the dosage if your dog seems uncomfortable.

Birch Bud Phytoembryonic Dosing Schedule

Size of Dog	Dose
Extra-small	1 diluted drop
Small	1 drop
Medium	2 drops
Large	3 drops
Extra-large	4 drops

Black currant phytoembryonic. Black currant helps support the immune system and adrenal glands and eases the inflammatory response associated with vaccination. Give once daily two weeks before vaccination and on the day of vaccination. Post-vaccination, administer twice daily for two weeks. Avoid in dogs with seizures.

Black Currant Phytoembryonic Dosing Schedule

Size of Dog	Dose
Extra-small	1 or 2 drops
Small	2 or 3 drops
Medium	3 or 4 drops
Large	5 or 6 drops
Extra-large	7 or 8 drops

Calendula or cleavers. Both calendula and cleavers are lymphatic herbs; they help lymph fluid flow and clean the lymphatics during this process. If you don't address the lymphatics, wastes can get trapped and circulate. Calendula is best for warm dogs and cleavers for cool dogs. Administer twice daily for one week before, on the day of vaccination, and for two weeks afterward. Lymphatic flow is a must during this protocol.

Calendula or Cleavers Dosing Schedule

Size of Dog	Dose
Extra-small	1–3 drops
Small	4–6 drops
Medium	7–10 drops
Large	11–15 drops
Extra-large	20–25 drops

Humic and fulvic acids. These minerals help remove heavy metals and other toxins from the body. Remember, more isn't better. Start at 1/4 of the manufacturer's suggested dose for your dog's weight and slowly increase. Give two weeks prior and six weeks after vaccination.

Juniper bud phytoembryonic. Juniper stem cells are anti-inflammatory and anti-pharmaceutical. Don't use this remedy if your dog is taking prescribed medications. This remedy supports the liver with detoxification, modifying ammonia so the body can excrete toxins through the kidneys and the liver. Juniper phytoembryonic therapy can cause rapid detoxification, so start out low and slow and expect mucus in the stools, increased urination, eye and ear discharge, and possibly a runny nose. These symptoms are temporary. Cut back on or discontinue the dosage if your dog seems uncomfortable. Give twice daily for eight weeks post-vaccination.

Do not exceed eight weeks. Start out with 1/4 of the dosage and increase slowly.

Juniper Bud Phytoembryonic Dosing Schedule

Size of Dog	Dose
Extra-small	1 diluted drop
Small	1 drop
Medium	2 drops
Large	3 drops
Extra-large	4 drops

Ledum 30C. Use twice on the day of the vaccine. Ledum helps avoid complications at the injection site.

Milk thistle seed tincture. Milk thistle seed increases glutathione levels and helps protect the liver while supporting the kidneys and pancreas. Administer twice daily for two weeks before the vaccination, on the day of vaccination, and for four weeks afterward.

Milk Thistle Seed Tincture Dosing Schedule

Size of Dog	Dose
Extra-small	2 drops
Small	4 drops
Medium	6 drops
Large	8 drops
Extra-large	10 drops

Skullcap tincture. Skullcap is a specific herb for the rabies vaccine and helps support the nervous system. It's useful for behavior-based side effects. Administer twice daily for two weeks before vaccination, on the day of vaccination, and for eight weeks afterward.

Skullcap Tincture Dosing Schedule

Size of Dog	Dose
Extra-small	2 drops
Small	4 drops
Medium	6 drops
Large	8 drops
Extra-large	10 drops

Thuja occidentalis 30C. Use once daily, three days prior to vaccine, the day of, and two days after the vaccine. Thuja helps with any potential reactions to vaccines as well as working with ledum to avoid excessive bruising, irritation, and hematoma (swelling) at the injection site.

Summary: Vaccination Preparation and Recovery Protocol

Pre-vaccination Schedule	
2 weeks before	Black currant phytoembryonic, once daily
	Milk thistle seed tincture, twice daily
	Skullcap tincture, twice daily
1 week before	Calendula tincture (for warm dogs) or cleavers tincture (for cool dogs), twice daily
3 days before	Homeopathic Thuja occidentalis 30C, once

Vaccination Day Schedule
Calendula tincture (for warm dogs) or cleavers tincture (for cool dogs), twice
Black currant phytoembryonic, once
Milk thistle seed tincture, twice
Skullcap tincture, twice
Homeopathic Ledum 30C, twice
Homeopathic Thuja occidentalis 30C, once

Post-vaccination Schedule	
For 2 days after	Homeopathic Thuja occidentalis 30C, once
For 2 weeks after	Calendula tincture (for warm dogs) or cleavers tincture (for cool dogs), twice daily
For 2 weeks after	Black currant phytoembryonic, twice daily
For 4 weeks after	Milk thistle seed tincture, twice daily
For 6 weeks after	Birch bud phytoembryonic, twice daily
For 8 weeks after	Juniper bud phytoembryonic, twice daily
	Skullcap tincture, twice daily

Injection Site Care

Have your veterinarian shave the vaccination site; injection into the right rear leg is preferable. When the vaccination is finished, *immediately* apply a paste of bentonite clay (just mix the clay with water to make a paste) to the area. Place a piece of gauze over the clay and press it into the injection site, allow it to settle, and let dry. When you get home, wipe away the clay with a warm washcloth, dispose of the used clay in the garbage, and repeat.

Heavy Metal Detoxification Protocol

Removing any heavy metals from your dog's body is important as they lead to chronic disease. Undertake this detoxification protocol two to three weeks after the vaccination protocol concludes. But, throughout that time, continue with either cleavers or calendula for added lymphatic stimulation.

When you are ready to begin the detoxification protocol, use the following.

Humic and fulvic acid. Return humic and fulvic acid to your dog's regimen to aid in releasing heavy metals from the body.

Fresh food and greens. Feed your dog fresh food during this protocol. Include mushroom broth, bone broth, raw milk, vegetables, and greens. If your dog is warm, give cooling greens like wheatgrass or chlorella. If your dog is cool, spirulina is a good choice, and consider adding warming immune boosters like an infusion of ginger.

Mountain pine phytoembryonic. Add mountain pine phytoembryonic to your dog's regimen. Mountain pine stimulates the lymphatic system and helps remove heavy metals. Like milk thistle seed, it increases glutathione levels and helps protect cells from heavy metal absorption. Give twice daily for four weeks. Cut back on or discontinue the dosage if your dog seems uncomfortable.

Mountain Pine Phytoembryonic Dosing Schedule

Size of Dog	Dose
Extra-small	2 drops
Small	4 drops
Medium	6 drops
Large	10 drops
Extra-large	12 drops

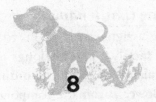

8

Plant and Fungi Monographs

As plants grow within, they take on a new form, operating through a new body, using us to fulfill their medicinal purpose. In one way, we use the plants to heal, and in another, they are using us.

SAJAH POPHAM,
EVOLUTIONARY HERBALISM

A monograph is a plant's resume, giving you a thorough understanding of its energetics, constituents, actions, and uses. There is much more to learn about each plant described in this chapter, of course; consider these monographs to be simply an introduction.

Herbs

Before we jump into the monographs for the fifty-five herbs featured in this chapter, we will walk through the structure of the monographs with explanations of each element. Remember that common names can change according to where you live. Latin names are universal and will tell you if you are using the correct plant.

🗡 Common name (*Latin name*)

Family: Taxonomy assigns each plant to a botanical family. Knowing which family a plant belongs to can often help you understand how plants are related according to their anatomical characteristics, flowers, aromatic components, medicinal properties, and energetics.

Energetics: As discussed in chapter 3, the energetics of a plant—whether it is warm or cool, dry or damp, relaxing or toning—is a key factor in its application. If you see the word *balancing*, it means that an herb can be modulating to affect both sides of the spectrum.

Energetic patterns indicating its use: These are the energetic patterns that the herb is used for.

Part used: This is the part(s) of the plant used for the applications described in this book. Note that different parts of these plants may have uses in other contexts.

Long-term use: "Long-term" in this context is generally defined as use of an herb for longer than 8 to 10 weeks.

Actions: These are the actions of the herb from the perspective of traditional herbalism. If any of the terms used here are unfamiliar to you, see appendix 1 for an explanation.

Constituents: These are the main constituents found in the herb, at the time the book was written and according to science.

Nutrients: These are the main nutrients found in the herb, according to science. If this section is missing from the monograph, it means that there isn't much research on this plant's specific nutrient value.

Cofactors: These are symptoms that are common with the herb's use; the more cofactors your dog has, the more strongly the herb is indicated. Cofactors can include both symptoms and conditions.

Flower essence: You'll find profiles of traditional flower essences at the end of this chapter. But some of the medicinal herbs also offer useful flower essences, and though they are not as common as those profiled later in this chapter, I have included them here, where applicable, with notes on their use for dogs.

Use for cats: Many of the herbs used with dogs can also be used with cats. This entry will tell you if this is the case for the herb in question. A cat would use the dosage recommended for an extra-small or small dog.

Applications

These are the ways in which we might use the herb to work with health conditions, support body systems, or address energetic imbalances. Note that this information is specific to canine health and limited to the scope of the discussions in this book. These herbs have many other uses, for animals and humans, that we will not examine here.

Preparation and Dosing Schedule

Here you'll find a table listing the types of remedies (tinctures, decoctions, dried herbs, and so on) I suggest for the herb within the context of this book. I include dosages based on the size of the dog, but please use this information in coordination with the discussion of dosages in chapter 6 (see page 133). There is much gray area in dosing. The suggested dosages are safe for most dogs. *Important:* Unless otherwise specified, the standard doses listed here should be given twice daily, and the acute doses should be given three to five times per day or every couple of hours depending on how acute the situation is.

Potential Concerns

Herb-drug interactions: Here you'll find a list of pharmaceuticals that the herb may have negative interactions with. Avoid using the herb in conjunction with these pharmaceuticals.

Cautions: Here you'll find any concerns or cautionary advice about the herb.

ᴄ Agrimony (*Agrimonia eupatoria*)

Family: Rosaceae
Energetics: cool and dry
Energetic patterns indicating its use: warmth, dryness, relaxation
Parts used: leaf and flower
Long-term use: yes
Actions: astringent, bitter tonic, cholagogue, diuretic, hemostatic, hepatic, vulnerary
Constituents: bitters, coumarins, flavonoids, nicotinic acid, phytosterols, silica, silicic acids, tannins, volatile oils
Nutrients: iron, vitamins B and K
Cofactors: bladder weakness, bloody diarrhea, bubbles in urine, chronic diarrhea, coughing, diarrhea with odor, early-stage kidney disease, excessive mucus, high blood pressure, high histamine levels, high pain threshold, incontinence, kennel cough, leaky gut, mucus in urine, poor appetite, relaxation in the kidneys, skin conditions
Flower essence: for skin eruptions, high pain threshold, restlessness at night, pacing, chewing of feet and sometimes entire body, tense body, high pain threshold, leaky gut, high histamine levels
Use for cats: yes

Applications

Diarrhea (acute): Mix 4 drops of agrimony with 2 drops of yarrow tincture in 1 ounce of filtered water. Give 60 ml of this solution for every 30 pounds of your dog's body weight, three times daily, until symptoms clear.

Diarrhea (chronic): Mix equal parts of agrimony tincture and blackberry leaf tincture. Give twice daily, using the tincture dose below.

Gastrointestinal system: Agrimony is a good source of tannins and a good anti-inflammatory, and it helps heal the gut with bitter compounds that regulate digestion and tone your dog's digestive tract. It is beneficial for leaky gut and stress-induced diarrhea with a strong odor.

Kidneys: When the kidneys are too relaxed, you'll see bladder weakness, a relaxed sphincter, and incontinence. Agrimony can help with all these issues and the beginning stages of kidney disease, especially when combined with nettle seed.

Nervous system: Useful for mitigating sympathetic excess. Relaxes the nervous system and releases tension that causes pain.

Respiratory system: Since the large intestine and the lungs are linked, agrimony's healing effects in the gastrointestinal system help dry out excessive mucus and support respiratory health.

Preparation and Dosing Schedule

	Extra-Small Dog	Small Dog	Medium Dog	Large Dog	Extra-Large Dog
Tincture	1 drop	2–3 drops	4–6 drops	8–10 drops	10–14 drops
Tincture for acute use	3 drops	6 drops	12 drops	20 drops	24 drops
Infusion	¼ teaspoon	½ teaspoon	1–2 teaspoons	1–2 tablespoons	3–6 tablespoons

Potential Concerns

Herb-drug interactions: none known

Cautions: Avoid in cases of constipation or excessive dryness.

⚹ Alfalfa (*Medicago sativa*)

Family: Fabaceae

Energetics: cool and damp

Energetic patterns indicating its use: warmth, dryness, tension

Part used: leaf (and for internal remedies, only the dried leaf)

Long-term use: safe in in small amounts

Actions: anticancer, antioxidant, antitumor, emollient (external), immunostimulant, nervine (mild), nutritive

Constituents: amino acids, carotenoids, chlorophyll, fiber, flavonoids, inositol, triterpenoid saponins

Nutrients: biotin, boron, calcium, chlorine, cobalt, folate, iron, magnesium, manganese, molybdenum, niacin, pantothenic acid, phosphorus, potassium, sulfur, vitamins (A, B-complex, C, D, E, K)

Cofactors: depleted immune system, early graying, high cholesterol, liver inflammation, splenectomy, surgery recovery, sympathetic excess, toxicity, trace mineral deficiency, weakness

Flower essence: for dogs who don't easily share or connect with other dogs, OCD behaviors

Use for cats: yes

Applications

Nervous system: Can be used to address sympathetic excess by relaxing the central nervous system (it's a CNS tonic) and releasing tension that causes pain. Supports neuron production in the brain and the heart.

Skin: Alfalfa is rich in antioxidants, vitamins, and minerals. This helps the liver improve the oxidation process and decrease oxidation levels in your dog's body. Alfalfa is also a good source of vitamin K, which is part of the reason it helps relieve inflammation of both the liver and the skin.

Preparation and Dosing Schedule

	Extra-Small Dog	Small Dog	Medium Dog	Large Dog	Extra-Large Dog
Tincture	1–2 drops	2–3 drops	4–6 drops	6–8 drops	8–10 drops
Infusion (dried leaf)	¼ teaspoon	½ teaspoon	1–2 teaspoons	1–2 tablespoons	3–6 tablespoons

Potential Concerns

Herb-drug interactions: anticoagulants

Cautions: For internal remedies, use only the dried leaf due to fresh alfalfa's high saponin content, which can cause diarrhea and nausea. Avoid large dosages. Do not give to dogs with lupus or autoimmune disorders. May cause gastrointestinal distress. Avoid alfalfa seeds. Alfalfa sprouts are nutritive and can be fed to dogs, but feed them in a rotation. Avoid conventional alfalfa; it is genetically modified (GMO). Always use organic.

⚹ Aloe (*Aloe vera*)

Family: Liliaceae

Energetics: cool and damp

Energetic patterns indicating its use: dryness, tension, warm to hot energetics

Part used: leaf gel and juice (fresh or dried/powdered)

Long-term use: dried and in a formula is acceptable

Actions: antibacterial, antifungal, anti-inflammatory, bitter, demulcent, emollient, immune modulator, vulnerary

Constituents: acemannan, amino acids, anthranoids, digestive enzymes, fatty acids, hormones, lignin, prostaglandins, resins, salicylic acid, saponins, sugars

Nutrients: aluminum, calcium, choline, chromium, cobalt, copper, fat, folate, iron, magnesium, manganese, niacin, phosphorus, potassium, protein, riboflavin, selenium, silicon, sodium, thiamine, vitamins (A,C, E, B_2, B_6, B_{12}), zinc

Use for cats: no

Cofactors: arthritis, bladder inflammation, burns, digestive insufficiency, dry joints, dryness, dry skin, ear infections, ear mites, gut inflammation, high blood sugar, irritated anal glands, kidney weakness, leaky gut, liver weakness, poor assimilation, ulcers, UTI, vitamin deficiencies, worms, yeast

Applications

Anal glands: Aloe reduces inflammation and soothes irritation. Use it combined with other herbs in a formula for anal gland conditions.

Gastrointestinal system: Aloe juice or gel helps soothe an inflamed gut and heal leaky gut because it helps tighten the junctions in a dog's gut lining. With its mucilage, aloe also feeds beneficial bacteria and so supports the microbiome. High in enzymes, it helps break down nutrients in the gut. Acemannan, an active constituent, is an effective deterrent of *Candida albicans*.

Skin: Aloe supports the skin internally by interacting with the gastrointestinal tract, lymphatics, moisture balance, and liver. It can also be used externally to help heal wounds and burns, soothe ears, and heal ear mite lesions (use gel).

Preparation and Dosing Schedule

External use: For external applications, use the fresh gel.

Internal use: Give small amounts of aloe juice for leaky gut and mild gastrointestinal distress. You can use powdered aloe in commercial dog-centered supplements or to rehydrate into juice.

Dosage: For internal use, mix 1 teaspoon of 100 percent aloe gel with 3 ounces of water or broth. If using dried powder, mix as directed. Give 1/2 teaspoon for every 20 pounds of bodyweight, once daily.

Potential Concerns

Herb-drug interactions: antiarrhythmic drugs, cardiac glycosides, corticosteroids, thiazide diuretics

Cautions: Do not use the latex (yellow-brown liquid between the outer coating and the inner gel) of aloe, as it can cause gastrointestinal distress and bloody diarrhea. Use only the gel or juice. When sourcing powder, ensure it is 100 percent dried powder of juice or gel—without latex or aloin.

Angelica (*Angelica archangelica*)

Family: Apiaceae

Energetics: warm and dry

Energetic patterns indicating its use: coolness, cold, dampness

Part used: dried root

Long-term use: only under the supervision of a holistic vet or herbalist

Actions: antibacterial, antispasmodic, bitter, carminative, cholagogue, diuretic

Constituents: coumarins, fructose, furanocoumarins, glucose, phenolic acids, sucrose, volatile oils

Nutrients: magnesium, potassium, riboflavin, thiamine, vitamin B_{12}

Cofactors: allergies, anal gland dryness, arthritis, bronchitis, constipation, cool energetics, digestive insufficiency, incontinence, itchiness, kidney weakness, lung mucus, malabsorption, nervousness, parasympathetic excess, poor appetite, poor circulation, skittishness, stiff joints, sympathetic excess

Flower essence: for dogs who are in the process of dying or for puppies following a difficult birth

Use for cats: yes

Applications

Angelica root can help wake up the vital force. It aids circulation and digestion, two key factors in balancing cold. Its upward movement provides circulation throughout the body to the periphery.

Kidneys: Stimulates kidney function and appetite and reduces bladder spasms.

Lipomas: Helps with systemic detoxification and elimination. Use in combination with other herbs as part of a formula, or pulse.

Lungs: Angelica warms, decreases inflammation, and improves circulation in the lungs. It's an expectorant, helping a dog bring up thick, stagnant mucus, and it also stimulates and modulates the immune system, making it helpful for coughs, bronchitis, and infections of the upper respiratory system.

Preparation and Dosing Schedule

	Extra-Small Dog	Small Dog	Medium Dog	Large Dog	Extra-Large Dog
Tincture	1 drop	2–3 drops	3–5 drops	6–8 drops	9–10 drops
Dried root	1/16 teaspoon	1/8 teaspoon	1/4 teaspoon	1/8 teaspoon	1/2 teaspoon

Potential Concerns

Herb-drug interactions: anticoagulants

Cautions: Don't confuse *Angelica archangelica* with *Angelica sinensis,* aka Chinese angelica; these herbs are *not* interchangeable. Do not give angelica in large doses. Do not give it to dogs with Cushing's disease, as it helps the body release cortisol and stimulates the adrenals.

⚘ Artichoke (*Cynara scolymus*)

Family: Asteraceae

Energetics: cool and dry

Energetic patterns indicating its use: warmth, dampness

Part used: leaf

Long-term use: yes

Actions: anticancer, antioxidant, bitter, cholagogue, diuretic, hepatoprotective

Constituents: cynaratriol, phenolic acid, silymarin

Nutrients: biotin, calcium, chromium, copper, folic acid, iron, magnesium, manganese, niacin, pantothenic acid, phosphorus, potassium, riboflavin, thiamine, vitamins (A, B_6, C, K), zinc

Cofactors: acid reflux, anemia, constipation alternating with diarrhea, difficulty digesting fats, digestive insufficiency, excessive heat, gallbladder sludge, high blood pressure, high liver enzymes, high toxic load, high triglycerides, IBD, IBS, insufficient bile flow, itchiness and scratching, kidney weakness, leaky gut, obesity, pancreatitis, poor appetite, poor microbiome health, skin conditions

Use for cats: yes

Flower essence: for solar plexus weakness, liver issues, aggression, trouble concentrating, training

Applications

Gastrointestinal system: Works with the gut immune system and supports a healthy microbiome. Helps regulate gastrointestinal inflammation, IBS, constipation alternating with diarrhea, and digestive insufficiency. Like burdock root, artichoke helps protect the liver and assists in the digestion of fats while increasing the assimilation of fat-soluble vitamins. It has an affinity for the gallbladder and can help remove and prevent gallstones.

Heart: Lowers cholesterol, regulates blood pressure, and decreases triglycerides.

Liver: Increases bile, supports detoxification through the liver, helps protect the liver against toxins, and reduces oxidative stress. May help regenerate liver cells, boost assimilation and antioxidant activity, and increase levels of catalase, glutathione, glutathione peroxidase, and superoxide dismutase. Helps decrease liver enzymes and process toxins from weight loss and excess fat around the liver. I use artichoke for dogs who are overweight and energetically warm to hot.

Preparation and Dosing Schedule

	Extra-Small Dog	Small Dog	Medium Dog	Large Dog	Extra-Large Dog
Tincture	1–2 drops	2–4 drops	4–6 drops	6–8 drops	8–10 drops
Dried herb	1/16 teaspoon	1/8 teaspoon	1/4 teaspoon	1/2 teaspoon	3/4 teaspoon

Potential Concerns

Herb-drug interactions: none known

Cautions: Artichoke will cause dogs to pee more. Avoid in cases of gallbladder obstruction.

◢ Ashwagandha (*Withania somnifera*)

Family: Solanaceae

Energetics: warm and dry

Energetic patterns indicating its use: coolness, dampness, tension

Part used: root

Long-term use: yes

Actions: adaptogen, analgesic, anti-inflammatory, antitumor, diuretic, immune modulator, nervine, reproductive tonic, tonic, trophorestorative

Constituents: alkaloids, antioxidants, flavonoids, saponins, steroidal lactones, withanine, withasomnine

Nutrients: calcium, carotene, iron, protein, vitamin C

Cofactors: adrenal depletion, anxiety, arthritis, cool energetics, depletion, geriatric condition, high stress levels, hypothyroidism, inflammation, low immune function, mast cell cancer, pain, respiratory symptoms, restlessness, stress, sympathetic excess, tension, weakness

Flower essence: for emotionally sensitive, whiny working dogs, or dogs with chronic stress, anxiety, and restlessness

Use for cats: yes

Applications

Kidneys: Helps tone and protect kidneys and increase circulation through the entire renal system.

Lipomas: Help regulate sympathetic activity, decrease stress and inflammation, and reduce tumors. Its anti-inflammatory effects and adrenal affinity help regulate stress hormones, improve circulation, and support the immune system.

Nervous system: Helps with sympathetic excess, high cortisol levels, and hyperactivity. Ashwagandha is a well-accepted adaptogen and can help your dog deal with stress.

Skin: High in antioxidants, ashwagandha reduces the oxidative stress that contributes to skin issues. It is also a good antimicrobial and can help balance your dog's dermal microbiome. It helps calm the skin and decrease inflammation.

Preparation and Dosing Schedule

	Extra-Small Dog	Small Dog	Medium Dog	Large Dog	Extra-Large Dog
Tincture	1–2 drops	2–4 drops	4–6 drops	6–8 drops	8–10 drops
Glycerin extract	4 drops	8 drops	12 drops	16 drops	20–25 drops

Preparation and Dosing Schedule (cont'd)

	Extra-Small Dog	Small Dog	Medium Dog	Large Dog	Extra-Large Dog
Decoction	¼ teaspoon	½ teaspoon	1 teaspoon	2 teaspoons	1 tablespoon
Dried root	¹⁄₁₆ teaspoon	⅛ teaspoon	¼ teaspoon	½ teaspoon	¾ teaspoon

Glycerin extract: Glycerin isn't appropriate for ashwagandha extraction, but ashwagandha is sometimes made and sold in "glycerite" form: It is extracted in alcohol, the alcohol is allowed to evaporate, and then the remaining extract is preserved in glycerin. If you are purchasing such a product, make sure the extraction was first done in alcohol.

Potential Concerns

Herb-drug interactions: antidepressants

Cautions: Avoid in cases of hyperthyroidism or deep-cold energetics. Ashwagandha elevates levels of GABA, so avoid large doses except for acute use. Don't give to dogs that are weak, skinny, and emaciated. Adaptogens can be too much for these types of dogs; wait until they get stronger.

⚹ Astragalus (*Astragalus membranaceus*)

Family: Fabaceae

Energetics: warm and dry

Energetic patterns indicating its use: coolness, tension, dampness, dryness

Part used: roots (at least 3 years old)

Long-term use: no, except under the guidance of a holistic vet or herbalist; use for no more than 8 weeks at a time, and give a 3- to 4-week break between cycles

Actions: antibacterial, antiviral, diuretic, immune stimulant, tonic, vasodilator

Constituents: amino acids, flavonoids, lignans, phytosterols, polysaccharides, triterpenoid saponins

Nutrients: copper, iron, manganese, potassium, selenium, zinc

Cofactors: anal gland relaxation, cancer, chemotherapy, chronic diarrhea, chronic viral load, cough, ear infections, environmental allergies, heart weakness, high histamine levels, inflammation, kennel cough, kidney disease, kidney weakness, labored breathing, lethargy, loss of appetite, lung weakness, splenectomy, steroid use

Flower essence: for dogs with trauma and scattered energy and dogs in need of grounding

Use for cats: yes

Applications

Allergies: Balances interleukins and brings down histamine levels, decreasing inflammation. Astragalus is high in antioxidants, supporting the liver by reducing oxidative stress. This takes pressure off the liver and eases environmental reactivity.

Cough: Astragalus is an effective antiviral and immune-stimulating herb that helps combat upper respiratory infections and strengthens the lungs. Helps shorten episodes of coughing and kennel cough. Restores moisture to the mucosa in the lungs, supporting the integrity of the lungs' elimination system.

Heart: Increases circulation, brings down inflammation, and, with its high flavonoid content, can help support heart health and increase interferon levels.

Immune: Astragalus is antiviral, increasing levels of immunoglobulin (an antibody) and white blood cells like T cells, NK cells, and macrophages.

Itchiness and scratching: Astragalus is a superb anti-inflammatory with high levels of antioxidants, and it positively affects the liver by helping it work more efficiently. All these effects can decrease a dog's itchiness.

Kidneys: Improves blood flow through the kidneys and decreases urine protein levels.

Leaky gut: Helps prevent histamine intolerance, which puts pressure on your dog's gut lining. Decreases inflammation and stimulates the immune system.

Nervous system: Helps dogs manage stress and balance sympathetic excess and anxiety. Mix with lion's mane mushroom to boost nerve regeneration capacities.

Preparation and Dosing Schedule

	Extra-Small Dog	Small Dog	Medium Dog	Large Dog	Extra-Large Dog
Tincture	1–2 drops	2–4 drops	4–6 drops	6–8 drops	8–10 drops
Glycerite	4 drops	8 drops	12 drops	16 drops	20 drops
Decoction	¼ teaspoon	½ teaspoon	2 teaspoons	2 tablespoons	5–6 tablespoons

Potential Concerns

Herb-drug interactions: steroids

Cautions: Not indicated for acute use or infections. Avoid in cases of auto-immune disease except under the guidance of a professional. Use only the *membranaceous* species; other astragalus species carry a risk of toxicity. Can cause selenium toxicity with long-term use.

◢ Bee Balm (*Monarda* spp.)

Family: Lamiaceae

Energetics: warm but balancing, stimulating/relaxing, dry

Energetic patterns indicating its use: coolness, cold, deep cold

Part used: leaf and flower

Long-term use: yes

Actions: analgesic, anti-inflammatory, antimicrobial, antiseptic, antispasmodic, bitter tonic, carminative, diaphoretic, diuretic, expectorant

Constituents: anthocyanins, flavonoids, luteolin, oleanolic acid, quercitrin, volatile oils (including camphene, carvacrol, linalool, and thymol)

Nutrients: fiber, vitamins C and K

Cofactors: anxiety, candida overgrowth, cough, diarrhea, ear infections, flu, fungal infection, gassiness, gastrointestinal inflammation, grief, inflammation, insomnia, kidney infection, leaky gut, nausea, respiratory tract infection, UTI

Flower essence: helps calm grief and bring joy

Use for cats: yes

Applications

Grief: The flower essence has an uplifting effect; use bee balm tincture or infusion if your dog is feeling nervous with grief.

Kidneys: Acts as an antiseptic and is useful for relieving UTIs and improving kidney tone.

Nausea: Bee balm is often overlooked as an effective tonic. It settles the stomach and has a tonic effect on the entire gastrointestinal tract. Give 1–5 drops of tincture diluted in water, two or three times per day.

Topical uses: can be used as a wash for swollen paws, bug bites, and skin irritations due to its anti-inflammatory and pain-relieving properties.

Preparation and Dosing Schedule

	Extra-Small Dog	Small Dog	Medium Dog	Large Dog	Extra-Large Dog
Tincture	1–2 drops	2–4 drops	4–6 drops	6–8 drops	8–10 drops
Infusion	⅛ teaspoon	½ teaspoon	1 teaspoon	2–3 teaspoons	1–2 tablespoons

Potential Concerns

Herb-drug interactions: none known

Cautions: Different varieties of bee balm have varying levels of stimulation.

◢ Blackberry (*Rubus fruticosus*)

Family: Rosaceae

Energetics: cool and dry

Energetic patterns indicating its use: warm to hot, dampness, relaxation

Part used: leaf

Long-term use: yes, but can cause excessive dryness when used long-term

Actions: antidiarrheal, anti-inflammatory, antimicrobial, antioxidant, astringent

Constituents: antioxidants, citric acid, flavonoids, fragarine, polysaccharides, tannins, triterpenes

Nutrients: calcium, iron, vitamins (C, E, K), magnesium

Cofactors: anal bleeding or infection, bladder gravel and stones, bladder infection, bladder relaxation, cat turd eating, diarrhea, giardiasis, IBD, IBS, inflammation, kidney weakness, leaky gut, liver stress, mouth inflammation, UTI

Flower essence: calms fear and builds confidence; for dogs that are hard to train, aging dogs, leaving the litter (meaning puppies; apply externally), dogs prone to diarrhea and leaky gut or suffering from illness; for throat chakra work

Use for cats: yes

Applications

Allergies: Blackberry leaf can help with seasonal allergies thanks to its normalizing influence on the gut and liver.

Anal gland infections: Use as a poultice for anal gland infections; its astringency will help tone the tissues.

Diarrhea: Blackberry leaf is excellent at clearing up bacteria-related diarrhea.

Gastrointestinal system: Reduces inflammation and combats pathogenic bacteria, making it helpful for diarrhea and pancreatitis, especially in severe acute cases. Especially helpful for damp dogs.

Kidneys: Helps tone the bladder and kidneys. Useful for UTIs and bladder infections. Combine with marshmallow root in an infusion for a soothing antibacterial remedy.

Preparation and Dosing Schedule

	Extra-Small Dog	Small Dog	Medium Dog	Large Dog	Extra-Large Dog
Tincture	2 drops	4–6 drops	6–8 drops	8–12 drops	10–16 drops
Tincture for acute use	4 drops	10 drops	16 drops	20–22 drops	22–30 drops
Infusion	½ teaspoon	1 teaspoon	3 teaspoons	2–3 tablespoons	4–6 tablespoons

Potential Concerns

Herb-drug interactions: none known

⚹ Burdock (*Arctium lappa*)

Family: Asteraceae

Energetics: slightly cool and damp, drying long-term

Energetic patterns indicating its use: warm to hot, dryness, tension

Part used: root

Long-term use: yes

Actions: adaptogen (mild), alterative, antibiotic, anti-inflammatory, antiseptic, appetite stimulant, bitter, decongestant, diaphoretic, digestive, diuretic, lymphatic, mild laxative, tonic, trophorestorative, vulnerary

Constituents: acetic acid, chlorogenic acid, inulin, lignans, mucilage, polysaccharides, resins, sesquiterpene lactones, steric acids, tannins, terpenes, triterpenes

Nutrients: calcium, chromium, cobalt, fiber, iron, magnesium, manganese, niacin, phosphorus, potassium, protein, riboflavin, selenium, silicon, thiamine, tin, vitamins A and C, zinc

Cofactors: acid reflux, arthritis, bloodshot eyes, chronic skin conditions, constipation, crusty skin, dandruff, difficulty digesting fats, difficulty getting up (better with movement), dry and crumbly stool, dry cough, dry skin, endocrine disorders, false heat, food sensitivities, hairless patches across the skin with dryness, high tolerance for pain, high toxic load, hot spots, hypothyroidism, inability to put on weight, inflammation, insufficient bile flow, leaky gut, liver insufficiency, low adrenal function, low digestive enzymes, low urine volume, nervousness, poor appetite, stagnant lymphatics, stiff joints, stiffness in hind end, tendency to pancreatitis, ulcers, warm energetics, yellow discharges

Flower essence: helps release anger, grief, sadness, and tension and tightness in the chest; impacts the emotions of the liver and lungs

Use for cats: yes

Applications

Allergies: Reduces a dog's chances of developing allergies due to its support for the gut and the liver.

Antibiotics recovery: Helps rebuild a healthy microbiome thanks to its prebiotic actions. It also supports assimilation, nutrient distribution, and all the systems of elimination, making it especially useful for recovery from antibiotics given after surgery.

Gastrointestinal system: Burdock root is a bitter; it increases bile production. It supports the liver in breaking down both fats and proteins and boosts levels of digestive enzymes. It revitalizes the gut's mucosal linings, increasing nutrient assimilation, strengthening weak tissues, and working to prevent leaky gut. Its inulin content serves as a prebiotic, helping to support the gut microbiome.

Kidneys: Though burdock root is mainly associated with the liver in conventional herbalism, it also supports elimination through the kidneys through its diuretic action, helping the kidneys filter more effectively.

Liver: High in antioxidants, burdock root helps protect the liver. It also stimulates bile production and helps the liver detoxify more efficiently, including detoxification of the blood.

Lymphatic system: Supports lymphatic movement and lipid transport and processing, relieving dryness and improving the assimilation of fat-soluble vitamins. In particular, burdock has influence over the lymphatic system inside the mammary glands, which are prone to infection in female dogs (mastitis). It also helps shrink lipomas.

Musculoskeletal system: Relieves stiffness in the back end, decreases heat, and helps revitalize dry joints.

Nervous system: Helps protect the myelin sheath and moisturizes the nervous system, helping nervous, anxious, and depleted dogs with dry energetics.

Skin: Burdock root is known for being a blood cleanser, and it's great in combination with herbs like yellow dock for skin conditions because it works on the liver-skin connection. Burdock supports the organs of elimination, like the liver, lymphatics, and kidneys, an action that in turn supports the skin, itself an organ of elimination. It also increases circulation, which helps clean and balance skin conditions.

Preparation and Dosing Schedule

	Extra-Small Dog	Small Dog	Medium Dog	Large Dog	Extra-Large Dog
Tincture	1–2 drops	2–4 drops	4–6 drops	6–8 drops	8–10 drops
Glycerite	4 drops	8 drops	12 drops	16 drops	20 drops
Decoction	1/8 cup	1/4 cup	1/2 cup	3/4–1 cup	1 1/2–2 cups
Dried root	1/16 teaspoon	1/8 teaspoon	1/4 teaspoon	1/2 teaspoon	1 teaspoon

Potential Concerns

Herb-drug interactions: none known

Cautions: Avoid burdock root in cases of SIBO. Burdock is a diaphoretic; it can bring what is within to the surface. You may see an increase in panting. Too high a dose can cause excessive itchiness.

✄ Calendula (*Calendula officinalis*)

Family: Asteraceae

Energetics: warm and dry

Energetic patterns indicating its use: coolness, cold, relaxation

Part used: flower with calyx

Long-term use: yes

Actions: alterative, anti-fungal, anti-inflammatory (gentle), antimicrobial, antiseptic, warming astringent, bitter, cholagogue, emollient, lymphatic, spasmodic, vulnerary

Constituents: antioxidants, calcium sulfate, carotenoids, chlorogenic acid, coumarins, flavonoids, flavonol glycosides, isoquercitrin, isorhamnetin, longispinogenin, lupeol, lutein, lycopene, mucilage, narcissin, neohesperidoside, phytosterols, polysaccharides, potassium chloride, quercetin, resin, rutin, saponins, sesquiterpenes, sterols, sulfate, triterpenes, tocopherols, volatile oils

Nutrients: calcium, magnesium, phosphorus, potassium, sodium, vitamins A and C

Cofactors: abrasions, bacterial infections of the skin, bruises, burns, candida overgrowth, cat turd eating, cold stomach, conjunctivitis, cough, damp and cold to neutral energetics that worsen in cold or damp weather, demodectic mange, depletion, diarrhea, digestive inflammation, digestive upset, dry skin, ear infections, elevated liver enzymes, excessive antibiotic use, irritated eyes, fatigue, food intolerance, frailty, grief, gum disease, hepatitis, hot spots, IBD, impacted anal glands, itchy skin, leaky gut, lethargy, lingering infections, nausea and vomiting, respiratory conditions, sarcoptic mange, sensitive stomach, sepsis, sprains, sunburn, thinness, ulcers, warts, yeast

Flower essence: for depression, deficiency, lack of bonding, weak digestion, reactivity to stimulus or weather, stiffness or rigidity

Use for cats: yes

Applications

Allergies: Calendula's actions on the liver, gastrointestinal tract, and lymphatic system can help resolve leaky gut, food intolerances, and excessive immune response.

Antibiotics recovery: Calendula is known as a bacteriostatic, meaning that it helps create an environment that isn't conducive to bacteria overgrowth. It doesn't kill bacteria; it adjusts the internal terrain so it's less hospitable to bacteria. This helps a dog's microbiome to repopulate in a balanced way after antibiotics use, a time when it is vulnerable to overgrowth by pathogenic microbes. Calendula is also antifungal, which can help specifically with preventing candida overgrowth in the digestive tract when dogs must use antibiotics. Combine calendula with *Saccharomyces boulardii* for this purpose.

Gastrointestinal system: Calms the digestive mucosa and inflamed intestinal linings through its demulcent action. Heals skin on the outside of the body and has the same effect inside the gastrointestinal tract, providing moisture and reducing inflammation. In regulating the terrain of the body's tissues, calendula supports a dog's microbiome.

Heart: In her book *The Complete Herbal Handbook for Farm and Stable*, herbalist Juliette de Bairacli Levy describes calendula as a mild tonic for the heart and arteries, pointing out its high antioxidant levels and anti-inflammatory properties.

Kidneys: Helps support elimination through the kidneys through its relationship with the lymphatic system. Has a downward movement in the body, helping fluids drain from the elimination channels like the intestines and kidneys.

Leaky gut: Calendula is excellent for leaky gut arising from cold energetics because it warms the core, helps repair the gut wall, and stimulates immune function.

Lipomas: By pushing through stagnation in the lymphatic system while warming internal tissues, calendula helps reduce lipomas.

Liver: Helps clear heat and stagnancy from the liver. Stimulates circulation in the portal vein, clearing out metabolic wastes and decreasing liver enzyme levels.

Lymphatic system: Gradually restores healthy lymphatic function, helping it process pathogens and avoid waste accumulation.

Skin: An excellent external wound healer (vulnerary), helping to prevent bacterial growth, reduce inflammation, and promote the healing of cells. Decreases swelling, discharge, and scarring from injuries like scrapes, burns, and abscesses. Makes an effective antiparasitic rinse for sarcoptic and demodectic mange. Mix with St. John's wort in an infusion or salve to help heal and soothe a hot spot. Helps disperse candida and other fungal infections of the skin.

Preparation and Dosing Schedule

	Extra-Small Dog	Small Dog	Medium Dog	Large Dog	Extra-Large Dog
Tincture	2 drops	4 drops	6 drops	8 drops	10–12 drops
Tincture as lymphatic stimulant	1 diluted drop	1 drop	2 drops	3 drops	4 drops

Preparation and Dosing Schedule (cont'd)

	Extra-Small Dog	Small Dog	Medium Dog	Large Dog	Extra-Large Dog
Glycerin extract	6 drops	12 drops	18 drops	24 drops	30 drops
Infusion	¼ teaspoon	½ teaspoon	1–2 teaspoons	1–2 tablespoons	3–6 tablespoons

Glycerin extract: Calendula's constituents do not extract well in glycerin. Make sure any "glycerite" of calendula was first extracted in alcohol and then preserved in glycerin.

Infusions: Let an infusion of calendula steep for 40 to 50 minutes. You can use the infusion internally, following the dosing schedule above, or externally as a rinse.

Potential Concerns

Herb-drug interactions: none

Cautions: Don't use with deep wounds involving pus, as its tremendous healing actions can seal the wound over the pus and cause infection. Calendula can bring on menses, so use caution with intact (unspayed) females. May cause a reaction in dogs allergic to other members of the Asteraceae family.

✌ Cayenne (*Capsicum annuum*)

Family: Solanaceae

Energetics: hot, pungent, stimulating, dry

Energetic patterns indicating its use: coolness, cold, deep cold, dampness

Part used: dried fruit

Long-term use: no

Actions: antioxidant, carminative, circulatory stimulant, stimulant

Constituents: amides, capsaicin, carotenoids, flavonoids, volatile oil

Nutrients: beta-carotene, calcium, cobalt, iron, magnesium, phosphorus, potassium, selenium, thiamine, tin, vitamins A and C

Cofactors: arthritis, asthma, cool to cold energetics, lack of appetite, pneumonia, poor circulation, poor digestion, secretions, weakness in the cardiac system

Use for cats: only in a cat-specific formula prepared by a holistic herbalist or herbal company

Applications

Circulation: Cayenne helps move things to the surface, clearing stagnation. It's excellent for cold conditions because it helps get the blood moving.

That said, it's helpful in both warm and cool conditions due its ability to balance circulation; in these cases it would be used in a formula where it is balanced by cooling herbs.

Preparation and Dosing Schedule

	Extra-Small Dog	Small Dog	Medium Dog	Large Dog	Extra-Large Dog
Tincture	1 diluted drop	1 drop	1–2 drops	2–3 drops	3–4 drops
Dried herb	Minute pinch	½ pinch	¾ pinch	1 pinch	Larger pinch

Cayenne should always be mixed with a fatty substance, goat milk, or butter. It is best used in a formula.

Potential Concerns

Herb-drug interactions: blood thinners

Cautions: Avoid cayenne for at least 10 days before surgery and in dogs with IBD, IBS, ulcers, or hot energetics. Do not use on broken skin or on any mucous membranes, including the eyes. Use a tincture to control dosage when possible.

✍ Chamomile (*Matricaria chamomilla*)

Family: Asteraceae

Energetics: cool and dry

Energetic patterns indicating its use: warm to hot energetics, dampness, tension

Part used: flower

Long-term use: yes

Actions: antiallergenic, anticatarrhal, antiemetic, anti-inflammatory, antimicrobial, antispasmodic, bitter, carminative, demulcent, diaphoretic, digestive, diuretic, nervine, relaxant, tonic, vulnerary

Constituents: amino acids, azulene, chamazulene, coumarins, flavonoids, glycosides, polysaccharides, quercetin, rutin, sesquiterpenes, tannins

Nutrients: calcium, chromium, iron, magnesium, manganese, phosphorus, potassium, selenium, silicon, thiamine, tin

Cofactors: acid reflux, agitation, allergies, anxiety, aversion to touch, biting, bullying behavior in groups, constipation, dampness, ear infections, ear pain, food sensitivities, gastrointestinal upset, heart excitability, high histamine levels, incontinence, insomnia, poor appetite, nausea, nervousness, pain, puking water, regurgitation, restlessness, roundworm, skin conditions, spasms, stress biting, stretching of the stomach across the floor, sympathetic excess, tension, vomiting water

Flower essence: for stress, hyperactivity, restlessness, anxiety, tension; helpful particularly for dogs that don't like to be touched or that have herding tendencies; for sacral chakra and solar plexus chakra work

Use for cats: yes

Applications

Anxiety: Helps calm the nervous system and adds moisture (short-term) for a dried-out nervous system. Calms nerve spasms, relieves sympathetic excess, and increases serotonin and dopamine levels.

Cough: Calms irritation, agitation, and spasms in the respiratory tract. It's a strong anti-inflammatory for delicate lung tissue. Use an infusion to help decrease coughing and spasms.

Gastrointestinal system: Relaxes the digestive tract, reduces gas, releases tension, and smooths muscle tissue. Its bitterness helps stimulate bile, decrease inflammation, and remove heat from the digestive system while calming the stomach lining. An infusion of dried German chamomile works well for upset stomach and nausea.

Histamine intolerance: Chamomile is a natural antihistamine. Prepare it as an infusion and pour it over your dog's food.

Liver: Supports the liver's detoxification pathways through its sesquiterpene lactone content. Decreases liver enzymes.

Nervous system: Helps modulate the nervous system; works as a relaxant for pain and upset in the nerves. Calms agitated or jumpy nerves.

Skin: With its antioxidants, anti-inflammatory action, and support for the liver, chamomile helps cool heat and reduce inflammation and irritation of the skin, leading to less itchiness and scratching. It's also a cooling antifungal, making it useful as a rinse for yeast infections of the skin.

Urinary system: Slightly diuretic, anti-inflammatory, and antibacterial, chamomile is good for dogs who hold their urine and suffer from bladder and urinary tract infections. It helps bring down blood pressure (systolic) and, in turn, decreases your dog's urine output, especially if it is excessive. As an infusion, it can help soothe irritated bladder membranes.

Preparation and Dosing Schedule

	Extra-Small Dog	Small Dog	Medium Dog	Large Dog	Extra-Large Dog
Tincture	1–2 drops	2–4 drops	4–6 drops	6–8 drops	8–10 drops
Tincture for acute use	4 drops	8 drops	12 drops	16 drops	20 drops
Glycerite	4 drops	8 drops	12 drops	16 drops	20–30 drops
Infusion	½ teaspoon	1 teaspoon	3 teaspoons	2–3 tablespoons	4–6 tablespoons

Potential Concerns

Herb-drug interactions: none known

Cautions: Some dogs (and cats) can be allergic to chamomile; give a very small dose to test.

⚔ Chickweed (*Stellaria media*)

Family: Caryophyllaceae

Energetics: cool and damp

Energetic patterns indicating its use: warm to hot energetics, excessive heat, dryness, tension

Parts used: leaf and flower

Long-term use: yes, but watch for dryness

Actions: alterative, anti-inflammatory, antibacterial, antiviral, appetite stimulant, demulcent, diuretic, emollient, lymphatic, nutritive, trophorestorative, vulnerary

Constituents: bioflavonoids, coumarins, gamma-linolenic acid, rutin, saponins, triterpenoids

Nutrients: calcium, copper, iron, magnesium, manganese, phosphorus, potassium, silicon, sodium, vitamins (A, B-complex, C, E), zinc

Cofactors: anal gland inflammation and stagnation, anxiety, asthma, blood poisoning, boils, bronchitis, cancer, CCL tears, colon problems, constipation, diabetes, diarrhea, excessive appetite, fear, gastritis, inflammation, itchy skin, lipomas, malabsorption, nervous stomach, nervousness, obesity, respiratory distress, skin problems, swellings, swollen lymph glands, tight muscles and tendons, ulcers

Flower essence: for dogs who don't share; for dogs that display aggression, food aggression, or barrier aggression (mix with violet flower essence for dogs that have been abused.

Use for cats: yes

Applications

Gastrointestinal system: High in polysaccharides, chickweed lubricates the intestines and soothes dry mucosa. It has a drawing nature both internally and externally, reducing systemic inflammation and removing stagnant metabolic wastes through the large intestine and lymphatic system. It helps keep the bowels moving, relieving constipation, and the anal glands lubricated.

Kidneys: Chickweed has an affinity for the kidneys. As an infusion, it is a nutritive tonic full of vitamins and minerals and helps minimize sodium reabsorption by the kidneys, which leads to the loss of fluids.

Liver: Supports the liver (and lymphatic system) in removing excess fats and metabolic wastes.

Lymphatic system: Chickweed has an affinity for the lymphatic system. It is cooling, bringing down heat in the gut, liver, endocrine system, and lymph. Its saponins increase cellular permeability and nutrient assimilation, which supports the cellular matrix, spleen, liver, small intestine, and lymph nodes. Chickweed helps break up congested lymphatics by flushing out the entire system. (This makes it an effective remedy for heat-associated lipomas.) It's a master of the water element and helps the body process fats and water.

Musculoskeletal system: Due to its action on the kidneys, chickweed has a supportive and moisturizing action on tendons and ligaments, reducing congestion and tension and improving elasticity.

Nervous system: Chickweed calms fear and anxiety arising from imbalance in the kidneys. It helps dogs with a nervous stomach and hyperexcited appetites who tend to have loose stools and irritated anal glands.

Skin: Through its support for the liver, chickweed can help improve skin conditions. You can also use chickweed as an anti-inflammatory rinse to relieve itching.

Preparation and Dosing Schedule

	Extra-Small Dog	Small Dog	Medium Dog	Large Dog	Extra-Large Dog
Tincture	1–2 drops	2–4 drops	4–8 drops	8–12 drops	10–16 drops
Glycerite	4 drops	8 drops	16 drops	24 drops	30–48 drops
Infusion	¼ teaspoon	½ teaspoon	1–2 teaspoons	1–2 tablespoons	3–6 tablespoons
Dried herb	50 mg per 25 pounds of your dog's body weight				

Infusion vs. dried herb: I don't recommend using the dried herb often. Chickweed is better used as an infusion, which is nutritive.

Potential Concerns
Herb-drug interactions: none known
Cautions: Avoid in dogs with cold energetics.

⚔ Cleavers (*Galium aparine*)
Family: Rubiaceae
Energetics: cool, damp, moisturizing
Energetic patterns indicating its use: dryness and dampness, excessive heat, tension (short-term)
Part used: flower and leaf before the plant has gone to seed
Long-term use: yes, in small amounts
Actions: adaptogen, alterative, anti-inflammatory, astringent, diuretic, laxative, lymphatic, vulnerary
Constituents: anthraquinones, asperuloside, caffeic acid, chlorophyll, citric acid, coumarins, flavonoids, gallotannin, glycosides, iridoids, polyphenols, quercetin, rutin, saponins, silicic acid, tannins
Nutrients: calcium, magnesium, potassium, vitamin (B₅, B₆, C)
Cofactors: bladder stones or gravel, calcifications, cancer, constipation, cystitis, decreased urination, doesn't want to be touched, ear infections, excessive uric acid from kidneys, excessive scratching, excitement, fibrous tissue, grief, hot spots, inflammation of the urinary tract, itchiness and scratching, lipomas, lymphatic stagnation, mammary cysts, neurological disorders, obesity, painful urination with crying out, prostate cancer, skin eruptions, swollen glands, warts, weakness in the pelvis

Flower essence: supports attachment and bonding; appropriate for dogs that have a hard time bonding with other dogs or a new family or for rescue dogs that are new to a family

Use for cats: yes, as a glycerite

Applications

Allergies: Cleavers helps Peyer's patches in the gastrointestinal tract absorb lymph fluid and settles the nervous system inside the gut; it helps move lymph fluid through the lymphatic system, calming sensitivities and processing toxins.

Kidneys: Tonifies the entire renal system, including the bladder and urinary tract. Helps clear heat from the kidneys. Helps bring down inflammation of the entire urinary tract. Combine with gravel root for bladder gravel and stones. Combine with marshmallow root for bladder infection accompanied by straining.

Lipomas: Cleavers stimulates the circulation of fluids, both lymph and blood, relieving stagnation and helping to remove water and toxins from the body. These actions can help shrink lipomas for dogs with warm energetics, especially when combined with liver support. It combines well with violet and chickweed for this purpose.

Liver: Clears heat from the liver. Use whenever you're working with the liver for a dog with warm-to-hot energetics. Helps protect the liver from toxic overload; can be combined with milk thistle seed or dandelion root to detoxify the liver.

Lymphatic system: Heat and stagnancy can build when the lymphatic system is dry, creating a cyclical backup. Cleaver's superpower is working with your dog's internal ocean and moisturizing the tissues, preventing and relieving heat and stagnation in the lymphatic system. Use short-term for this purpose.

Skin: Helps dissolve warts. Quells itchiness and scratching. Prepare cleavers as a cold infusion and use as a rinse to dispel heat and inflammation and shrink skin malignancies, mast cell tumors, and wounds. The cold infusion also makes a good antiseptic rinse for fresh wounds.

Surgery recovery: Use cleavers after surgery to break up congestion and help move toxins out through the kidneys. It helps minimize and shrink fibrous scar tissue.

Preparation and Dosing Schedule

	Extra-Small Dog	Small Dog	Medium Dog	Large Dog	Extra-Large Dog
Tincture	1–2 drops	2–4 drops	4–6 drops	6–8 drops	8–10 drops
Tincture for acute use	4 drops	8 drops	12 drops	16 drops	20–30 drops
Tincture for lymphatic stimulation	1 drop	2 drops	3 drops	4 drops	5 drops
Glycerite	2–6 drops	4–10 drops	8–16 drops	12–24 drops	20–32 drops
Infusion	2 fluid ounces per 20 pounds of your dog's body weight				

Infusion: Prepare fresh cleavers as a cold infusion, using 2 tablespoons of the chopped fresh leaf per cup of cold water and letting it steep for 8 to 12 hours. Prepare dried cleavers as a standard hot water infusion, using 1 tablespoon of the dried herb per cup of almost-boiling water and letting it steep for 30 to 45 minutes. Cleavers is sensitive to heat, and a cold infusion is best for utilizing its water-soluble constituents.

Potential Concerns

Herb-drug interactions: lithium, blood-thinning medications

Cautions: Cleavers are diuretic; when dogs consume this herb, they will pee and drink more. Excessive handling of the fresh herb may cause skin irritation. Don't use with dogs that have high blood pressure. Don't use cleavers with dogs that have heart- or kidney-related edema or diabetes. In the long term, medium to high dosages will be drying.

⚹ Couch Grass (*Elymus repens*, syn. *Agropyron repens*)

Family: Poaceae

Energetics: cool and damp, balancing

Energetic patterns indicating its use: warmth, heat, dryness

Parts used: rhizomes or roots

Long-term use: yes, in small doses

Actions: antimicrobial, demulcent, diuretic, urinary demulcent

Constituents: agropyrene, amino acids, flavonoids, glycoside, inositol, inulin, mannitol, mucilage, saponins, triticin

Nutrients: calcium, carotene, fiber, iron, magnesium, phosphorus, vitamins (A, B$_6$, C, E, K), zinc

Cofactors: arthritis, bladder gravel, bladder infection, bladder inflammation, bronchitis, CCL tears, chronic skin conditions, chronic vomiting, constipation, eczema, enlarged prostate, eye weakness, gout, high cholesterol, hot urine, incontinence, kidney dryness, kidney stones, lymphatic stagnation, nervous system weakness, pain in the urinary system, protein in the urine, spleen weakness, ulcer, urination with crying out, UTI, weakness in the lower back, worms

Use for cats: yes

Applications

Kidneys: Helps diminish urinary fire, heal urinary tract and bladder infections, dissolve kidney stones, and clear up kidney gravel. Reduces bladder irritation and pain and helps resolve incontinence. Its high mucilage content soothes a dog's urinary passages and dissipates heat. Especially good for urination with crying out.

Preparation and Dosing Schedule

	Extra-Small Dog	Small Dog	Medium Dog	Large Dog	Extra-Large Dog
Tincture	1–2 drops	2–4 drops	4–6 drops	6–8 drops	8–10 drops
Tincture for acute use	4–6 drops	6–10 drops	10–12 drops	14–20 drops	20–25 drops
Glycerite	4 drops	8 drops	12 drops	16 drops	20 drops
Infusion	¼ teaspoon	½ teaspoon	1–2 teaspoons	1–2 tablespoons	3–6 tablespoons

Tincture: Use a tincture of the fresh rhizome of couch grass if possible.

Potential Concerns

Herb-drug interactions: prescription diuretics

Cautions: Avoid using couch grass for dogs with SIBO or cardiac edema.

🌿 Dandelion (*Taraxacum officinale*)

Family: Asteraceae

Energetics: cool and dry

Energetic patterns indicating its use: warmth, heat, dampness, relaxation

Parts used: root, flower, and leaf

Long-term use: yes

Actions: adaptogen, alterative, anticatarrhal, appetite stimulant, bitter, blood cleanser, bowel tonic, cholagogue, digestive, diuretic, laxative, tonic, trophorestorative, vulnerary

Constituents: *leaf and flower*—carotenoids, chlorophyll, coumarins, inulin, lactucopicrin, latex, lecithin, myristic acid, phenolic acids, tannins, taraxacerin, taraxacin; *root*—fructose (in spring), inulin (in fall), laevulin (in spring to early summer), lecithin, phenolic acids, taraxacoside

Nutrients: beta-carotene, calcium, choline, iron, magnesium, manganese, phosphorus, potassium, riboflavin, selenium, silicon, sodium, thiamine, vitamins (A, B1, C, D, E)

. . . .

Tip! Dandelion flowers contain approximately 7,000 IUs of vitamin A per ounce.

. . . .

Cofactors: cancer, chronic constipation, chronic skin conditions, arthritis, bile insufficiency, dampness, diabetes (under supervision of a veterinarian), edema, food allergies, gallstones, hormone-based incontinence, indigestion, itchy skin, lipomas, liver congestion and toxicity, liver weakness, poor assimilation

Flower essence: for the loyal or restless dog who is always on the job or has excessive prey drive; for senior dogs who are unaware of their body functions

Use for cats: yes

Applications

Antibiotics recovery: Add fresh or dried dandelion root, an excellent source of prebiotic inulin, to your dog's food while giving antibiotics to help feed the microbiome and protect commensal bacteria. Dandelion also supports detoxification through the liver, which can be helpful during and after antibiotics use.

Blood and lymph: The leaf helps clear the lymphatics and blood, especially when a high toxic load is associated with heat, inflammation, and lipoma formation. It contains a full spectrum of mineral salts that support blood detoxification.

Gastrointestinal system: Dandelion's bitterness stimulates digestion by increasing stomach acid and pancreatic enzyme production. It promotes bile flow, helping with the digestion of fats. Dandelion acts as a tonic for the spleen, intestines, and pancreas, thereby contributing to healthy stool formation and preventing constipation and allergies from built-up toxins. It also stimulates appetite; I find it particularly useful with geriatric dogs who have difficulty keeping up their appetites.

Heart: Dandelions are a good source of potassium, decrease heart-related edema, and decrease blood lipids (fats) such as cholesterol and triglycerides.

Kidneys: Dandelion leaf is diuretic, but unlike pharmaceutical diuretics, it doesn't deplete potassium when it stimulates kidney elimination because it is itself a good source of potassium. Dandelion is also a wonderful remedy for inflammatory UTIs and female hormone-based incontinence.

Liver: It's useful for both acute and chronic liver imbalances, helping to disperse and reduce heat. With its ability to stimulate the gallbladder and bile, it can keep fluids moving when your dog is too hot, especially in elevated temperatures.

Skin: Dandelion moves wastes through the kidney and liver, which cleanses the skin. Combine it with burdock root or yellow dock root for chronic skin issues and itchiness. Remember that liver herbs can at first cause itching as detoxification progresses. Start with a low dosage and slowly work your way up. Dandelion-infused vinegar makes a good rinse to promote balanced skin.

Preparation and Dosing Schedule

	Extra-Small Dog	Small Dog	Medium Dog	Large Dog	Extra-Large Dog
Tincture	1–2 drops	2–4 drops	4–6 drops	6–8 drops	8–12 drops
Glycerite	5 drops	10 drops	15 drops	25 drops	30–40 drops
Infusion (leaf)	¼ teaspoon	½ teaspoon	1–2 teaspoons	1–2 tablespoons	3–6 tablespoons

Preparation and Dosing Schedule (cont'd)

	Extra-Small Dog	Small Dog	Medium Dog	Large Dog	Extra-Large Dog
Decoction (root)	¼ teaspoon	½ teaspoon	1–2 teaspoons	1–2 tablespoons	3–6 tablespoons
Dried root or leaf	1/16 teaspoon	⅛ teaspoon	¼ teaspoon	½ teaspoon	¾–1 teaspoon

Potential Concerns

Herb-drug interactions: blood pressure medications, diuretics; avoid in combination with ciprofloxacin and levofloxacin

Cautions: May cause digestive upset, including diarrhea. Can cause an allergic reaction in some individuals and may lower blood pressure. If nausea occurs, decrease the dosage. Dandelion can be drying, so avoid long-term use in dogs with a dry constitution.

⚹ Echinacea (*Echinacea purpurea, E. angustifolia*)

Family: Asteracea/Compositae

Energetics: cool but balancing, dry, stimulating

Energetic patterns indicating its use: warm to hot energetics, excessive heat, cold, false heat, dampness, stagnation (can be used for both hot and cold tissue states, from lack of stimulation)

Part used: root, flower, and leaf

Long-term use: no; limit to 6 weeks, then take a 3-week break

Actions: alterative, analgesic, antibacterial, anticatarrhal, antifungal (leaves and flowers), anti-inflammatory, antimicrobial, antiseptic, antiviral, appetite stimulant, diaphoretic, immune stimulant (mostly the root), lymphatic

Constituents: alkylamides, arabinogalactan, cynarin, chicoric acid, dichroic acid (*E. purpurea* only), echinacin (*E. angustifolia* only), flavonoids, heteroxylans, inulin, polysaccharides, volatile oils

Nutrients: chromium, iron, magnesium, manganese, niacin, riboflavin, potassium, selenium, silicon, vitamins C and E, zinc

Cofactors: bacterial overgrowth, candida, CCL tears, chronic skin conditions, chronic UTIs, deep cold energetics, dull eyes, ear infections, environmental allergies, excessive heat, grief, high histamine levels, hot spots, infection, kidney weakness, leaky gut, lethargy, lipomas, low immune function, reactivity, sepsis, snakebites, spider bites, stagnant lymphatics, stings, stomatitis, ulcers, warts, weak connective tissue, yeast

Flower essence: boosts the immune and nervous systems; for recovery, stagnation, transitions

Use for cats: yes

Applications

Echinacea, like burdock root, is a blood purifier and works on the entire dog-as-ecosystem. Working through the channels of elimination, it helps clean the lymph, blood, and interstitial fluid. Though it shouldn't be used for long periods of time, it's an herbal alterative.

Kidneys: Echinacea has an influence on kidney function through its support for elimination. Stimulating and toxin clearing, it helps move metabolic wastes and improves the eliminative functions of the interstitial fluid, lymphatic system, gut, kidneys, and entire liver and skin system

Liver: Echinacea provides fast-acting cellular support, clearing away metabolic wastes and supporting systemic organ function, in turn, taking pressure off the liver.

Lymphatic system: Helps move lymph fluid and supports lymph node function.

Respiratory system: Helps stimulate the immune system and reduces inflammation in the upper respiratory system. Usually used as part of a formula or protocol for serious lung conditions like pneumonia.

Skin: Anti-inflammatory, antioxidant, and antimicrobial, echinacea can be used internally and externally to help support a dog's skin. In fact, most herbs that support the liver (as echinacea does) support the skin. Echinacea decreases free radical production by reducing oxidation, which helps prevent early aging. It also helps support your dog's production of natural skin oil.

Yeast: Naturally antifungal, echinacea can help control candida when used as a part of a comprehensive protocol for candida overgrowth. Be sure to cycle it, working it in and out of your dog's regimen.

Preparation and Dosing Schedule

	Extra-Small Dog	Small Dog	Medium Dog	Large Dog	Extra-Large Dog
Tincture	1–2 drops	2–4 drops	4–6 drops	6–8 drops	10–12 drops
Tincture for acute use	4 drops	8 drops	10–12 drops	12–16 drops	16–25 drops
Glycerite	2–4 drops	16 drops	20 drops	25 drops	30 drops

Glycerin extract: Echinacea's constituents do not extract well in glycerin. Make sure any "glycerite" of echinacea was first extracted in alcohol and then preserved in glycerin.

Potential Concerns

Herb-drug interactions: corticosteroids, cyclosporine

Cautions: Can have gastrointestinal side effects. May cause a reaction in dogs allergic to other members of the Asteraceae family. Don't use in large doses except for acute situations in which it is well indicated. Use with caution for dogs with anemia or general weakness. Avoid for dogs with lupus. Avoid using the root with dogs who have autoimmune conditions or low white blood cell counts.

⚔ Elecampane (*Inula helenium*)

Family: Asteraceae

Energetics: warm and dry

Energetic patterns indicating its use: coolness, cold, dampness, dryness, relaxation

Part used: root

Long-term use: yes

Actions: antibacterial, antiseptic, astringent, expectorant

Constituents: bitter principles, helenalin, helenin, inulin, phytosterols, polyacetylenes, polysaccharides, triterpenes, volatile oils

Nutrients: calcium, chromium, fiber, iron, magnesium, manganese, niacin, phosphorus, potassium, riboflavin, selenium, silicon, vitamins A and C

Cofactors: anal gland congestion, asthma, bacterial infections, bronchitis, cataracts, chronic lung conditions, crusty skin, deficiency, dental problems (loose teeth, tooth decay), dry skin, fever, high histamine levels, kennel cough, leaky gut, lethargy, loss of appetite, mast cell tumors, pneumonia, poor absorption, stagnant fluids, surgery recovery, thick mucus, worms

Flower essence: brings sunshine and creates harmony; helps establish the self when it has been lost; good for rescue, trauma, abuse, and PTSD

Use for cats: yes

Applications

Antibiotics recovery: Due to its positive effects on the liver and digestive system, in addition to its prebiotic contributions, elecampane is excellent for facilitating recovery from antibiotics when used for a period of 6 to 8 weeks.

Digestive system: Provides prebiotics and thins fluids, making it good for leaky gut, especially when it is accompanied by poor appetite. Influences the liver and gallbladder, helping stimulate bile flow due to its bitterness.

Lungs: Helps clear thick mucus from the respiratory system. Its astringent qualities help dry up wet conditions, stagnant secretions, and fluid infections. It soothes bronchial linings and helps relieve congestion. Elecampane helps quell coughing through its relaxation of smooth muscle tissue.

Preparation and Dosing Schedule

	Extra-Small Dog	Small Dog	Medium Dog	Large Dog	Extra-Large Dog
Tincture	1 drop	4 drops	6 drops	8 drops	10–12 drops
Tincture for acute use	2–4 drops	8 drops	12 drops	16 drops	20–24 drops
Decoction	¼ teaspoon	½ teaspoon	1–2 teaspoons	1–2 tablespoons	3–6 tablespoons

Potential Concerns

Herb-drug interactions: none known

Cautions: Avoid in cases of SIBO. May cause mild reactions in dogs sensitive to other members of the Asteraceae family. Avoid in dogs with low blood sugar and hypertension.

✺ Fennel (*Foeniculum vulgare*)

Family: Apiaceae

Energetics: slightly warm, dry

Energetic patterns indicating its use: coolness, warmth, dampness

Part used: seed

Long-term use: yes, but not usually needed

Actions: antacid, antiemetic, anti-inflammatory, antispasmodic, appetite stimulant, carminative, digestive, diuretic, expectorant, parasiticide

Constituents: alpha-pinene, apigenin, beta-myrcene, beta-pinene, coumarins, flavonoids, kaempferol glycosides, quercetin, rosmarinic acid, rutin

Nutrients: calcium, copper, fiber, iron, manganese, niacin, phosphorus, potassium, vitamins A and C, zinc

Cofactors: conjunctivitis, constipation, dementia, excessive gas/farting, high histamine levels, IBS, inability to keep water down, kidney stones, nausea, poor appetite, vomiting water

Flower essence: for dogs with parasites, dementia, or (when mixed with fireweed flower essence) chronic disease

Use for cats: yes

Applications

Digestive system: Fennel's downward-moving energy makes it a good remedy for nausea and gas. It helps relax a dog's stomach, increases appetite, and improves slow digestion. Fennel works with the entire digestive and liver system, including the gallbladder, liver, and spleen. I like to make an infusion with 1 teaspoon of ground fennel seed at the first sign of nausea and have it on standby. Fennel and ginger are classic herbs for digestive upset, but ginger is hot and fennel is much cooler (on the heat spectrum). Since many dogs are prone to excessive heat, I tend to recommend fennel for nausea and vomiting more than I would ginger. It's indicated when dogs can't keep water down and obstruction has been ruled out.

Preparation and Dosing Schedule

	Extra-Small Dog	Small Dog	Medium Dog	Large Dog	Extra-Large Dog
Tincture	1 drop	2 drops	3 drops	4 drops	5 drops
Glycerite	2 drops	4 drops	6 drops	8 drops	10 drops

Preparation and Dosing Schedule (cont'd)

	Extra-Small Dog	Small Dog	Medium Dog	Large Dog	Extra-Large Dog
Decoction	¼ teaspoon	½ teaspoon	I teaspoon	I tablespoon	2 tablespoons
Dried ground seed	1/16 teaspoon	⅛ teaspoon	¼ teaspoon	½ teaspoon	I teaspoon

Potential Concerns

Herb-drug interactions: none known

Cautions: Avoid using large doses. Can cause reactions of the skin and respiratory tract. Can raise estrogen (estragole) levels. Avoid in cases of active pancreatitis as it can stimulate pancreatic secretions.

🌿 Ginger (*Zingiber officinale*)

Family: Orchidaceae

Energetics: warm to hot

Energetic patterns indicating its use: coolness, cold, deep cold, dampness; for cool dogs, ginger can be used to heat up more cooling formulas for better tolerance

Part used: root

Long-term use: yes

Actions: alterative, analgesic, antibacterial, anticatarrhal, antiemetic, antimicrobial, antiviral, appetite stimulant, bitter, carminative, diaphoretic, expectorant, immune modulator, stimulant

Constituents: bisabolene, gingerols, shogaols (dried root), volatile oil, zingiberene

Nutrients: aluminum, calcium, chromium, cobalt, fiber, iron, magnesium, manganese, niacin, phosphorus, protein, riboflavin, selenium, sodium, thiamine, vitamins (A, B-complex, C)

Cofactors: allergies, arthritis, aversion to cold, cool to cold energetics, coughing, diarrhea, digestive insufficiency, excessive saliva, heart weakness, high levels of heavy metals, high toxic load, high histamine levels, inflammation, leaky gut, lipomas, low circulation, lung weakness, lymph stagnation, nausea, obesity, poor circulation, food sensitivities, shivering, slow digestion, stiff joints, ulcers, vaccines, vomiting

Use for cats: yes

Applications

Gastrointestinal system: Fresh ginger is a good source of enzymes and is a wonderful digestive tonic for cold dogs that need warming from the core. Prepare it as an infusion and dilute it 1:1 with water. Powdered dried ginger can relieve motion sickness and nausea for dogs; use it in capsule form and administer 30 minutes prior to a car ride. Use only for dogs who are cool to cold. A glycerite of ginger might also be helpful for this purpose. For general vomiting: prepare an infusion using 1/4 inch of the root, shredded, and steeping it in almost boiling water for 5–10 minutes. Use ginger for cool to cold dogs with excessive saliva.

Heart: Helps support circulation and is a strong anti-inflammatory. It helps lower blood lipids (like cholesterol) and blood pressure and supports a healthy weight.

Kidneys: Improves circulation and blood flow to the kidneys, which improves systemic health, including the liver-kidney connection, as it also supports the liver. It helps lower creatine levels and can be a good addition to kidney disease support protocols. Healthy kidneys need minerals to function properly. Ginger provides ample warmth and minerals to kidney tissues, which brings down inflammation and stabilizes filtration. This helps prevent UTIs and decrease bladder inflammation.

Liver: A powerful antioxidant, ginger helps reduce free radical production and oxidation rates. This improves liver function and elimination.

Lungs: Decreases inflammation and opens the bronchial passageways. Helps the body thin, break down, and expel mucus from the lungs.

Lymphatic system: Stimulates lymph circulation and opens the channels of elimination for systemic filtration.

Yeast: Can help control yeast overgrowth in the gastrointestinal tract through its antifungal and pungent properties.

. . . .

Tip! You can combine ginger with cooling herbs to warm them up, if needed. (But ear-test ginger for your dog first; see page 150.)

. . . .

Preparation and Dosing Schedule

	Extra-Small Dog	Small Dog	Medium Dog	Large Dog	Extra-Large Dog
Infusion	⅛ teaspoon	¼ teaspoon	1 teaspoon	1 tablespoon	2 tablespoons
Dried root	1/16 teaspoon	⅛ teaspoon	¼ teaspoon	½ teaspoon	¾ teaspoon

Ginger is best as an infusion rather than a tincture, which would compound its heat.

Potential Concerns

Herb-drug interactions: blood-thinning medications, aspirin (and willow, the original source of aspirin)

Cautions: Avoid in cases of ulcers, bleeding, and high fever. Avoid in dogs with gallstones. Don't apply to open wounds or inflamed skin.

🌿 Goldenrod (*Solidago* spp.)

Family: Asteraceae

Energetics: warm and dry

Energetic patterns indicating its use: coolness, cold, deep cold, dampness

Parts used: flower and leaf

Long-term use: no, and rarely needed

Actions: anticatarrhal, antifungal (mild), anti-inflammatory, antimicrobial, antioxidant, antiseptic, astringent, carminative, diuretic, vulnerary

Constituents: amino acids, antioxidants, astragalin, carotenoids, flavonoids, glycosides, hyperoside, quercetin, rutin, saponins, tannins, volatile oils

Nutrients: vitamin C

Cofactors: allergies, bladder infection, bloodshot eyes, cool to deep cold energetics, crusty skin, dark urine, dryness, food sensitivities, hot spots, kidney weakness, musculoskeletal weakness, prostate weakness, slow digestion, undigested food in the stool, weakness in the back end

Flower essence: for kidney weakness, shyness in groups, sixth chakra work, or recovery after a long illness or rescue situation

Use for cats: yes

Applications

Kidneys: Has an affinity for the kidneys and the digestive system, with a concentration on the lower part of the dog. Addresses chronic weakness in the kidneys at the beginning stages of disease. Indicated for dogs with crusty skin, weakness in the back and hind legs, allergies, and chronic bladder infections. Goldenrod is a restorative herb that tones and balances the kidneys and entire kidney (renal) system. Even though it has warmth, it is wonderful for dryness in the kidneys.

Preparation and Dosing Schedule

	Extra-Small Dog	Small Dog	Medium Dog	Large Dog	Extra-Large Dog
Tincture	1 drop	2–3 drops	4–6 drops	6–8 drops	8–10 drops
Tincture for acute use	3 drops	9 drops	18 drops	24 drops	30 drops
Glycerite	3 drops	6 drops	12 drops	16–20 drops	20–30 drops
Infusion	1 teaspoon per 10 pounds of your dog's body weight				

Infusion: Let goldenrod steep in hot water for 45 minutes to an hour.

Potential Concerns

Herb-drug interactions: none known

Cautions: Avoid in late-stage kidney disease or failure. Make sure your dog is getting enough hydration when using goldenrod. May cause a reaction in dogs allergic to other members of the Asteraceae family. Avoid in cases of edema.

⚰ Goldenseal (*Hydrastis canadensis*)

Family: Ranunculaceae

Energetics: neutral to cool, dry

Energetic patterns indicating its use: relaxation

Part used: root

Long-term use: no, except under the supervision of a holistic vet or herbalist; limit to 7 days, then take a 10-day break

Actions: anticatarrhal, anti-inflammatory, antimicrobial, antiparasitic, antiseptic, antiviral, alterative, astringent, bitter, hemostatic, laxative, vulnerary

Constituents: alkaloids (phthalide isoquinoline), berberastine, berberine, canadine, chlorogenic acid, hydrastine, isoquinoline, phenolic acids, resin

Nutrients: iron, manganese, selenium, silicon, vitamins A and C, zinc

Cofactors: arthritis, bacterial overgrowth, biofilm in the gut, bloody diarrhea, candida overgrowth, cat turd eating, dental problems (bleeding gums, cavities, loose teeth, periodontitis), CCL tears, ear infections, esophagitis, giardia, hot spots, Lyme or other tick-born disease, parasites, poor appetite, stomatitis

Use for cats: yes, with supervision from a holistic vet or herbalist

Applications

Immune support: Goldenseal helps increase white blood cells, strengthen the immune system, and fight bacteria overgrowth. It offer systemic immune support but has an affinity for the lungs and can help resolve coughs.

Kidneys: High in berberine, goldenseal can help with UTIs.

Yeast: Goldenseal is a strong antimicrobial and can help rebalance candida populations. I recommend using it with *Saccharomyces boulardii* and a soil-based probiotic.

Preparation and Dosing Schedule

	Extra-Small Dog	Small Dog	Medium Dog	Large Dog	Extra-Large Dog
Tincture for acute use	1 drop	2–3 drops	4–6 drops	6–8 drops	8–10 drops
Glycerite for acute use	3 drops	6 drops	12 drops	16 drops	20 drops
Decoction	¼ teaspoon	½ teaspoon	1 teaspoon	2 teaspoons	1 tablespoon

Potential Concerns

Herb-drug interactions: has been known to interfere with the liver's P450 detoxification pathway; use with care in conjunction with any pharmaceutical medications

Cautions: May cause excessive salivation, especially in cats. Don't use for more than a week. Do *not* use with puppies. Do *not* use excessive dosing. Can cause diarrhea, dizziness, low blood sugar, nausea, and vomiting. Don't use externally on a wound or hot spot with infection or pus. Avoid in cases of liver disease or high liver enzymes. Can cause excessive bile production by overstimulating the liver.

Note: Goldenseal is endangered; be sure to obtain it only from ethical suppliers.

⚘ Gotu Kola (*Centella asiatica*)

Family: Apiaceae

Energetics: cool, slightly dry

Energetic patterns indicating its use: warmth, heat, excessive heat, dampness, relaxation

Part used: leaf

Long-term use: yes

Actions: alterative, antioxidant, astringent, trophorestorative

Constituents: alkaloids, asiatic acid, asiaticoside, ester glycosides, fatty acids, flavonoids, madecassoside, phenols, phytosterols, resins, tannins, triterpenes, triterpenoid saponins, sterols, volatile oils

Nutrients: calcium, iron, magnesium, manganese, phosphorus, selenium, silicon, sodium, vitamins (A, C, B), zinc

Cofactors: acid reflux, adrenal weakness, anal gland conditions, anxiety, arthritis, CCL tears, chronic digestive conditions, cognitive decline, connective tissue weakness, dementia, diarrhea, edema, fever, heart weakness, hernia, high blood pressure, high cholesterol, high toxic load, hypothyroid, leaky gut, nervousness, obesity, skin inflammation, stagnancy, stress, ulcers, weakness

Use for cats: yes

Applications

Gastrointestinal system: Supports the digestive system by clearing liver heat and bringing down excessive oxidation. Helps with stress and anxiety through your dog's gut-based nervous system. This is especially helpful for dogs with chronic digestive insufficiency, which can leave them worn out. It strengthens connective tissues in the gut, making it an effective supportive herb for leaky gut.

Heart: Helps with venous flexibility and strength and increases circulation throughout the dog-as-ecosystem. Helps protect nerve tissue inside the heart, which is important because the heart contains a high level of neurons and its own mini nervous system, referred to as the heart brain because it signals the brain more than the brain signals the heart. Together with the vagus nerve, your dog's heart continually interacts with the brain, including the amygdala, cerebral cortex, and hypothalamus. Heart health is brain health. Everything is connected.

Musculoskeletal system: Supports connective tissues, like tendons and ligaments.

Skin: Supports collagen production and increases circulation to the skin. Can reduce inflammation in the skin when used consistently.

Preparation and Dosing Schedule

	Extra-Small Dog	Small Dog	Medium Dog	Large Dog	Extra-Large Dog
Tincture	1–3 drops	2–5 drops	4–8 drops	6–12 drops	10–16 drops
Infusion	¼ teaspoon	½ teaspoon	1–2 teaspoons	1–2 tablespoons	3–6 tablespoons

Potential Concerns

Herb-drug interactions: antihypertensive drugs, cholesterol drugs, NSAIDs

Cautions: Don't use in large doses long-term. Can have a sedating effect, especially in tincture form. Avoid in cases of hypoglycemia.

Note: Gotu kola is endangered in the wild; look for cultivated sources of this herb.

🌿 Gravel Root (*Eupatorium purpureum*)

Family: Asteraceae

Energetics: neutral, dry

Part used: root

Long-term use: no

Actions: anti-inflammatory, antimicrobial, astringent, diaphoretic, diuretic

Constituents: cistifolin, euparin, euparone, eupurpurin, flavonoids, pyrrolizidine alkaloids, resins, silica, volatile oils

Nutrients: calcium, iron, potassium, sodium

Cofactors: arthritis, bladder gravel and stones, bloody urine, CCL tears, cloudy urine, dampness, difficulty with urination, hip dysplasia, infections in the lower half of the body, infection in the paws, kidney stones, lower back weakness, lung weakness, poor circulation, pus in the vagina or penis, pyometra, urination with crying out, UTIs, weak connective tissues

Flower essence: for loner dogs that don't connect with others, have separation anxiety, and have destructive chewing when left alone

Use for cats: yes

Applications

Kidneys: Gravel root is one of my favorite herbal remedies for kidney issues, especially for cooler dogs. However, I also use it in warmer dogs, balancing it with a few cooling herbs. Gravel root helps dissolve solids in the body, including bladder stones, bladder gravel, kidney stones, and arthritic deposits related to the kidneys. I like to combine it with marshmallow root (which is cooling) for warm dogs that need to pass stones through the kidneys or bladder.

Preparation and Dosing Schedule

	Extra-Small Dog	Small Dog	Medium Dog	Large Dog	Extra-Large Dog
Tincture for acute use	1 drop	2 drops	3 drops	4 drops	5 drops
Glycerite for acute use	3 drops	6 drops	9 drops	12 drops	15 drops
Decoction	½ teaspoon	1 teaspoon	2 teaspoons	1 tablespoon	2 tablespoons

Glycerin extract: Gravel root's constituents do not extract well in glycerin. Make sure any "glycerite" of gravel root was first extracted in alcohol and then preserved in glycerin.

Potential Concerns

Herb-drug interactions: none known

Cautions: Use in small amounts; don't use large dosages for more than a few days. Avoid in cases of kidney disease and cardiac-related edema.

⚞ Hawthorn (*Crataegus* spp.)

Family: Rosacea

Energetics: *berry*—slightly warm, slightly dry; *leaf and flower*—cool and dry

Energetic patterns indicating its use: warm to hot energetics, dampness, relaxation

Part used: dried berry, leaf, and flower

Long-term use: yes

Actions: antispasmodic, appetite stimulant, carminative, diuretic, stimulant, trophorestorative, vasodilator

Constituents: *berry*—acetylcholine, aesculin, ascorbic acid, botulin, cardiotonic amines, caffeic acid, choline, chlorogenic acid, citric acid, daucosterol, flavonoids, hyperin, hyperoside, oxalic acid, palmitic acid, pectin, polymeric procyanidin, quercetin, triterpene acid, tyramine; *leaf and flower*—acetylcholine, adenine, ancatolic acid, amines, amygdalin, asorbic acid, caffeic acid, choline, chlorogenic acid, flavonoids, fructose, hyperin, hyperoside, luteolin, neotegolic acid, oleanolic acid, oligomeric proanthocyanidins, pectin, quercetin, rutin, triterpenes, tyramine, ursolic acid

Nutrients: aluminum, calcium, chromium, cobalt, iron, magnesium, manganese, niacin, phosphorus, potassium, selenium, silicon, vitamins (A, B-complex, C), zinc

Cofactors: agitation, anxiety, autoimmune diseases, difficulty digesting protein, difficulty processing fats, food allergies, grief, heart murmur, heat excitation, heat in the cardiovascular system, high cholesterol, high triglycerides, history of pancreatitis, inability to pay attention, irregular heart rhythm, low or high blood pressure, nervousness, nervous stomach, poor appetite with panting, restlessness, stagnant lymphatics, undigested food in the stool

Flower essence: for heart weakness, heart chakra work, grief, extreme behavior, fearfulness

Use for cats: yes

Applications

Anxiety: Calms sympathetic excess and brings about parasympathetic activity.

Heart: Cools the heart and cardiac system. The berry is a good source of heart-healthy antioxidants and rutin (flavonoid). When there is congestion and heat in the cardiac center, dogs can be a bit anxious, agitated, or restless, usually accompanied by excess panting. Hawthorn is a slow-and-steady-wins-the-race tonic herb. When oxidation increases, hawthorn helps fight free radicals in the body. It clears weakness and congestion in the cardiac system. It strengthens the entire vasculature, including tissues, veins, capillaries, and heart muscle.

Lymphatic system: Hawthorn supports the lymphatic system by aiding in the digestion of fats. It also clears lymphatic heat (and does the same for respiratory heat).

Preparation and Dosing Schedule

	Extra-Small Dog	Small Dog	Medium Dog	Large Dog	Extra-Large Dog
Tincture	1 drop	2–3 drops	3–4 drops	4–5 drops	5–6 drops
Glycerite	2 drops	6 drops	8 drops	10 drops	12 drops
Decoction (dried berry)	1 tablespoon	2 tablespoons	3 tablespoons	4 tablespoons	5 tablespoons
Dried berry, leaf, and flower	1/16 teaspoon	1/4 teaspoon	1/2 teaspoon	1 teaspoon	2 teaspoons

Potential Concerns

Herb-drug interactions: Avoid using hawthorn in conjunction with digoxin; be careful with other heart medications.

Cautions: Avoid for dogs with ulcers. Do not use for acute heart conditions.

🌿 Juniper Berry (*Juniperus communis*)

Family: Cupressaceae

Energetics: warm and dry

Energetic patterns indicating its use: coolness, cold, dampness

Part used: berry

Long-term use: no

Actions: analgesic, antibacterial, antifungal, antioxidant, antiseptic, antispasmodic, bactericidal, carminative, diaphoretic, disinfectant, diuretic, expectorant

Constituents: alpha-eudesmol, alpha-pinene, beta-pinene, borneol, cadinene, camphor, camphene, caryophyllene, germacrene, limonene, myrcene, pectin, resin, sabinene, tannins, terpinen-4-ol, volatile oil

Nutrients: calcium, iron, magnesium, manganese, niacin, phosphorus, potassium, silicon, sulfur, vitamins A and C

Cofactors: bile insufficiency, bladder infection, dark-colored urine, digestive insufficiency, fungal infection, heart weakness, high blood pressure, lethargy, lower back pain, not wanting to be touched on the abdomen, poor appetite, poor assimilation, skin rash, skin tags, stomatitis, UTI, warts, worms

Use for cats: yes

Applications

Kidneys: Juniper berries are female seeds but look like little blueberries. Their polyphenolic bioflavonoids reduce oxidative stress, which helps reduce the load of the liver. This, in turn, assists the kidneys. Juniper berries also help increase glutathione and superoxide dismutase levels. In the urinary tract, the berries help increase urine flow, which cleans a dog's kidneys, removes wastes, flushes bacteria out of the bladder and urinary tract, and prevents UTIs.

Preparation and Dosing Schedule

	Extra-Small Dog	Small Dog	Medium Dog	Large Dog	Extra-Large Dog
Tincture for acute use	1 drop	2–3 drops	3–6 drops	6–9 drops	8–12 drops
Decoction for acute use	⅛ teaspoon	½ teaspoon	1–2 teaspoons	1–1½ tablespoons	3–6 tablespoons

Potential Concerns

Herb-drug interactions: lithium

Cautions: High doses can cause kidney damage. Avoid in cases of kidney disease, kidney stones, and heart-related edema. Never use long-term or in large dosages.

🙠 Lemon Balm (*Melissa officinalis*)

Family: Lamiaceae

Energetics: cool and dry

Energetic patterns indicating its use: warm to hot energetics, excessive heat, dampness, tension

Part used: leaf

Long-term use: yes

Actions: anticatarrhal, antiemetic, antihistamine, antimicrobial, antispasmodic, antiviral, appetite stimulant, cardioprotective, carminative, diaphoretic, nervine, relaxant, sedative, trophorestorative

Constituents: bioflavonoids, caryophyllene oxide, caffeic acid, citral, citronellal, flavonoids, linalool, phenolic acids, polyphenolics, pomolic acid, rosmarinic acid, tannins, terpenes, triterpenic acids, ursolic acid, volatile oil

Nutrients: boron, calcium, chromium, copper, iron, magnesium, manganese, molybdenum, potassium, protein, selenium, thiamine, vitamin C

Cofactors: acid reflux, anxiety, bladder infections, bulging eyes, candida overgrowth, cognitive decline, congested anal glands, diarrhea, digestive upset, ear infections, excessive gas, food sensitivities, heart weakness, heat in the cardiovascular system, high blood pressure, high histamine levels, hot spot, hyperadrenalism, hyperthyroidism, low vagal tone, lymphatic stagnation, nausea, nervous pooping, hyperexcited nervous system, poor appetite, restlessness, seizures, SIBO, stomach cramping, stress, stress pooping, sympathetic excess, thinness with heat, underweight, UTI

Flower essence: for hyperthyroidism, depletion, leathery skin, long bouts of chronic disease, dissociation, dementia, aging difficulties, PTSD

Use for cats: yes

Applications

Lemon balm helps decrease thyroid function making it a superlative remedy for hyperthyroidism when taken long-term.

Gastrointestinal system: As a carminative, lemon balm relieves slow digestion, spasm, and nervous stomach. It helps normalize histamine levels, vagal tone, and overall digestion and minimize acid reflux by calming nerve receptors in a dog's gut, thereby decreasing reactivity.

Kidneys: Anti-inflammatory and antioxidant, lemon balm helps detoxify the entire renal system, including the bladder. It reduces bladder inflammation and helps decrease the incidence of UTIs.

Nervous system: Calms the entire nervous system, including the nerves that govern the cardiac system, helping with anxiety, restlessness, and cognitive decline. It's great for dogs with hair-trigger aggressive reactivity and sympathetic excess, especially in working dogs. Use as an infusion for this purpose.

Preparation and Dosing Schedule

	Extra-Small Dog	Small Dog	Medium Dog	Large Dog	Extra-Large Dog
Tincture	1 drop	2 drops	4 drops	6 drops	10 drops
Glycerite	3 drops	6 drops	12 drops	18 drops	30 drops
Infusion	⅛ cup	¼ cup	½ cup	¾–1 cup	1½–2 cups
Dried herb	1/16 teaspoon	¼ teaspoon	½ teaspoon	1 teaspoon	2 teaspoons

Potential Concerns

Herb-drug interactions: barbiturates, benzodiazepines, synthetic thyroid hormones, sedatives

Cautions: Use caution with hypothyroidism.

⚴ Licorice (*Glycyrrhiza glabra*)

Family: Leguminosae

Energetics: neutral and damp

Energetic patterns indicating its use: cool to warm to hot energetics, dryness, tension

Part used: root

Long-term use: choose deglycyrrhizinated licorice root for long-term use; limit regular licorice to 2 weeks, then take a 3-week break. Medical herbalist Paul Bergner warns against its negative effect on the adrenal glands with continued use.

Actions: adaptogen, anticatarrhal, anti-inflammatory, antimicrobial, antioxidant, antiseptic, antiviral, appetite stimulant, demulcent, expectorant, hepatoprotective, immune modulator, immune stimulant, tonic, trophorestorative

Constituents: chalcones, coumarins, flavonoids, formononetin, glabridin, glycyrrhizin, hispaglabridin A and B, isoflavones, licoricidin, licoflavono, phytosterols, polysaccharides, triterpenoid saponins

Nutrients: biotin, calcium, iron, lecithin, magnesium, manganese, pantothenic acid, potassium, selenium, silicon, sodium, vitamins (A, B-complex, C), zinc

Cofactors: acid reflux, arthritis, bronchitis, burping, constipation, cough, digestive dryness, digestive heat, dry constitution, dry cough, flea allergy, inflammation, itchiness, kennel cough, leaky gut, liver disease, lung inflammation, nervous system weakness, pain, poor assimilation, skin disorders, ulcers, upper respiratory infection

Use for cats: yes

Applications

You'll see licorice in many formulas; it helps bring balance since it is energetically neutral.

Gastrointestinal system: Licorice is excellent for digestive dryness because it has an influence on the gut lining, providing moisture and nutrition and expelling heat. Its anti-inflammatory action in the gut helps decrease immune hypersensitivity and reactivity, which can combat food sensitivities, and acid reflux, and help the gut and its microbiome recover from damage caused by pharmaceuticals, including antibiotics. All these actions contribute toward resolution of leaky gut.

Kidneys: It influences the urinary tract, kidneys, and adrenal glands. As an anti-inflammatory and demulcent, it has an affinity for the bladder, decreasing inflammation and irritation, which helps recovery from UTIs and incontinence.

Lungs: Moisturizes delicate lung tissue and mucosa, counteracting dryness and reducing inflammation.

. . . .

Tip! Deglycyrrhizinated licorice can be added to drying formulas for balance.

. . . .

Preparation and Dosing Schedule

	Extra-Small Dog	Small Dog	Medium Dog	Large Dog	Extra-Large Dog
Tincture	1 drop	2 drops	3 drops	4 drops	5 drops

Preparation and Dosing Schedule (cont'd)

	Extra-Small Dog	Small Dog	Medium Dog	Large Dog	Extra-Large Dog
Glycerite	3 drops	6 drops	9 drops	12 drops	15 drops
Decoction	1 teaspoon	2 teaspoons	2–3 teaspoons	¼ cup	½ cup
Dried powdered herb	1/16 teaspoon	⅛ teaspoon	¼ teaspoon	¾ teaspoon	1 teaspoon

Recommended use: The preferred method of use for dogs is tinctures and glycerites. A diluted decoction can be used to soothe the gut.

Potential Concerns

Herb-drug interactions: prescription diuretics

Cautions: Use in moderation only. If diarrhea occurs, cut back on the dosage. If you are a novice herbalist, use only the deglycyrrhizinated form. Avoid using the non-deglycyrrhizinated form in dogs with heart disease, congestive heart failure, hypertension, diabetes, liver disease, or kidney disease. To use licorice for periods longer than 2 weeks, consult an herbalist or holistic vet; if using licorice for more than 6 weeks, use the deglycyrrhizinated form.

⚘ Marshmallow (*Althaea officinalis*)

Family: Malvaceae

Energetics: cool and damp

Energetic patterns indicating its use: warm to hot energetics, dryness, tension

Part used: root

Long-term use: yes

Actions: antacid, antioxidant, antispasmodic, demulcent, diuretic, emollient, expectorant, laxative, nutritive, relaxant, tonic, vulnerary

Constituents: antioxidants, arabinans, arabinogalactans, asparagine, flavonoids, galacturonorhamnans, mucilage, pectin, phenolic acids, polysaccharides, sucrose

Nutrients: calcium, iron, magnesium, niacin, phosphorus, potassium, selenium, silicon, vitamins (A, B_1, B_2, C), zinc

Cofactors: acid reflux, arthritis, blood in the stool, cancer, constipation, diarrhea, dry mouth, excessive burping, food sensitivities, gravel in the bladder, high toxic load, high urine volume, immune hyperactivity, inflamed anal glands, inflamed joints, inflamed stomach, leaky gut, low immune function, low saliva volume, low urine volume, pharmaceutical-based diarrhea, stagnant lymphatics, ulcers, urinary stones, warm paws and skin

Flower essence: for anxiety, aggression, nervousness

Use for cats: yes

Applications

Marshmallow is well indicated for heat and dryness in many areas, but especially the gastrointestinal and urinary systems. For extra-dry constitutions, combine marshmallow with deglycyrrhizinated licorice.

Gastrointestinal system: Dispels heat; is soothing and cooling for the entire system. One indication of the need to use marshmallow root is the presence of mucous-filled stools. It's my go-to remedy for constipation in dogs, as it moistens the stool body and lubricates the mucous membranes of the intestines. Marshmallow can pull heat out of the upper and lower intestines and stomach, which is balancing and thus good for both diarrhea and constipation. Because it reduces inflammation and protects and tightens gut junctions, it's indicated for use with leaky gut.

Kidneys: Can address dryness in the kidneys and bladder. Increases elimination through the kidneys. Works as a balancer, helping both dogs who urinate too much and dogs who urinate too little. Good for resolving stones and gravel, inflammation, urinary tract and bladder infections, and irritation of the mucous membranes within the urinary system. A salty diuretic, marshmallow's properties help detoxify the kidneys and cleanse the bladder.

Liver: Marshmallow is high in antioxidants, which help combat oxidation and free radicals, thus reducing the load of the liver. (It also improves health systemically and reduces the risk of cancer.) Marshmallow decreases cell adhesions, supports interstitial fluid (matrix), and promotes pathogenic cell death. It supports healthy immune function through phagocytosis, which processes and detoxifies damaged cells.

Lungs and Cough: With its anti-inflammatory, antispasmodic, and moisturizing properties marshmallow works well to relieve a dry cough and soothe irritation and dryness in the lungs. It's safe for long-term use and can add support for systemic inflammation and heat.

. . . .

Tip! An infusion of marshmallow leaf is wonderful for dried-out skin and dandruff on a dog's rump.

. . . .

Yeast: Marshmallow root is a broad-spectrum antimicrobial and can dispel yeast, including candida. Use a combination of dried marshmallow in capsules and a strong decoction of the root or infusion of the powdered root. For an external wash: rinse your dog's yeasty areas, massage infusion or decoction into skin, and let dry.

Preparation and Dosing Schedule

	Extra-Small Dog	Small Dog	Medium Dog	Large Dog	Extra-Large Dog
Glycerite	3–6 drops	6–8 drops	10–15 drops	15–25 drops	25–30 drops
Cold-water decoction	½ teaspoon	1 teaspoon	1 tablespoon	3 tablespoons	6 tablespoons
Dried powdered root	⅛ teaspoon	¼ teaspoon	½ teaspoon	1 teaspoon	1½ teaspoons

Potential Concerns

Herb-drug interactions: none known

Cautions: Take any pharmaceuticals 2 hours away from a marshmallow dose. Can lower blood sugar.

✍ Meadowsweet (*Filipendula ulmaria*)

Family: Rosaceae

Energetics: neutral to warm

Energetic patterns indicating its use: relaxation

Part used: leaf and flower

Long-term use: yes, in the small doses noted here (use large doses only under the supervision of a holistic vet or herbalist)

Actions: analgesic, antacid, antibacterial, anti-inflammatory, antiseptic, antispasmodic, astringent, cardiotonic, carminative, digestive, diuretic, stomachic, trophorestorative

Constituents: antioxidants, citric acid, coumarin, flavonoids, iridoid glycosides, methyl-salicylate, mucilage, phenol glycosides, quercetin, salicin, salicylic aldehyde, tannins, volatile oil

Nutrients: calcium, iron, magnesium, vitamin C

Cofactors: acid reflux, arthritis, bladder stones, burping, cystitis, diarrhea, edema, gastrointestinal upset, high liver load, high uric acid levels, history of chronic UTI, immune weakness, indigestion, inflammation, joint pain, leaky gut, lung phlegm, lung weakness, nausea, pain, panting, poor circulation, skin inflammation, systemic inflammation, ulcers

Flower essence: for restlessness, neediness, inability to settle, anxiety, possible pain

Use for cats: no

Applications

Arthritis and pain: A good source of salicylic acid, meadowsweet is an effective anti-inflammatory and pain reliever. Helps dogs with arthritis by relieving pressure and calcifications in the joints. Use it as a part of a dog's pain and inflammation regimen.

Gastrointestinal system: Reduces pain and inflammation in the intestinal tract and helps heal the lining of the stomach and intestines. Helps normalize the gastrointestinal tract. A natural antacid that doesn't negatively affect your dog's stomach acid levels. Helps with diarrhea through its astringency. Use it in cases of severe leaky gut where dogs have pain, inflammation, and reactivity.

Urinary system: Meadowsweet's effects extend to the urinary system. Can help remove bladder gravel and reduce pain.

Preparation and Dosing Schedule

	Extra-Small Dog	Small Dog	Medium Dog	Large Dog	Extra-Large Dog
Tincture	1–3 drop	2–5 drops	4–8 drops	6–12 drops	10–16 drops
Glycerite	6 drops	10 drops	16 drops	24 drops	32 drops
Infusion	½ teaspoon	1 teaspoon	2 teaspoons	1 tablespoon	2 tablespoons
Dried powdered herb	1/16 teaspoon	1/8 teaspoon	1/4 teaspoon	1/2 teaspoon	3/4–1 teaspoon

Potential Concerns

Herb-drug interactions: aspirin, hydrocodone, morphine, narcotics

Cautions: Don't use if your dog is allergic to aspirin, as the herb contains salicylic acid. Avoid in large doses, as it can cause nausea and vomiting.

⚹ Milk Thistle (*Silybum marianum*)

Family: Asteraceae

Energetics: neutral

Energetic patterns indicating its use: heat, dryness, dampness

Part used: seed

Long-term use: yes (but only for the seeds, not the standardized extract)

Actions: antihistamine, anti-inflammatory, antioxidant, appetite stimulant, astringent (mild), bitter, diaphoretic, digestive, diuretic, emmenagogue, hepatoprotective, tonic, trophorestorative

Constituents: amines, amino acids (arginine, cysteine, glutamic acid, glycine, isoleucine, leucine, methionine, phenylalanine, proline, serine, tyrosine), betaine, bitter principles, campesterol, flavolignans, fixed oils, gamma linoleic acid, isosilybinin, lignans, mucilage, silybin, silychristin, silydianin (silymarin), sterols, tyramine

Nutrients: calcium, copper, iron, magnesium, manganese, potassium, sodium, zinc

Cofactors: agitation, aggression, anal gland issues, bladder gravel, candida "die-off" reactions, chronic diarrhea, cold paws and head, constipation, cool or warm energetics, dampness, deficiency, diarrhea from pharmaceutical use, difficulty with training (training won't "stick"), dryness, excitement (jumping out of its skin), high anxiety, high histamine levels, high liver enzymes, high use of pharmaceuticals, inflammation, leptospirosis, lipomas, nausea, nose punching, parvo, poor appetite, pushy and in-your-face behavior, use of pharmaceutical flea and tick prevention, vaccines, warts, weakness

Flower essence: releases anger and liver heat; for dogs who are easily agitated, frustrated, insecure, trying to please too much; for work with the heart chakra

Use for cats: yes

Applications

Gastrointestinal system: milk thistle seed is sweet, making it a nutritive tonic, and has an affinity for the liver system, including the gastrointestinal tract. It's moistening and soothing due to its oily nature, but also bitter, and it softens dry stool associated with low bile levels. Milk thistle is a great support for dogs taking antibiotics; it protects the complete gastrointestinal tract and system, including the liver, gallbladder, spleen, and pancreas.

Heart: Supports circulation and drainage in the cardiac system. Can be combined with hawthorn for 5 to 6 weeks in late spring and early summer to help support the heart and detoxification of the circulatory system.

Kidneys: Milk thistle is a mild kidney tonic that helps break up and remove kidney stones.

Liver: Assists the liver in breaking down metabolic wastes. Increases glutathione levels, helps cleanse the blood, reduces the body's toxic load, reduces free radicals and oxidation, and boosts circulation, including through the portal vein, helping push through stagnancy while decreasing inflammation and supporting liver function. Helps restore liver cells and reduces liver enzymes, supporting phase 1 and 2 liver detoxification. Give milk thistle seed to any dog using steroids or flea, heartworm, and tick medications.

Skin: Helps the liver detoxify, opening elimination pathways and increasing nutrient assimilation, which supports healthy skin. Can increase moisture, which can help dogs with chronic skin conditions. Be aware that milk thistle can initially increase itchiness, especially if the dosage is too high.

Vaccine recovery: A specific for vaccination. Milk thistle increases glutathione levels and supports the liver, kidneys, and pancreas. It helps the body process and metabolize pharmaceuticals through the liver while protecting it.

Yeast: Helps the body deal with the symptoms of yeast die-off and the stagnating wastes they create.

Preparation and Dosing Schedule

	Extra-Small Dog	Small Dog	Medium Dog	Large Dog	Extra-Large Dog
Tincture	1–2 drops	2–3 drops	4–6 drops	6–8 drops	8–10 drops
Tincture for acute use	1 diluted drop per 1 pound of your dog's body weight, given as needed two to five times daily				
Glycerin extract	6 drops	9 drops	18 drops	24 drops	30 drops
Infusion	½ teaspoon	1 teaspoon	2 teaspoons	1–3 tablespoons	¼ cup
Freshly ground seed	⅛ teaspoon	¼ teaspoon	½ teaspoon	1 teaspoon	2 teaspoons–1 tablespoon
Powdered seed	¼ teaspoon	½ teaspoon	1 teaspoon	2 teaspoons	1 tablespoon
Standardized extract	150 mg	250–300 mg	300–500 mg	500–800 mg	800–1,200 mg

Tincture: Give away from food.

Glycerin extracts: Milk thistle seed's constituents do not extract well in glycerin. Make sure any "glycerite" of milk thistle seed was first extracted in alcohol and then preserved in glycerin.

Infusion: Steep 1 teaspoon of lightly ground seeds in 8 ounces of almost boiling water for 30 minutes. However, water is not the best solvent for extracting milk thistle seed's constituents. The infusion will have a mild effect.

Ground or powdered seeds: Give these doses twice daily with food.

Standardized extract: Don't give standardized extract for more than 8 weeks except under supervision of your holistic vet; it has a high level of the active ingredient. This extract can be used in combination with the plain seed when you have a dog with high liver enzymes.

· ·

Tip! For liver support, give milk thistle seed in spring and fall for eight weeks in capsule, powder, or drop doses of tincture.

· ·

Potential Concerns

Herb-drug interactions: diabetic drugs, anxiety drugs, blood thinners, cholesterol drugs, statins, insulin, metronidazole (Flagyl), Denamarin

Cautions: Can cause aggression. If this happens, switch to powdered milk thistle (nonstandardized) giving one-quarter of the current dosage. If this is still too much, move to the milk thistle flower essence. When the aggression clears, you can slowly increase the dose. Milk thistle seed (nonstandardized) should not be taken for more than 8 to 12 months; the standardized extract should not be taken for more than a few months. I recommend using this herb seasonally as a preventive and when well indicated.

🌿 Milky Oats (*Avena sativa*)

Family: Poaceae

Energetics: neutral to cool and damp

Energetic patterns indicating its use: warm to hot energetics, dryness, tension

Part used: fresh "milky" seed

Long-term use: yes

Actions: adaptogen, demulcent, nervine, nervine trophorestorative, nutritive, tonic, vulnerary

Constituents: avenine, cellulose, lipids, phytosterols, proteins, saponins, silicic acid, starch, steroidal saponins, sterols, trigonelline

Nutrients: iron, manganese, phosphorus, potassium, selenium, silicon, sodium, vitamins (A, B-complex, E), zinc

Cofactors: acid reflux, aggression, anxiety, brittle nails, chronic stress, deficient constitution, dementia, dryness, excessive humping, exhaustion, fear of noises, grief, hair-trigger reactivity, heart weakness, high histamine levels, hypersensitive nervous system, hypertension, low immune function, marking or peeing in the house, low vagal tone, nervous tension, poor assimilation, PTSD, trauma, weak connective tissues, poor recovery, poor skin and coat, restlessness, sympathetic excess, ulcers

Use for cats: yes

Applications

Heart: Has an affinity for the cardiac nervous system. Reduces inflammation, decreases cardiac cytokine levels, increases arterial flexibility, and supports neurons and neural transmission from the heart to the brain.

Nervous system and anxiety: Milky oat has strong affinity to the nervous system. It's a gentle nervine that helps dogs with depleted nervous systems and chronic illness. It's good for dogs who won't stop humping or have sympathetic excess, low vagal tone, PTSD, trauma, grief, and chronic stress. Milky oats helps ease anxiety, restlessness, aggression, and fear. They are well indicated for dogs that have experienced prolonged or chronic stress and suffer from nervous system exhaustion. In his monograph on this herb, herbalist Sajah Popham writes, "Milky Oats assist in this generalized nervous system exhaustion pattern by moving through the brain and nervous system, rebuilding, restoring, and strengthening the entire system. I like to think of this plant as increasing our resilience factor, meaning that we become stronger in our nervous tone and aren't quite as easily triggered or stressed out by life circumstances." I find this to be true of its use with dogs as well— especially with those sympathetic-dominant hair-trigger dogs who react to everything.

Preparation and Dosing Schedule

	Extra-Small Dog	Small Dog	Medium Dog	Large Dog	Extra-Large Dog
Tincture (fresh milky oats)	1–3 drops	2–5 drops	4–8 drops	6–12 drops	10–20 drops
Infusion	½ teaspoon	1 teaspoon	1 tablespoon	¼ cup	½ cup

Tincture: Milky oats is a good addition to tincture formulas that contain drying herbs, as it can moisturize them; it is especially good in formulas designed to support the nervous system.
Infusion: For medicinal effect, milky oats are best used as a tincture, but for their nutritive value, they can be given as an infusion.

Potential Concerns
Herb-drug interactions: none known
Cautions: Can cause gas and bloating in some dogs, especially in large dosages.

◢ Mullein (*Verbascum thapsus*)
Family: Scrophulariaceae
Energetics: *leaf*—cool, damp, sweet; *root*—slightly warm to neutral, slightly dry; *flower*—cool to neutral

Energetic patterns indicating its use: warm to hot energetics, dryness, tension

Parts used: leaf, flower, and root

Long-term use: yes

Actions: anti-inflammatory, antispasmodic, antiviral, demulcent, expectorant, hemostatic, immune modulator, nervine relaxant, trophorestorative

Constituents: antioxidants, aucubin, flavonoids, glycosides, hesperidin, iridoid compounds, mucilage, polysaccharides, terpenoids, triterpenoid saponins, tannins, thapsic acid, verbascoside, volatile oils

Nutrients: beta-carotene, calcium, iron, magnesium, manganese, potassium, selenium, silicon, sodium, sulfur, vitamin C, zinc

Cofactors: anal gland conditions, bronchitis, candidiasis, cartilage damage, colon inflammation, cough, deficient constitution, diarrhea, dryness, fear of noises, grief, hyperadrenalism, incontinence, low immune function, lung weakness, nervousness, pain, pneumonia, spinal conditions, swollen lymph, swollen prostate, sympathetic excess, weak connective tissues, wounds, yeast overgrowth

Flower essence: for help finding inner peace, clarity, hidden potential, courage, joy; for help with training; to relieve grief, spinal conditions, trauma, hair-trigger stress

Use for cats: yes

Applications

Lungs and cough: Antispasmodic and moisturizing, mullein can help ease dry coughs and relieve spasms. It helps remove excess mucus and soothe hacking. As an infusion, mullein leaf coats tissues and decreases inflammation. It's relaxing as well as cleansing. You can use it for kennel cough and dryness, irritated respiratory conditions, and trachea inflammation.

Musculoskeletal system: Mullein root helps decongest and moisturize the spine. It's anti-inflammatory and supports a healthy nervous system. Mullein brings moisture to joints and helps balance synovial fluid.

Urinary system: Helps stop non-hormonal-related incontinence. Helps stop bladder and urinary spasms by interacting with the bladder nerve. Mullein root decreases inflammation and, combined with the leaf, brings moisture to the entire urinary tract without overdoing it due to its astringency. It can help tone leaky mucous membranes without overstimulation.

Yeast: Mullein leaf is antifungal and can be used to address yeast (candida) in the gastrointestinal tract and bladder and externally (as a wash or infused oil) on the skin.

Preparation and Dosing Schedule

	Extra-Small Dog	Small Dog	Medium Dog	Large Dog	Extra-Large Dog
Tincture (leaf)	2 drops	6 drops	8 drops	10 drops	15 drops
Tincture (root)	2 drops	4 drops	6 drops	8 drops	10 drops
Tincture (leaf) for acute use	4 drops	8 drops	10 drops	20 drops	30 drops
Glycerite	4 drops	10–12 drops	16 drops	20 drops	30 drops
Infusion	¼ teaspoon	½ teaspoon	1–2 teaspoons	1–2 tablespoons	3–6 tablespoons

Potential Concerns

Herb-drug interactions: none known

Cautions: Wear a mask and gloves when handling dried mullein leaf to prevent contact with and inhalation of its fine hairs. Strain finely when preparing the leaf as an infusion.

⚕ Nettle (*Urtica dioica*)

Family: Urticaceae

Energetics: *leaf*—cool, dry; *seed*—slightly warm, balancing; nettles can be used with most energetics because they are not too cool and their stimulating action helps with lack of function

Energetic patterns indicating its use: warmth, heat, coolness, cold, dampness, damp heat, stagnation, relaxation

Parts used: leaf and seed

Long-term use: yes, but can become drying

Actions: adaptogen, alternative, antiemetic, antihistamine, anti-inflammatory, antioxidant, diuretic, nutritive tonic, stimulant, styptic, trophorestorative, vulnerary

Constituents: 5-hydroxytryptamine, acetylcholine, amines, amino acids, ascorbic acid, carbonic acid, carotenoids, chlorophyll, choline, flavonoids, formic acid, glucoquinone, linoleic acid, lutein, lycopene, mucilage, oleic acid, omega-3 fatty acids, palmitic acid, quercetin, serotonin, saponins, stearic acid, sterols, tannins

Nutrients: *leaf*—alpha-carotene, boron, bromine, calcium, chlorine, chromium, copper, iodine, iron, magnesium, phosphorus, potassium, selenium, silica, silicon, sulfur, vitamins (A, B-complex, C, E, F, K), zinc; *seed*—beta-carotene, calcium, folic acid, iron, magnesium, manganese, phosphorus, potassium, silicon, vitamins (A, B, C, E, K)

Cofactors: adrenal gland weakness, allergies, arthritis, chronic skin conditions, crying out during urination, depleted ecosystem, diarrhea, ear infections, environmental allergies, food sensitivities, high histamine levels, hypothyroidism, inability to break down proteins, incontinence, inflamed tissues, itchiness and scratching, kidney weakness, leaky gut syndrome, musculoskeletal weakness, prolapsed anal glands, uric acid buildup, weakness in the back end, wet skin

Flower essence: for the runt of a litter (given externally), dogs who are picked on, street dogs in rescue, displaced dogs, dogs suffering from deficiency, or dogs that have just been spayed or neutered; for inability to gain weight, arthritis, allergies, immune weakness, and mast cell activation/tumors

Use for cats: yes

Applications

Anxiety: Nettle seed is an adaptogen, helping your dog deal with stress. It strengthens the adrenal glands, increases serotonin levels, and helps relieve restlessness and anxiety.

Gastrointestinal system: Helps regulate the entire gastrointestinal tract, including a dog's anal glands. Helps calm gastrointestinal overreactivity and restore function. Reduces hyper histamine responses and bacterial imbalances. Use nettles as an infusion for best results with gastrointestinal issues.

Kidneys: The kidneys are where nettle shines, and especially the seed. The seed is my first go-to when kidney function wanes. Damp accumulation can occur in the renal system, usually manifesting as cloudy urine.

(This can be kind of hard to notice in dogs, but if you suspect that dampness in the urinary tract is an issue, then try to collect a urine sample for viewing.) Dampness can also cause pain in the urinary tract, which results in crying out at the beginning or the end of urination. Nettles can help with this situation; they offer detoxification and nutrition and encourage a gradual draining downward to the kidneys. They are drying and filling, meaning they can help with membranes that are too permeable, which plays a key role in helping with leaky gut for those dogs with heat and stagnation. They can help ease food and environmental sensitivities and allergies as well. Their action isn't quick, but slow and steady wins the race.

Liver: Both the leaves and seeds are rich in minerals, giving the liver what it needs for detoxification. The herb's strong support for the kidneys reduces the load on the liver. Nettle can help with high levels of hydrogen peroxide, free radicals, and heavy metals. It decreases high liver enzymes and cholesterol levels and is hepatoprotective.

Musculoskeletal system: Your dog's kidneys influence healthy bone formation (mineralization) due to their interaction and influence on the water element and minerals, especially calcium and phosphorus. They also produce a hormone called calcitriol that interacts with vitamin D, keeping bones strong. Thus, since mineral-rich nettles improve kidney function, they also influence the musculoskeletal system, strengthening bones, connective tissues, tendons, and ligaments.

Skin: As noted throughout, herbs that support the liver also support the skin (liver-skin connection), and that's true for nettles. They are great for addressing itchiness, dryness, inflammation, and allergic reactions from insect bites. Use dried nettles as a rinse for a dog's itching skin.

Tonic effects: Nettle leaves are high in minerals and act as a tonic or alterative for the dog-as-ecosystem, helping increase both elimination and nutrition. They help the body wake up and function better as they clean the blood and remove stagnancy. Nettles help astringe tissues and have a tightening effect on relaxed tissues, including blood vessels—another way they help provide nutrition throughout the body. Nettles support the lymphatic system and help clear fluids, including edema. They fortify and strengthen the entire body.

Preparation and Dosing Schedule

	Extra-Small Dog	Small Dog	Medium Dog	Large Dog	Extra-Large Dog
Tincture (seed)	I drop	2 drops	3 drops	4 drops	5 drops
Tincture (leaf)	3 drops	10 drops	15 drops	20 drops	25–30 drops
Glycerite (leaf)	6 drops	20 drops	30 drops	40 drops	50–60 drops
Infusion	¼ teaspoon	½ teaspoon	1–2 teaspoons	1–2 tablespoons	3–6 tablespoons
Dried herb	100 mg per 10 pounds of your dog's body weight, given with food				

Leaf tincture: For food sensitivities and allergies, give the leaf tincture with quercetin (100 mg for every 30 pounds of your dog's weight, twice daily with food). For cool dogs, include bromelain (25 mg for every 15 pounds of your dog's weight, twice daily with food). However, if bromelain causes itchiness, nausea, or vomiting, use the nettles and quercetin combination; this reaction can indicate that your dog is too warm.

Potential Concerns

Herb-drug interactions: diuretics

Cautions: Avoid touching fresh nettle leaves; use the dried leaf, a dried leaf infusion, or a tincture only.

. . . .

Tip! St. John's wort salve takes away the sting of nettle.

. . . .

🌢 Olive (*Olea europaea*)

Family: Oleaceae

Energetics: neutral to warm, slightly dry

Energetic patterns indicating its use: coolness, cold, dampness

Part used: flower, leaf, root

Long-term use: yes

Actions: antibacterial, antifungal, antihistamine, anti-inflammatory, antimicrobial, antioxidant, antiseptic, antiviral, astringent, hypotensive, neuroprotective, styptic, vulnerary

Constituents: apigenin-7-glucoside, beta-carotene, diosmin, flavonoids, hydroxytyrosol, luteolin-7-glucoside, secoiridoid monoterpenes, oleanolic acid, oleuropein, phenolics, polyphenols, rutin, triterpenoids, tyrosol, verbascoside

Nutrients: calcium, chromium, iron, magnesium, potassium, selenium, vitamins C and D, zinc

Cofactors: allergies, antibiotic use, antibiotics damage, arthritis, bacterial infections, candida overgrowth, cartilage degradation, chronic pain, chronic skin conditions, chronic UTIs, cognitive decline, constipation, cough, dental infections, ear infections, food sensitivities, gastrointestinal reactivity, high blood pressure, high toxic load, high viral load, history of antibiotics use, hypertension, inflammation, joint pain, kennel cough, liver weakness, low immune function, lung weakness, Lyme and other tick-borne disease, osteoarthritis, plaque, swollen joints, tumors, viral infections, X-ray exposure

Flower essence: for pain, exhaustion, adrenal fatigue, allergies, kidney support, organ weakness, helpful for working dogs and elder dogs; often used after a seizure, helpful during crate training

Use for cats: yes

Applications

Antimicrobial: With a minimum 12 percent concentration of oleuropein, olive leaf is an excellent eradicator of biofilm and bacteria, yeasts, and viruses. It's specifically indicated for Lyme disease and its coinfections. It increases white blood cell counts and helps the immune system destroy viruses by preventing them from replicating. It kills yeasts and helps prevent biofilm formation. It's antiviral and can be used for kennel cough. It also offers support for the lungs and constipation. (Remember, the lungs and large intestine are linked and support each other or share weaknesses.)

Preparation and Dosing Schedule

	Extra-Small Dog	Small Dog	Medium Dog	Large Dog	Extra-Large Dog
Tincture	3 drops	6 drops	8–10 drops	10–15 drops	12–20 drops
Glycerite	6 drops	12 drops	20 drops	30 drops	30–45 drops
Infusion	¼ teaspoon	½ teaspoon	1–2 teaspoons	1–2 tablespoons	3–6 tablespoons
Dried herb	¹/₁₆ teaspoon	⅛ teaspoon	¼ teaspoon	½ teaspoon	¾–1 teaspoon

Potential Concerns

Herb-drug interactions: blood pressure medications, blood thinners

Cautions: Can cause vomiting and nausea; always give with food. Use phytoembryonic olive if vomiting occurs.

◢ Oregon Grape Root (*Berberis aquifolium*)

Family: Berberidaceae

Energetics: cold and dry

Energetic patterns indicating its use: warm to hot energetics, heat, excessive heat, dampness

Part used: root

Long-term use: no

Actions: alterative, antibacterial, antiemetic, antifungal, antimicrobial, astringent, bitter, cholagogue, diuretic, hemostatic, hepatic

Constituents: berberine, corydine, isoquinoline alkaloids

Nutrients: manganese, silicon, sodium, vitamins (C, D, E), zinc

Cofactors: acid reflux, arthritis, biofilm, candida overgrowth, cat turd eating, constipation, cough, diarrhea, digestive inflammation, ear infections, ear mites, gastritis, giardiasis, hot spots, impacted anal glands, liver congestion, moist lung conditions, pharmaceutical-based constipation, poor appetite, poor assimilation, stagnant lymphatics, tick-born disease, undigested food in the stool, weak immune system

Flower essence: for dogs who can't trust others, dogs going to new homes, liver imbalances, dogs who are picked on, feelings of being unsafe

Use for cats: yes

Applications

Cough: Oregon grape root is a strong antiviral, offering support to the immune system and helping to heal lungs with stagnant mucus.

Elimination and nutrition: Helps clean both blood and lymph, thereby positively influencing the dog-as-ecosystem through the dual channels of nutrition and elimination. Through its influence on the liver, Oregon grape root improves the assimilation of nutrients in the gastrointestinal tract.

Immune system: Helps stimulate the lymphatic system, supporting immune function through elimination.

Kidneys: Oregon grape root helps normalize a dog's inner terrain through its positive effects on the digestive system, which in turn has a positive influence over the kidneys and urinary system. Its antimicrobial action can help address urinary and bladder infections, and it tones mucous membranes in the renal system as well.

Preparation and Dosing Schedule

	Extra-Small Dog	Small Dog	Medium Dog	Large Dog	Extra-Large Dog
Tincture for acute use	1 drop	2–4 drops	4–6 drops	6–8 drops	10–12 drops
Decoction	¼ teaspoon	½ teaspoon	1–2 teaspoons	1–2 tablespoons	3–6 tablespoons
Dried powdered herb	Used externally as needed				

Potential Concerns

Herb-drug interactions: avoid with pharmaceuticals

Cautions: Do not use long-term. Avoid use in dogs with cold conditions or liver disease.

Note: Oregon grape is endangered; be sure to obtain its root only from ethical suppliers.

⚖ Parsley (*Petroselinum crispum*)

Family: Apiaceae

Energetics: warm and dry

Energetic patterns indicating its use: coolness, cold, relaxation

Part used: leaf

Long-term use: yes

Actions: antibacterial, antifungal, antihistamine, antispasmodic, appetite stimulant, bitter, carminative, diuretic

Constituents: antioxidants, apiole, chlorophyll, coumarins, flavonoids, mucilage, myristicin, volatile oil

Nutrients: calcium, iron, potassium, phosphorus, selenium, silicon, sulfur, vitamins (A, B-complex, C), zinc

Cofactors: abscess, allergies, anemia, arthritis, bad breath, bladder gravel, calcifications, chronic bladder infections, chronic UTIs, constipation,

stretching across the floor after eating, ear infections, edema, fleas (repellent), high blood sugar levels, high liver enzymes, IBD, inflammation, inflammation of the bladder, kidney stones, kidney weakness, liver congestion, low adrenal function, low appetite, low blood pressure, low urine output, mucus in the urine, stagnation in the anal glands, swellings, thickening of the bladder lining, urination with crying out, wasting, weak digestion, weight loss

Flower essence: for dogs who hold their urine, are obstinate, are hard to train, are going through potty training, or mark in the house

Use for cats: yes

Applications

Gastrointestinal system: Helps stimulate appetite, reduces intestinal inflammation and IBD symptoms, and relieves bad breath, excess gas, constipation, nausea, and discomfort after eating. Its high vitamin C content helps support gut immune function and health. Its high vitamin B content helps with folate absorption and methylation through the liver.

Kidneys: Supports the liver and kidneys, balances sodium levels, supports the adrenals, and reduces inflammation throughout the renal system. It helps dogs with hot urine, pain, infections, and protein in urine.

Preparation and Dosing Schedule

	Extra-Small Dog	Small Dog	Medium Dog	Large Dog	Extra-Large Dog
Tincture	1–3 drops	2–5 drops	4–8 drops	6–12 drops	10–16 drops
Infusion	¼ teaspoon	½ teaspoon	1–2 teaspoons	1–2 tablespoons	3–6 tablespoons

Infusion: The infusion can be made from either fresh or dried parsley.

Potential Concerns

Herb-drug interactions: none known

Cautions: Avoid in cases of acute kidney inflammation and kidney disease. With excessive use, it can cause uterine contractions.

⚔ Passionflower (*Passiflora incarnata*)

Family: Passifloraceae

Energetics: cool to neutral, dry

Energetic patterns indicating its use: tension

Part used: flower

Long-term use: yes

Actions: analgesic, antispasmodic, nervine, pain reliever, relaxant, sedative

Constituents: alkaloids, amino acids, apigenin-C-glycosides, coumarins, cyanotic glucosides, flavonoids, glycoproteins, harman alkaloids, harmane, harmaline, harmol, isovitexin, laricinic acid, lycopene, malt, phenolic acids, phytosterols, quercetin, rutin, schaftoside, volatile oil

Nutrients: calcium, vitamins A and C

Cofactors: adrenal weakness, alternating constipation with diarrhea, anxiety, epilepsy, fear, grief, heart weakness, insomnia, muscle pain, muscle spasm, nervous symptoms that come and go, nervousness, rapid breathing, seizures, spasmodic cough, stress, tension, twitching, worry

Flower essence: for grief or for dogs that are rehoming, boarding, or kenneling

Use for cats: yes

Applications

Anxiety and nervousness: Passionflower increases GABA levels in the brain, which helps calm the nervous system. It helps reduce anxiety and nervousness. It's an antispasmodic muscle relaxer and can help with twitching, hyperactivity, inflammation, and nerve-related pain. It helps restless, fearful, and nervous dogs at night. Combined with other nerviness, passionflower can help control seizures, as it depresses the central nervous system.

Preparation and Dosing Schedule

	Extra-Small Dog	Small Dog	Medium Dog	Large Dog	Extra-Large Dog
Tincture	1–2 drops	2–4 drops	4–6 drops	6–12 drops	10–16 drops
Glycerite	4 drops	8 drops	12 drops	20 drops	30 drops
Infusion	¼ teaspoon	½ teaspoon	1–2 teaspoons	1–2 tablespoons	3–6 tablespoons

Glycerite: The glycerite dosage is double the tincture dosage, but beginning at the low end. Work up as needed.

Potential Concerns

Herb-drug interactions: sedatives, lithium, MAOs, central nervous system depressants

Cautions: Start with a small dose to see how this herb affects your dog.

⚔ Pau d'Arco (*Handroanthus impetiginosus*)

Family: Bignoniaceae

Energetics: slightly warm and dry

Energetic patterns indicating its use: cool to cold conditions, dampness, relaxation

Part used: inner bark

Long-term use: no

Actions: analgesic, antibacterial, antifungal, anti-inflammatory, antimicrobial, antioxidant, antiviral, astringent, cytotoxic, immune modulator, immune stimulant, tonic

Constituents: antioxidants, beta-lapachone, calcium oxalate, carnosol, catechins, coumarins, flavonoids, iridoids, lapachol, lapachone, phenolic acids, tannins, veratric acid, xyloidone

Nutrients: calcium, iron, potassium, selenium, sodium, vitamins (A, B, C), zinc

Cofactors: active viral infection, arthritis, cancer, candida overgrowth, fever, high toxic load, inflammation, osteoarthritis, pain, prostate inflammation, stagnant lymphatics, ulcers, yeast

Use for cats: yes

Applications

Yeast: Pau d'arco is highly antioxidant and antimicrobial. It's used for yeast infections/overgrowth and inflammation. In small dosages, pau d'arco can help modulate immune system reactivity and inflammation, reducing the effects of candida-related leaky gut. It detoxifies the digestive tract and has influence over toxins and liver congestion through its positive effect on digestive lymphatics.

Preparation and Dosing Schedule

	Extra-Small Dog	Small Dog	Medium Dog	Large Dog	Extra-Large Dog
Tincture	1 drop	2–4 drops	4–8 drops	6–12 drops	10–12 drops
Dried herb	1/16 teaspoon	1/8 teaspoon	1/4 teaspoon	1/2 teaspoon	3/4 teaspoon

Potential Concerns

Herb-drug interactions: anticoagulants, antiplatelet medicines

Cautions: High in selenium. Excess use can cause diarrhea, dizziness, nausea, vomiting, and in rare cases internal bleeding. Avoid with bleeding disorders. Don't use in high doses.

✿ Plantain (*Plantago major*)

Family: Plantaginaceae

Energetics: cool, damp

Energetic patterns indicating its use: warmth, heat, excessive heat, dryness, relaxation

Part used: leaf

Long-term use: yes

Actions: alterative, antibacterial, anticatarrhal, antidiarrheal, anti-inflammatory, antiseptic, astringent, demulcent, diuretic, expectorant, hemostatic, hepatoprotective, immune modulator, inflammation modulator, vulnerary

Constituents: alkaloids, apigenin, arabinose, asperuloside, aucubin, baicalein, catalpol, chlorogenic acid, galactose, glucose, hispidulin, iridoid glycosides, luteolin, mucilage, nepetin, phenolic acids, plantamajoside, polysaccharides, tannins, xylose

Nutrients: iron, potassium, vitamins A and C, zinc

Cofactors: abscess, acid reflux, allergies, anal gland issues, antibiotics use, antibiotics damage, bloodshot eyes, bloody stool, cataracts, conjunctivitis, constipation, dry lungs, dry stool, food sensitivities, gastrointestinal pain, glyphosate exposure, gut sensitivity, incontinence, inflammation, intestinal infection, kennel cough, kidney dryness, mouth sores, water retention, wounds

Use for cats: yes

Applications

Cough: Plantain lubricates and moisturizes lung tissues, soothing dry coughs. It is versatile and balancing because of its astringency. You can use it for dry and moist respiratory conditions and random coughs.

Gastrointestinal system: Like slippery elm, plantain can help with both diarrhea and constipation. It also helps with leaky gut, food intolerances (bitter), glyphosate sensitivity, and antibiotic damage. Plantain's anti-inflammatory action helps heal any wounds in the gastro-intestinal tract. It works with the liver to detoxify small and large intestine wastes, supporting a dog's microbiome and gut-mediated immune system.

Skin: Plantain is a powerful external wound healer. It's antibacterial and antiseptic and should be part of your emergency kit as it draws and stimulates surface immunity. Internally, it can help stop itchiness.

Urinary system: Diuretic, demulcent, and astringent, plantain helps soothe irritation in the bladder and urinary tissues and relieve pain and heat. It can be used for blood in the urine and assists with clearing up any urinary infections.

Preparation and Dosing Schedule

	Extra-Small Dog	Small Dog	Medium Dog	Large Dog	Extra-Large Dog
Tincture	2–3 drops	4–6 drops	5–10 drops	8–15 drops	10–20 drops
Glycerite	6 drops	12 drops	20 drops	30 drops	40 drops
Infusion	⅛ cup	¼ cup	½ cup	¾ cup	1 cup
Dried leaf	⅛ teaspoon	¼ teaspoon	½ teaspoon	¾ teaspoon	1 teaspoon

Glycerite: Plantain works well as a glycerite.

Potential Concerns

Herb-drug interactions: blood thinners, digoxin, lithium

Cautions: Avoid in dogs with kidney disease.

⚹ Red Clover (*Trifolium pratense*)

Family: Fabaceae

Energetics: cool and slightly damp, balancing

Energetic patterns indicating its use: warm to hot energetics, excessive heat, dryness, tension

Part used: flower

Long-term use: yes

Actions: alterative, demulcent, expectorant, lymphatic, nutritive, antispasmodic

Constituents: amino acids, antioxidants, biochanin A, coumarins, daidzein, genistein, formononetin, isoflavones, polysaccharides, pratensein, resins, salicylic acid, saponins, trifoside, volatile oils

Nutrients: calcium, chromium, magnesium, niacin, phosphorus, potassium, thiamine, vitamins (A, B, C), zinc

Cofactors: chronic skin conditions, cognitive decline, cysts, dementia, dry cough, dry eye, dry lungs, dry skin, hacking cough, high toxic load, lipomas, liver weakness, lung weakness, lymph congestion, mammary tumors, mast cell tumors, mastitis, tumors, warts, weak immune system

Flower essence: for restoring balance after surgery; a Rescue Remedy alternative for fear or shock; for debility and weakness

Use for cats: yes, in 1–2 drop dosages due to salicylic acid content

Applications

Gastrointestinal and lymphatic: Helps increase lymphatic function in the gut and works with gut flora to turn its isoflavone content into viable hormones to help balance and support female dogs after a spay.

Heart: Red clover helps with arterial flexibility, increasing circulation and thinning your dog's blood. Its isoflavones can balance estrogen levels, which supports healthy heart function.

Kidneys: Increases urine, balances moisture, and helps excrete excess mucus, metabolic wastes, and toxins. Its high mineral content helps nourish the kidneys and protect them from excessive stimulation.

Lipomas, cysts, and tumors: Red clover can help dissolve cysts and lipomas as it works with the liver and lymph system. Red clover and violet together can help dissolve mammary tumors. I once rescued a pug, named Elouise, who was given a few months to live with mammary tumors; on a regimen of red clover and violet, she lived an additional 33 months.

Skin: Red clover is anti-inflammatory, boosts collagen levels, and balances estrogen. It also increases circulation and relieves dryness. These actions can prevent early aging, mitigate systemic inflammation, and contribute to healthy skin.

. . . .

Tip! A formula combining red clover, bilberry, and eyebright in equal parts can help balance dry eyes and moisturize ocular tissues.

. . . .

Preparation and Dosing Schedule

	Extra-Small Dog	Small Dog	Medium Dog	Large Dog	Extra-Large Dog
Tincture	2 drops	4 drops	6–8 drops	8–15 drops	10–20 drops
Glycerite	4 drops	8 drops	16 drops	25 drops	30 drops
Infusion	¼ teaspoon	½ teaspoon	1–2 teaspoons	1–2 tablespoons	3–6 tablespoons

Potential Concerns

Herb-drug interactions: blood thinners

Cautions: Avoid using red clover in dogs with clotting disorders or internal/external bleeding. Avoid for at least 2 weeks after surgery.

◢ Rose (*Rosa* spp.)

Family: Rosaceae

Energetics: *hips*—cold and dry; *petals*—cool and damp

Energetic patterns indicating its use: warm to hot energetics, dampness, dryness, tension, relaxation

Part used: rose hip, petals from the flower

Long-term use: yes

Actions: *petals*—alterative, antibacterial, anti-inflammatory, antispasmodic, astringent, nervine, nutritive, tonic; *hips*—antibacterial, anti-inflammatory, antioxidant, antispasmodic, astringent, carminative, hemostatic, nutritive, tonic

Constituents: antioxidants, carotene, citric acid, fatty acids, flavonoids, linoleic acid, lutein, nicotinamide, pectin, polyphenols, retinoids, saponins, tannins

Nutrients: calcium, folic acid, iron, magnesium, manganese, potassium, quercetin, silicon, sodium, sulfur, vitamins (A, B, C, D, E, K), zinc*

Cofactors: allergies, arthritis, autoimmune disorders, chronic yeast infections, cough, grief, heat, high histamine levels, high toxic load, hip dysplasia, ill-formed stool, immune deficiency, inflammation, irritated mucous membranes, kennel cough, leaky gut, lethargy, liver stress, low immune function, lymphatic stagnation, mast cell tumor,

---

*Most of the nutrition is in the rose hips.

nervous system disorders, red and runny nose, stiffness, weak connective tissues

Flower essence: calming; balances energy; reduces stress and anxiety; for heart chakra work and grief

Use for cats: yes

Applications

Gastrointestinal system: Rose hips decrease heat in the lymphatic system and gastrointestinal tract, which can help with inflammation, diarrhea, and runny stool. They are also an effective prebiotic. This makes them an excellent addition to an antibiotics recovery protocol; you can give them during antibiotics use and afterward for support.

Heart: Decreases heat in the cardiovascular system, working through the nervous system to ease heart irregularities.

Immune system: High in vitamin C and other vitamins, rose hips are great for the immune system, and the flower petals are antiviral. The petals and hips together can help ease a cough; use in a formula with other herbs for warm to hot dogs.

Kidneys: Disperses heat from the kidneys and clears toxins from the renal system.

Nervous system: Soothing and relaxing, rose helps calm the nervous system. It's good for dogs with sympathetic excess and PTSD and can help dogs with restlessness, anxiety, grief, and fright. I like rose flower essence mixed with comfrey for trauma.

Preparation and Dosing Schedule

	Extra-Small Dog	Small Dog	Medium Dog	Large Dog	Extra-Large Dog
Tincture	2 drops	3–6 drops	6–8 drops	10–15 drops	12–20 drops
Glycerite	4 drops	6–12 drops	12–16 drops	20–30 drops	24–40 drops
Infusion	¼ teaspoon	½ teaspoon	1–2 teaspoons	1–2 tablespoons	3–6 tablespoons
Dried and powdered rose hips	⅛ teaspoon	¼ teaspoon	½ teaspoon	¾ teaspoon	1 teaspoon

Dried and powdered rose hips: Be sure that the dried rose hips are organic.

Potential Concerns

Herb-drug interactions: none known

Cautions: The hairs in rose hips can irritate the intestines. Use high-quality, well-sifted powder only. Avoid rose with cold dogs and limit with cool dogs. Rose hips can be drying long-term; you may have to use them with a demulcent.

⚞ Rosemary (*Rosmarinus officinalis*)

Family: Lamiaceae

Energetics: warm, dry, stimulating

Energetic patterns indicating its use: coolness, cold, dampness, tension, relaxation

Part used: leaf and flower

Long-term use: yes

Actions: anti-inflammatory, antifungal, antimicrobial, antioxidant, antiviral, carminative, cholagogue, diaphoretic, nervine, spasmolytic

Constituents: alpha-pinene, antioxidants, borneol, bornyl acetate, camphene, cineol, flavonoids, luteolin, oleanolic acid, rosmarinic acid, tannins, triterpenes, salicylates, ursolic acid, volatile oil

Nutrients: calcium, copper, folic acid, iron, magnesium, manganese, pantothenic acid, potassium, pyridoxine, riboflavin, vitamins A, B_6, and C

Cofactors: alopecia, anxiety, asthma, burping, cognition issues, deficiency, dementia, high cortisol levels, hyperactivity, indigestion, liver congestion, nervousness, pain, poor circulation, restlessness, spleen weakness, stagnation, weak digestion

Flower essence: for sympathetic excess, weakness, heart weakness, and lethargy; useful for adopted dogs, rescue dogs, and geriatric dogs

Use for cats: yes, in small amounts due to the salicylic acid content

Applications

Antibiotics recovery: Helps strengthen the gastrointestinal tract and control pathogens, giving the microbiome space to recover after antibiotics treatment.

Circulation: Like cooling yarrow, rosemary helps with circulation, which is key everywhere blood and lymph flow in the dog-as-ecosystem. It relaxes, tones, and stimulates the venous system and lymph vessels while decreasing oxidation rates.

Gastrointestinal system: Like burdock root and hawthorn, rosemary helps stimulate bile production from the liver and thus assists with the digestion of fats. Stimulating, it warms the core to the periphery. Over the long term rosemary is drying, but in the short term, used acutely, it can increase moisture, especially in the digestive system.

Liver: Increases bile through stimulation of the liver and gallbladder; can help detoxify your dog's liver, decrease oxidation rates, and lower liver enzymes.

Nervous system: Rosemary's fat content (its volatile oils) feeds the myelin sheath covering nerves, supporting their basic function and thus enhancing brain cognition. This can be helpful for dogs with dementia. While it has a tonic effect on the tissues, it is slightly relaxant to the sympathetic nervous system (it increases parasympathetic activity).

Preparation and Dosing Schedule

	Extra-Small Dog	Small Dog	Medium Dog	Large Dog	Extra-Large Dog
Tincture	1–2 drops	2–4 drops	4–8 drops	6–12 drops	10–16 drops
Glycerite	2 drops	4 drops	8 drops	12 drops	20 drops
Infusion	¼ teaspoon	½ teaspoon	1–2 teaspoons	1–2 tablespoons	3–6 tablespoons

Glycerite: The glycerite dosage is double the tincture dosage, but beginning at the low end. Work up as needed.

Potential Concerns

Herb-drug interactions: none known

Cautions: Avoid high dosages unless well indicated. For dogs that have seizures, avoid high dosages of rosemary in any form, and avoid rosemary essential oil altogether; infusions, diluted decoctions, and drop dosages of the tincture are fine to use. . If you are afraid of using this plant with your dog, then don't.

⤫ Skullcap (*Scutellaria lateriflora*)

Family: Lamiaceae

Energetics: cool and dry (long-term)

Energetic patterns indicating its use: excessive heat, dryness, dampness, tension (but dogs with cool energetics can use short-term, in a formula or pulsed, if well indicated)

Part used: leaf and flower

Long-term use: yes

Actions: analgesic, anti-inflammatory, antispasmodic, astringent (mild), bitter, euphoric, nervine, relaxant, sedative, tonic, trophorestorative

Constituents: baicalein, cellulose, chrysin-7-glucuronide, fiber, iridoids, resins, rosmarinic acid, scutellarin, scutellonin, tannins, volatile oil

Nutrients: calcium, chromium, iron, magnesium, manganese, niacin, phosphorus, potassium, protein, riboflavin, silicon, sodium, thiamine, vitamins A and C, zinc

Cofactors: aggression, agitation, barrier aggression, CCL tears, emotionally driven insomnia, hair-trigger aggression, heat in the lymphatic system, heat in the nervous system, heat in the small intestine, hyperthyroidism, intense behaviors, muscle tightness, muscle twitching, nervous diarrhea, pain in the gastrointestinal tract, rabies vaccine, restlessness, sensitivity to noise (mix with nettle seed), stress, sympathetic excess, tendency toward overstimulation, tension, tightness, trauma, twitching, vaccine reactions, weakness

Flower essence: to calm panic, fear, anxiety, and sensitivity to noise; for cardiac support; for rescue dogs who are disconnected from people; for root and crown chakra work

Use for cats: yes

Applications

Cough: Relaxes smooth muscle and decreases spasms, making it useful for easing a cough.

Liver: Skullcap's bitterness stimulates the liver and gallbladder, encouraging bile production and relaxed digestion.

Musculoskeletal system: Excels as a relaxant and, in many cases, pain reliever through its action of calming smooth muscles throughout the body. Eases muscle twitching and restlessness. Useful for recovery from CCL tears.

Nervous system: Nourishes and strengthens the nervous system, easing sympathetic excess, relaxing tension, pushing through stagnation, and healing damaged nerves. Can help dogs who tend toward sympathetic excess switch back and forth between parasympathetic and sympathetic states. Skullcap is a great remedy for dogs who are depleted and exhausted from trauma and stress as well as anxious, hard-to-settle dogs, including those displaying panic, fright, and excitement.

Vaccine recovery: Useful for behavior-based side effects specific to the rabies vaccine. Give twice daily for 10 weeks after vaccination.

Preparation and Dosing Schedule

	Extra-Small Dog	Small Dog	Medium Dog	Large Dog	Extra-Large Dog
Tincture	1–3 drops	2–5 drops	4–8 drops	6–12 drops	10–16 drops
Tincture for acute use	6 drops	10 drops	16 drops	24 drops	32 drops
Glycerite for chronic conditions	6 drops	10 drops	16 drops	24 drops	32 drops
Glycerite for acute conditions	9 drops	15 drops	24 drops	36 drops	48 drops
Infusion	¼ teaspoon	½ teaspoon	1–2 teaspoons	1–2 tablespoons	3–6 tablespoons

All remedies: Use fresh skullcap to prepare these remedies when possible.
Glycerite for acute conditions: This dosage is triple the standard tincture dosage. Give this dose three or four times daily until symptoms ease.

Potential Concerns

Herb-drug interactions: central nervous system depressants, sedatives

Cautions: When skullcap isn't working for a dog, it can sometimes cause excitement. (I had a case where a dog took skullcap and started humping everything.) Avoid with pharmaceutical sedatives. Overdose symptoms are dizziness and confusion.

Note: Purchase skullcap only from companies or growers you trust, as commercial supplies of skullcap can be adulterated with germander, a plant that can be harmful to dogs.

❧ Slippery Elm (*Ulmus rubra*)

Family: Ulmaceae
Energetics: neutral to cool, damp

Energetic patterns indicating its use: warm to hot energetics, heat, dryness, tension

Part used: inner bark

Long-term use: yes

Actions: antacid, anti-inflammatory, antioxidant, astringent (mild), demulcent, emollient, expectorant, nutritive, vulnerary

Constituents: D-galactose, D-galacturonic acid, fiber, lignin, mucilage, palmitic acid, pectin, polyphenols, polysaccharides, tannins

Nutrients: calcium, magnesium, potassium

Cofactors: acid reflux, collapsed trachea, constipation, diarrhea, dry cough, esophageal conditions, gastrointestinal upset, hot spots, urinary tract infection, ulcers, IBD, IBS, sluggish anal glands, inflammation, liver weakness, wounds

Use for cats: yes

Applications

Gastrointestinal system: Nourishes the microbiome as a prebiotic and supports the entire gastrointestinal tract (and it's good for dry lungs too). Can help with acid reflux, ulcers, and both constipation and diarrhea. Slippery elm is good for dogs with megaesophagus as it reduces inflammation and helps food pass through relaxed esophageal tissue.

Preparation and Dosing Schedule

	Extra-Small Dog	Small Dog	Medium Dog	Large Dog	Extra-Large Dog
Glycerite	4 drops	8 drops	12 drops	15–20 drops	20–25 drops
Slurry	I Tablespoon for every 25 pounds of bodyweight				
Infusion	I Tablespoon for every 25 pounds of bodyweight				
Dried powdered bark	⅛ teaspoon	¼ teaspoon	½ teaspoon	¾ teaspoon	I teaspoon

Slurry Instructions and Dosage: stir 1/2 teaspoon of slippery elm powder into 1/2 cup of cold water. Simmer, constantly stirring for 2–3 minutes until thick. Add more powder for added thickness. Let cool and syringe into mouth.

Cold Infusion: 2 tablespoons of herbs per 8 ounces of almost cool water. Cover and let sit overnight—strain in the morning. Will last 3 days in refrigerator.

Note: If giving slippery elm for purposes other than an emergency, limit slippery elm to once daily 3 hours away from pharmaceuticals.

Potential Concerns

Herb-drug interactions: may interfere with absorption of pharmaceuticals

Cautions: Avoid in cases of edema and severe lung congestion. Can cause contact dermatitis. Though it's moisturizing, slippery elm can be drying when used for too long; use it only for short periods of time. It can interfere with absorption; give away from medication and food by at least 3 hours when used daily.

Note: Slippery elm bark is endangered; be sure to obtain it only from ethical suppliers. You can use Siberian elm (*Ulmus pumila*) interchangeably.

🌿 Solomon's Seal (*Polygonatum* spp.)

Family: Asparagaceae

Energetics: cool and damp

Energetic patterns indicating its use: warm to hot energetics, heat, dryness, tension

Part used: root

Long-term use: yes

Actions: anti-inflammatory, astringent, cardiotonic, demulcent, expectorant, tonic, vulnerary

Constituents: allantoin, amino acids, cardiac glycosides (low), L-azetidine-2-carboxylic acid, mucilaginous polysaccharides, steroidal saponins

Cofactors: arthritis, blood in the urine, bone spurs, calcifications, CCL tears, diarrhea, disc conditions, dryness in the anal glands, dry and creaky joints, dry cough, fatty liver, gastrointestinal inflammation, heart weakness, high blood pressure, inflammation, leaky gut, liver weakness, lung inflammation, musculoskeletal inflammation, musculoskeletal weakness, repetitive stress injuries, stagnant lymphatics, tight ligaments and tendons, uterine prolapse

Flower essence: for aggression, irritation, fighting, inflexibility

Use for cats: yes

Applications

Musculoskeletal system: Solomon's seal is a lubricant for the musculoskeletal system. It helps lubricate joints and relax ligaments and tendons. Use it in a formula or as a decoction leading up to winter to help keep your dog's musculoskeletal system moist and pliable through spring.

Preparation and Dosing Schedule

	Extra-Small Dog	Small Dog	Medium Dog	Large Dog	Extra-Large Dog
Tincture	1–3 drops	2–5 drops	4–8 drops	6–12 drops	10–16 drops
Tincture for acute use	6 drops	10 drops	16 drops	24 drops	32 drops
Decoction	¼ teaspoon	½ teaspoon	1–2 teaspoons	1–2 tablespoons	3–6 tablespoons

Potential Concerns

Herb-drug interactions: digitalis

Cautions: Avoid high doses unless using acutely. Use only the root. Can cause nausea and vomiting.

🌿 St. John's Wort (*Hypericum perforatum*)

Family: Hypericaceae

Energetics: slightly warm and dry

Energetic patterns indicating its use: coolness, cold, deep cold, dryness, tension

Part used: leaf and flower

Long-term use: yes

Actions: alterative, analgesics, astringent, antiviral, antimicrobial, anti-inflammatory, bitter, disinfectant, diuretic, hepatoprotective, immune modulator, neuroprotective, nervine, nerve trophorestorative, relaxant, tonic, vulnerary

Constituents: 2-methyloctane, alpha- and beta-pinene, carotene, carotenoids, caryophyllene, catechins, decanal, flavonoids, glycosides, hyperforin, hypericin, hyperoside, naphthodianthrones, nonane, octanal, pectin, phloroglucinols, rutin, tannins, volatile oils, xanthine derivatives

Nutrients: vitamins A and C

Cofactors: adrenal excess, aggression, anxiety, CCL tears, chronic inflammation, excessive disruptive dreaming, grief, hair-trigger reactivity, hypothyroidism, intact (unspayed) female, leaky gut, liver stagnation, irritation, lethargy, nerve damage, poor microbiome health, pain, redness and heat, skin conditions, slow digestion, stagnation, sympathetic excess, ulcers, weak gut-brain connection, weakness

Flower essence: for calming an overprotective or jealous dog (useful during training); encourages better sleep and eases winter blues

Use for cats: yes

Applications

Gastrointestinal system: St. John's wort can help with nervous stomach, leaky gut, and stomach irritation. It's an underused remedy for intestinal permeability. Supportive for gut-brain communication, vagal tone, and nervous dogs who are affected by nervous tension or reactivity. Its astringency and antimicrobial action help clean up the small intestine and increase assimilation and elimination with the help of the liver.

Grief: An excellent remedy for dogs having a difficult time dealing with grief, including dogs displaying sensitive, withdrawn behaviors. Can use the flower essence for this purpose.

Skin: St. John's wort can help clean and disinfect wounds and decrease inflammation and heat. Use it for hot spots and mange.

Preparation and Dosing Schedule

	Extra-Small Dog	Small Dog	Medium Dog	Large Dog	Extra-Large Dog
Tincture	1–3 drops	2–5 drops	4–8 drops	6–12 drops	10–16 drops
Tincture for acute use	6 drops	10 drops	16 drops	24 drops	32 drops
Cold infusion	¼ teaspoon	½ teaspoon	1–2 teaspoons	1–2 tablespoons	3–6 tablespoons

Potential Concerns

Herb-drug interactions: all pharmaceuticals (if your dog is using any kind of pharmaceutical, use homeopathic St. John's wort instead of an herbal remedy)

Cautions: High doses can cause phototoxicity in humans, though I've never had this issue with dogs.

🌢 Turmeric (*Curcuma longa*)

Family: Zingiberaceae

Energetics: warm and dry

Energetic patterns indicating its use: cool, cold, dampness, relaxation, stagnation

Part used: rhizome

Long-term use: yes

Actions: analgesic, antibacterial, anticancer, antifungal, antihistamine, anti-inflammatory, antioxidant, antiseptic, antispasmodic, antiviral, astringent, bitter, carminative, cholagogue, circulatory stimulant, expectorant, immune modulator, vulnerary

Constituents: 1,8-cineole, alpha-linolenic acid, alpha- and gamma-atlantone, alpha-phellandrene, antioxidants, berberine, borneol, dehydroturmerone, curcuminoids, d-sabinene, monodesmethoxycurcumin, p-coumaroylferuloylmethane, di-p-coumaroylmethane, polysaccharides, turmerone, zingiberene

Nutrients: calcium, chromium, cobalt, iron, magnesium, manganese, niacin, phosphorus, potassium, protein, riboflavin, selenium, silicon, proteins, sodium, thiamine, vitamins A and C, zinc

Cofactors: anemia, arthritis aggravated by cold weather, chronic respiratory distress, cool energetics, cough, excess gas, high blood pressure, high histamine levels, inflammation, joint pain, lipomas with cool energetics, low bile production, low immune function, low vital force, lung weakness, mange, mast cell tumor, nausea, pain, poor circulation, senior dog, skin disorders, stagnant digestion, stagnation, thick blood, tick-borne disease, vomiting, worms

Use for cats: yes

Applications

Gastrointestinal system: Turmeric is stimulating but anti-inflammatory in the gastrointestinal tract. It supports the microbiome as a prebiotic, and it boosts beneficial bifidobacteria and butyrate-producing bacteria. This supports its immune-modulating properties and dominoes into support for other organ systems, especially the renal system. Turmeric is also a natural antihistamine that helps with leaky gut and food sensitivities.

Heart: Increases circulation and relaxes tension in the blood vessels, which reduces inflammation in the body. This, in turn, improves cognitive function.

Lipomas: Stimulates the lymphatic system, helping clear stagnation. This, together with its support for liver detoxification and anti-inflammatory properties, makes it useful for addressing lipomas. I use it internally and externally (as a paste) for lipomas. Turmeric will stain everything it comes in contact with. If using externally, you may want to confine your dog to a crate or indoor pen to limit their movement and exposure.

Liver: Stimulates the liver, increasing bile production, and balances phase 1 and phase 2 liver detoxification pathways. Decreases liver enzymes and triglycerides, helps modulate oxidation, provides antioxidants, and increases glutathione and superoxide dismutase, all of which helps prevent early aging, reduce inflammation, and support detoxification.

Lungs: Improves lung function by decreasing inflammation and protecting delicate lung tissues from pollutants by modulating immune responses. Helps the body break down stagnant mucus, which eases coughs and opens air passages.

Skin: Works through the liver-skin connection to balance skin conditions associated with poor circulation and stagnation. Circulation is the key to helping decrease inflammation. Turmeric stimulates circulation as well as relieves blood stagnation. You can use turmeric paste topically to reduce the inflammation of wounds, but be careful as it stains everything orange!

Urinary tract infections (prevention): Turmeric is antibacterial against both *E.coli* and staphylococcus bacteria. Though it isn't a viable solution for acute UTIs, it is a good herb for UTI prevention, correcting imbalance before infection begins. It does this by interfering with quorum sensing (how pathogens communicate).

Yeast: Turmeric is a good antifungal that can balance *Candida albicans* populations in the body, preventing and resolving yeast overgrowth.

Preparation and Dosing Schedule

	Extra-Small Dog	Small Dog	Medium Dog	Large Dog	Extra-Large Dog
Decoction	¼ teaspoon	½ teaspoon	1–2 teaspoons	1–2 tablespoons	3–6 tablespoons

Preparation and Dosing Schedule (cont'd)

	Extra-Small Dog	Small Dog	Medium Dog	Large Dog	Extra-Large Dog
Dried powdered rhizome	1/16 teaspoon	1/8 teaspoon	1/4 teaspoon	1/2 teaspoon	1 teaspoon

Enhancing bioavailability: Give turmeric together with some kind of fat to increase the bioavailability of its constituents. Turmeric products for humans often include an extract of black pepper for this purpose, but I don't recommend black pepper for dogs as it can irritate the gut lining.

Potential Concerns

Herb-drug interactions: blood-thinning medications

Cautions: Avoid in cases of hepatitis, jaundice, gallstones, or bile duct obstruction. Large doses of curcumin extract can leach iron out of the blood. Can act as a uterine stimulant. Can upset the gastrointestinal tract, especially in warm to hot dogs.

◢ Usnea (*Usnea barbata*)

Family: Usneaceae

Energetics: cool and neutral

Energetic patterns indicating its use: warm to hot energetics, dampness, dryness

Part used: whole lichen

Long-term use: no

Actions: analgesic, antibacterial, antifungal, antimicrobial, antiparasitic, antiviral, astringent, expectorant, immune stimulant, immune modulator, vulnerary

Constituents: alpha-linolenic acid, bitters, diffractaic acid, fatty acids, flavonoids, isolichenin, lichenic acid, lichenin, linoleic acid, mucilage, phytosterols, polysaccharides, protolichesterinic acid, starch, tannins, usnic acid

Nutrients: iron, magnesium, phosphorus, potassium, silicon, sodium, selenium, vitamins (A, B, E, K), zinc

Cofactors: acute and chronic pain, asthma, bacterial infections, black mold exposure, bronchitis, candidiasis, cat turd eating, cough (dry or damp), cramping, giardiasis, inflammation, low urine volume, lung congestion, poor appetite, ringworm, spasm, stagnant lymph tissue, tumors, ulcers, UTIs, viral infections

Use for cats: yes

Applications

Candida: Helps clear heat from the gastrointestinal tract and combats yeast overgrowth.

Cough: Supports immune function in the lungs and reduces cough through its mucilage (dry cough) and astringency (damp cough), making it balancing.

Immune system: Usnea is cool and stimulating, and it moves lymph, clears toxins, and decreases inflammation. Usnea is among the rare plants that are helpful for acute infections because it is both antimicrobial and immune stimulating.

UTIs: Antiseptic and immune supportive, usnea can help clear UTIs and prevent recurring infections.

Preparation and Dosing Schedule

	Extra-Small Dog	Small Dog	Medium Dog	Large Dog	Extra-Large Dog
Tincture	1–3 drops	2–5 drops	4–8 drops	6–12 drops	10–16 drops
Decoction	¼ teaspoon	½ teaspoon	1–2 teaspoons	1–2 tablespoons	3–6 tablespoons

Potential Concerns

Herb-drug interactions: none known

Cautions: Limit usnea use to 3 weeks; take a 2-week break between cycles. Be sure to use only *Usnea barbata,* and not other species, due to toxicity concerns.

⚶ Uva-Ursi (*Arctostaphylos uva-ursi*)

Family: Ericaceae

Energetics: cool, dry, stimulating

Energetic patterns indicating its use: warm to hot energetics, excessive heat, dryness, relaxation (NOT tension)

Part used: leaf (runners)

Long-term use: no; acute use only

Actions: antimicrobial, antiseptic, astringent, diuretic, immune modulator, tonic

Constituents: arbutin, bitters, flavonoids, hyperin, hydroquinone glucosides, phenolic acids, phenol glycosides, tannins, triterpenes

Nutrients: iron, magnesium, manganese, potassium, phosphorus, selenium, silicon, sodium, vitamins A and C, zinc

Cofactors: acidic urine, arthritis, bile insufficiency, biofilm, bladder infection, bronchitis, chronic diarrhea, digestive infection, heart weakness, incontinence, inflammation, lower back weakness, low pancreatic enzyme levels, Lyme disease, mucus in urine, nausea, prostate inflammation, protein in the urine, SIBO, stones, ulcer, upper respiratory infection, urination with crying out, UTIs

Flower essence: for dogs who have experienced abandonment or whose bonded mate or caregiver has died; for deep trauma situations with abuse; for heart chakra work

Use for cats: yes

Applications

Kidneys: Uva-ursi is a urinary stimulant; it increases urine flow. It is also antiseptic, reducing bacteria in the urinary tract and bladder. It astringes urinary membranes, which helps with incontinence, helping to control urinary leakage while also stimulating the kidneys for higher output. When dogs are on the cold spectrum, stimulating herbs like uva-ursi are beneficial because dogs moving toward cold are at a higher risk of infection.

Preparation and Dosing Schedule

	Extra-Small Dog	Small Dog	Medium Dog	Large Dog	Extra-Large Dog
Tincture	1 drop	2 drops	3 drops	4 drops	5 drops
Tincture for acute use	2 drops	5 drops	8–10 drops	10–15 drops	12–20 drops
Glycerite	2 drops	4 drops	6 drops	8 drops	10 drops
Infusion	¼ teaspoon	½ teaspoon	1–2 teaspoons	1–2 tablespoons	3–6 tablespoons

Potential Concerns

Herb-drug interactions: lithium

Cautions: Uva-ursi is highly astringent; it causes irritation of the tissues, which is why it should be used only for a short period of time, and care must be taken when using it for dogs with excessive tension. Avoid in cases of kidney disease or kidney failure. May cause constipation, nausea, and vomiting; overuse can cause liver injury (due to the hydro-quinone) and retinal thinning. Acute use in a balanced formula that can help decrease its astringency is recommended. Avoid in conjunction with cranberry.

⚝ Violet (*Viola* spp.)

Family: Violaceae

Energetics: cool and damp

Energetic patterns indicating its use: warmth, heat, excessive heat, dryness, tension

Part used: flower and leaf

Long-term use: yes

Actions: alterative, astringent (slight), demulcent, diuretic, expectorant, lymphatic, nutritive, vulnerary

Constituents: flavonoids, gaultherin, mucilage, myosin, phenolic glycosides, rutin, odoratin, saponins, salicylic acid, tannins, violarutin, violin

Nutrients: calcium, magnesium

Cofactors: abscess, asthma, bronchitis, congested anal glands, constipation, cysts, damp stagnation, dry cough, dry lungs, dry mucosa, dryness in the gastrointestinal tract, dry skin, heat or excessive heat, grief, high histamine levels, high toxic load, inflammation, inflammation of trachea, lipomas, mammary cancer, mammary tumors, mast cell tumors, poor assimilation, poor circulation, stagnation in the digestive system, surgery recovery, swollen lymph nodes, weakened immune system

Flower essence: for dogs that are timid, unsocial, rigid, stoic, unable to relax, or staring too much

Use for cats: yes, as a glycerite and in low doses due to the salicylic acid content

Applications

Gastrointestinal system: Violet, especially the leaf, provides mucilage, which is responsible for its demulcent qualities and provides a form of prebiotic soluble fiber, which feeds the gut microbiome. Violet provides anti-inflammatory support to tissues while coating the mucosa and pushing through stagnation.

Lymphatics: Violet gives the lymphatics breath. It supports the ebb and flow of proper lymphatic function. It's a versatile herb helping the lymphatics nourish and cleanse the dog-as-ecosystem.

· ·

Tip! When using violet for the intestines and lymphatics, it's best to use an infusion of violet rather than a tincture or glycerite. The mucilaginous water works to coat and soothe the whole digestive tract.

· ·

Nervous system: Violet is a gentle nervine for energetically warm to hot dogs with excessive nervousness and reactivity. I find it useful for stoic dogs who can't relax.

Preparation and Dosing Schedule

	Extra-Small Dog	Small Dog	Medium Dog	Large Dog	Extra-Large Dog
Tincture	2 drops	5 drops	8 drops	12 drops	15 drops
Glycerite	4 drops	10 drops	16 drops	24 drops	30 drops
Infusion	2 teaspoons	1½ tablespoons	¼ cup	½ cup	¾–1 cup

Potential Concerns

Herb-drug interactions: none known

Cautions: Avoid violet in dogs who are cold, deficient, and weak. Violet can have a mild laxative effect; if diarrhea or loose stool occur, decrease the dosage. However, violet might be an effective choice if a dog has constipation and suspected lymphatic stagnation because it coats the intestines and helps lubricate the stool.

⚹ Wood Betony (*Stachys officinalis*)

Family: Lamiaceae

Energetics: slightly warm, balancing, dry

Energetic patterns indicating its use: dampness, atrophy, relaxation, tension

Parts used: leaf and flower

Long-term use: yes

Actions: antispasmodic, astringent, bitter, carminative, expectorant, nervine, stimulant, trophorestorative, vulnerary

Constituents: alkaloids, betaine, flavonoids, iridoids, phenylethanoid glycosides, rosmarinic acid, tannins, volatile oils

Nutritional Profile: calcium, choline, magnesium, manganese, phosphorus, potassium

Cofactors: adrenal exhaustion, aging dogs, anemia, anxiety, bile insufficiency, cognitive decline, constipation, dementia, diarrhea, excessive flatulence, gallbladder weakness, head trauma, IBD, insomnia, leaky gut, liver congestion, nausea, nervous pooping, nervousness, parasites, poor appetite, poor assimilation, poor circulation, protein sensitivity, PTSD, restlessness, spleen weakness, stomach discomfort, stomach spasm, stress, sympathetic excess, tension, trauma, ulcers

Flower essence: helpful for nervous pooping or peeing; helpful for agility work and training; helpful for developing trust with a new dog

Use for cats: yes

Applications

Gastrointestinal system: Bitter and carminative (warming and cooling), wood betony helps with food allergies and sensitivities, leaky gut, and gut trauma by stimulating secretions through the liver, pancreas, and stomach. It works with the gut-brain to release tension and support healthy vagus function.

Nervous system: Wood betony reduces nervous tension and sympathetic excess and helps calm your dog's nervous system, including the brain, which increases cerebral circulation. This herb is perfect for geriatric dogs with nervous system imbalances and waning cognitive function. It's good for those dogs who are hard to train or constantly (secretly) yelling "Squirrel!" It calms a low hum of anxiety and restlessness. I like to combine 50 percent wood betony, 35 percent milky oats, and 15 percent skullcap to make a nice, calming nervine formula for warm dogs.

Preparation and Dosing Schedule

	Extra-Small Dog	Small Dog	Medium Dog	Large Dog	Extra-Large Dog
Tincture	2 drops	2–3 drops	6 drops	8–10 drops	10–15 drops
Infusion	¼ teaspoon	½ teaspoon	1–2 teaspoons	1–2 tablespoons	3–6 tablespoons

Potential Concerns

Herb-drug interactions: none known

Cautions: Avoid wood betony with dry conditions (except for acute use). Can be mixed with moisturizing herbs for longer use.

Note: Wood betony is endangered in the wild; be sure to obtain it from ethically wildcrafted or cultivated sources.

🍂 Yarrow (*Achillea millefolium*)

Family: Asteraceae

Energetics: cool, balancing, stimulating

Energetic patterns indicating its use: warmth, coolness, cold, heat, tension, relaxation

Part used: leaf and flower

Long-term use: yes

Actions: alterative, antimicrobial, antiseptic, antispasmodic, astringent, bitter, diaphoretic, diuretic, emmenagogue, hemostatic, hypotensive, immune modulator, vulnerary

Constituents: alkaloids, alkamides, apigenin, azulene, bioflavonoids, borneol, caffeic acid, camphor, carotenoids, chamazulene, cineole, coumarins, fatty acids, flavonoids, furanocoumarins, inositol, limonene, linalool, luteolin, phenolic acids, polyacetylenes, rutin, salicylic acid, sesquiterpene lactones, succinic acid, tannins, thujone, volatile oil

Nutrients: choline, iron, magnesium, manganese, phosphorus, potassium, selenium, silicon, sodium, vitamins (A, B-complex, C, E, K), zinc

Cofactors: acute bruising, anal gland leakage, arthritis, bleeding anal glands, bleeding gums, blood in stool or urine, diarrhea (acute or chronic), dry and scaly skin, excessive menstrual bleeding, food sensitivities, high histamine levels, hot skin, hot stool, intestinal inflammation, itchiness, leaky gut from heat, pneumonia, poor appetite, systemic heat (in the cardiovascular, digestive, liver, lymphatic, respiratory, and urinary systems), UTI, UTI with blood

Flower essence: gives strength; for separation anxiety, anxiety, food sensitivities, and overwhelm; for EMF exposure; for dogs who sit in the corner at day care or who are empathetic

Use for cats: yes, but avoid the tincture

Applications

Gastrointestinal system: Yarrow is a multifaceted balancing herb that provides both stimulation and relaxation. It removes congestion in the portal vein, clearing the way for nutrition and detoxification. This helps move blood and fluid through the process of circulation, which is integral to good digestion. Use yarrow for hot dogs with leaky gut as yarrow helps with gut membrane permeability.

Kidneys: Antiseptic and stimulating, yarrow helps heal UTIs and reduce inflammation. It's especially good for hot, painful, and bloody urine. Yarrow excels at easing heat, redness, swelling, and sensitivity to touch.

Preparation and Dosing Schedule

	Extra-Small Dog	Small Dog	Medium Dog	Large Dog	Extra-Large Dog
Tincture	1–2 drops	2–4 drops	4–6 drops	6–8 drops	8–10 drops
Tincture for acute use	3 drops	6 drops	10 drops	12–15 drops	15–20 drops
Glycerite	4 drops	8 drops	12 drops	16 drops	20 drops
Infusion	¼ teaspoon	½ teaspoon	1–2 teaspoons	1–2 tablespoons	3–6 tablespoons

Potential Concerns

Herb-drug interactions: none known

Cautions: Give yarrow 2 hours away from any pharmaceuticals. May cause a reaction in dogs allergic to other members of the Asteraceae family.

🍂 Yellow Dock (*Rumex crispus*)

Family: Polygonaceae

Energetics: cool and dry

Energetic patterns indicating its use: warmth, heat, dampness, stagnation, relaxation

Part used: root

Long-term use: no, unless drop dosing

Actions: alterative, astringent, bitter, cholagogue, choleretic, digestive, laxative, lymphatic, nutritive, tonic

Constituents: 1,8-dihydroxy-3-methyl-9-anthrone, anthraquinones, bitters, brassidinic acid, calcium oxalate, chrysophanein, chrysophanic acid, chrysophanin, emodin, erucic acid, nepodin, oxalic acid, physcion, rheochrysin, rumicin, quinone, tannins

Nutrients: aluminum, calcium, cobalt, iron, magnesium, manganese, niacin, phosphorus, potassium, riboflavin, selenium, silicon, sodium, thiamine, tin, vitamins (A, B, C)

Cofactors: acid reflux, alternating constipation with diarrhea, anal itchiness, anemia, arthritis, congested anal glands, damp skin conditions, diarrhea, dry skin conditions, easily irritated anal glands, emotional and physical irritation, excessive saliva, heat in the digestive system, high histamine levels, high toxic load, hot diarrhea, hot spots, ill-formed stool, inability to finish bowel movement, itchiness, leaky anal glands, leaky gut, painful joints, poor assimilation, ravenous appetite, skin conditions, undigested food in stool, warm and itchy skin, white-coated tongue, yellow discharge from eyes, yellowish skin conditions

Use for cats: yes

Applications

Gastrointestinal system: Helps clear heat and tighten tissues for rapid transit through the colon. It is well indicated when dogs seem unable to poop completely or have ill-formed stool with heat. Yellow dock is balancing, as it can help with both constipation and diarrhea. It can help with acid reflux and excessive saliva production too.

Liver: Yellow dock contains glycosides that help protect liver function, stimulate detoxification, and increase bile production. It is indicated for dogs who are emotionally and physically irritated from heat.

Skin: Yellow dock helps with heat and itchiness when used externally as a rinse and internally.

Preparation and Dosing Schedule

	Extra-Small Dog	Small Dog	Medium Dog	Large Dog	Extra-Large Dog
Tincture	1 drop	2 drops	3 drops	4 drops	5 drops
Tincture for acute use	2 drops	4 drops	6 drops	8 drops	8–10 drops
Decoction	¼ teaspoon	½ teaspoon	1 teaspoon	2 tablespoons	3 tablespoons

Potential Concerns

Herb-drug interactions: antiarrhythmics, cardiac glycosides, diuretics, potassium-lowering drugs

Cautions: Avoid large doses, which can cause diarrhea, nausea, and vomiting. Avoid in cases of diabetes, gout, kidney stones, IBD, and intestinal bleeding. Use only drop doses; do *not* give in material dosages.

Medicinal Mushrooms

Mushrooms can be highly beneficial to your dog's diet and health as long as they are cooked or extracted. For nutritional purposes, you can gently cook and dehydrate mushrooms and make dried mushroom powders. For medicinal purposes, you'll want to purchase a powdered or liquid extract. Do your research when buying mushrooms; you'll want to use an organically grown or ethically wildcrafted source.

Extracts are predominantly extracted in hot water or in hot water and alcohol (double extraction). Some manufacturers triple extract (spagyric) their mushrooms by adding the plant's ashen salts back into the extraction, which is also appropriate for dogs. For dried powdered extracts, the alcohol is evaporated and the mushrooms and their extracted constituents are dried as a powder. For liquid extracts for dogs, the alcohol is evaporated and the mushrooms' extracted constituents are preserved with glycerine.

To access the water-soluble constituents of mushrooms, you can make a decoction at home, but make sure you simmer your mushrooms for at least 2–4 hours. For every cup of mushrooms, add 4 cups of water.

Below are introductory monographs about the mushrooms I mention in this book. Use them as a guide. ***Important:*** I've included supportive dosage recommendations—to be given twice daily. For mushroom powders in capsules, the minimal dosage is 200 mg for every 15 pounds of body weight. Mushroom dosages can fluctuate greatly depending on why you are using a specific mushroom or mushroom combination. For example, cancer and lipomas will need a much higher dose than those for general support.

⚞ Chaga (*Inonotus obliquus*)

Family: Hymenochaetaceae

Part used: canker

Energetics: neutral, dry

Energetic patterns indicating its use: warm to hot energetics, tension

Long-term use: yes

Actions: adaptogen, antiallergy, antibacterial, anticancer, anti-inflammatory, antioxidant, antiviral, immune modulator, tonic

Constituents: amino acids, antioxidants, betulin, beta-d-glucans, inotodiol (found only in chaga), lanosterol, lanostanes, melanin, phelligridin, polyphenols, triterpenes (many)*

Nutrients: calcium, copper, iron, magnesium, vitamins (A, C, D, E), zinc

Cofactors: anxiety, biofilm, cancer, digestive insufficiency, early aging, high cholesterol, high histamine levels, history of antibiotics use, IBD, IBS, inflammation, interdigital cysts (external), leaky gut, liver weakness, low immune function, mast cell cancer, mast cell tumors, papillomas, ulcers, warts

Use for cats: yes

Applications

Cough: Helps ward off viruses by modulating and supporting the immune system. Chaga stimulates cytokines that act as messenger relays when dogs cough or have kennel cough. It reduces inflammation and decreases pain.

Histamine: Chaga (as a hot water and alcohol extraction) is an important active mast cell tumor remedy. It's anti-inflammatory and immunomodulating, and its proven ability to stabilize systemic histamine response is impressive. Decreasing histamine can help decrease mast cell tumors, which are related to high histamine.

Warts: Chaga works with immune function to help break down the virus that causes warts and papillomas.

---

*The outer black part of the fungus contains more betulin, and the inner red part more lanostanes.

Preparation and Dosing Schedule

	Extra-Small Dog	Small Dog	Medium Dog	Large Dog	Extra-Large Dog
Extracted dried powder	1/16 teaspoon	1/8 teaspoon	1/4 teaspoon	1/2 teaspoon	3/4 teaspoon
Glycerite	0.5 ml per every 10 pounds of your dog's body weight, given before feeding				
Decoction	1/4 teaspoon	1/2 teaspoon	1–2 teaspoons	1–2 tablespoons	3–6 tablespoons

Potential Concerns

Herb-drug interactions: none

Cautions: Avoid using chaga with dogs prone to oxalate stones, or ask if the product/batch has been tested for oxalates.

. . . .

Tip! You sometimes see chaga products described as "full spectrum" chaga that purports to mix wild chaga fruiting body with lab-grown mycelium. This is deceitful marketing. Chaga is a parasite to a birch tree. Chaga doesn't have a fruiting body!

. . . .

⚹ Cordyceps (*Cordyceps militaris*)

Family: Cordycipitaceae

Energetics: warm to hot

Energetic patterns indicating its use: coolness, cold, false heat, tension

Part used: fruiting body

Long-term use: yes, if well indicated and under the supervision of a holistic vet or herbalist or as part of a balanced formula

Actions: adaptogenic, adrenal tonic, anti-inflammatory, antihistamine, antioxidant, antitumor, expectorant, immune modulator, immune stimulant

Constituents: adenine, adenosine, amino acids, antioxidants, beta-glucan, cordycepin (fruiting body only), D-mannitol, ergosterol, glutamic acid, histidine, palmitic acid, polysaccharides, proline, sterols, tyrosine, valine

Nutrients: iron, magnesium, selenium, vitamin B_{12}

Cofactors: adrenal depletion, arthritis, asthma, bloody cough, chronic fatigue, chronic loose stool, cold to cool energetics, endocrine disorders, fatty liver, hepatitis, infertility, inflammation, kennel cough, kidney weakness, leaky gut, low immune function, lung weakness, lupus, obesity, poor appetite, kidney failure, stress, thin stools, tumors, weakness
Use for cats: yes

Applications

Cancer: In nonestrogenic cancers, cordyceps helps promote apoptosis (cancer cell death) and helps prevent metastasis (cancer cell spread) and can be used during chemotherapy helping protect the kidneys and liver.

Gastrointestinal system: Cordyceps is good for cool dogs with leaky gut as it is anti-inflammatory and high in polysaccharides. Helps bring down inflammation in large intestine and supports a balanced histamine response.

Heart: Benefits the entire vascular system by regulating blood pressure, strengthening the heart muscle, and improving circulation. This helps improve blood flow to other organs like the liver and kidneys.

Immune system: Like most mushrooms, cordyceps is immunomodulating. It strengthens the immune system by increasing the number of NK (natural killer) cells, which defend the body against bacteria and viruses.

Kidneys: Restores kidney function after damage caused by toxicity; can be helpful in cases of kidney failure. Protect the kidneys and liver by improving blood flow, which helps defend against disease. Trophorestorative to the kidneys.

Liver: Increases glutathione and superoxide dismutase levels, reducing inflammatory oxidation. Can help decrease liver enzymes. Combined with burdock root, it helps reduce liver fat caused by eating a processed diet.

Lungs: Dilates the airways, increasing blood oxygen levels. Every cell is enriched by this process, enhancing energy levels and heightening cell function. It especially benefits dogs suffering from kennel cough, asthma, and bronchitis.

Nervous system: Relieves stress and helps activate parasympathetic activity, reducing inflammation and balancing hormones.

Preparation and Dosing Schedule

	Extra-Small Dog	Small Dog	Medium Dog	Large Dog	Extra-Large Dog
Extracted dried powder	¹⁄₁₆ teaspoon	⅛ teaspoon	¼ teaspoon	½ teaspoon	½–¾ teaspoon
Glycerite	I drop per pound of your dog's body weight				
Decoction	I teaspoon	I tablespoon	¼ cup	½ cup	I cup

Recommended use: Use the powder in combination with the glycerite for cold to deep cold conditions.

Potential Concerns

Herb-drug interactions: blood thinners, diabetes medications

Cautions: Cordyceps is warm to hot energetically and can deplete the adrenals if used long-term and without being well indicated. When using it for conditions with warm energetics, combine it with cooling herbs or mushrooms to help balance it out. Don't use in dogs with estrogen-based cancers. Can cause aggression, restlessness, agitation, and excessive humping or peeing. If any side effects occur, discontinue.

Note: *Cordyceps sinensis* is a popular species of cordyceps, but it grows inside the bat moth and is hard to source and expensive. *C. militaris* is cultivated cordyceps.

⚲ Lion's Mane (*Hericium erinaceus*)

Family: Hericiaceae

Energetics: neutral to cool, damp

Energetic patterns indicating its use: warm to hot and cool energetics, dryness, tension

Parts used: fruiting body and mycelium

Long-term use: yes

Actions: antibacterial, antifungal, anti-inflammatory, antimicrobial, antioxidant, antitumor, immune modulator, neuroprotective

Constituents: adenosine, beta-D-glucans, ergosterol (provitamin D2), cyathane derivatives, erinacines, hericenones, galactoxyloglucan, glucoxylan, mannoglucoxylan, nerve growth factor, oleanolic acids, oligosaccharides, protein, xylan

Nutrients: iron, manganese, niacin, potassium, riboflavin, thiamine, vitamin B_{12}, zinc

Cofactors: anxiety, bronchitis, dementia, flea and tick medications, gastric ulcers, gut inflammation, heart weakness, leaky gut, low immune function, Lyme disease and coinfections, muscle twitching, nerve damage, nervous conditions, nervousness, restlessness, sympathetic excess, yeast overgrowth

Use for cats: yes

Applications

Gastrointestinal system: Helps strengthen the intestinal lining and reduces inflammation in the gut.

Immune system: Contains five polysaccharides and polypeptides, making it a powerful immune enhancer and immune modulator. These anti-inflammatory substances help balance your dog's immune system by providing a high level of antioxidants, which mitigates oxidative stress.

Nervous system: Lion's mane has strong nerve-regenerating properties. The fruiting bodies protect and regenerate neuronal cells and help the body produce NGF (nerve growth factor), which is required for sensory neurons to function properly. The mycelium produces a substance called erinacines A that supports NGF synthesis. This is important in nerve injury, with special implications for brain injuries. Lion's mane also supports and strengthens the myelin sheath that coats nerves. Use the mycelium in combination with the fruiting body for serious nerve damage.

Preparation and Dosing Schedule

	Extra-Small Dog	Small Dog	Medium Dog	Large Dog	Extra-Large Dog
Extracted dried powder	1/16 teaspoon	1/8 teaspoon	1/4 teaspoon	1/2 teaspoon	3/4 teaspoon
Glycerite	5–6 drops	5–10 drops	10–20 drops	15–30 drops	20–35 drops
Decoction	1 teaspoon	1 tablespoon	1/4 cup	1/2 cup	1 cup

Potential Concerns

Herb-drug interactions: none

Cautions: Start out with a low dosage of this mushroom and slowly work your way up.

✄ Maitake (*Grifola frondosa*)

Family: Meripilaceae

Part used: fruiting body and mycelium

Energetics: neutral to cool

Energetic patterns indicating its use: warm to hot energetics, cool energetics, tension

Long-term use: yes

Actions: adaptogen, antiaging, antiallergy, antibacterial, anticancer, antidiabetic, anti-inflammatory, antimicrobial, antioxidant, antitumor, antiviral, chemoprotective, COX-1 and COX-2 inhibitors, hepatoprotective, immune boosting, immune modulator, tonic

Constituents: amino acids, antioxidants, beta-glucan, ergosterol, flavonoids, grifolan, lectins, phenolic acids, polysaccharides, triterpenes

Nutrients: fiber, magnesium, manganese, phosphorus, potassium, protein, selenium, vitamins (C, D, B_1, B_2, B_3, B_5, B_6), zinc

Cofactors: anal gland congestion, anxiety, arthritis, antibiotic use, autoimmune disorders, cancer, cognitive decline, dementia, depression, diabetes, dry lungs, fever, heart weakness, hepatitis, high blood pressure, high cholesterol, lipoma, low circulation, liver weakness, lung weakness, lymphoma, mammary cancer, nervous system conditions, obesity, pain, restlessness, spleen weakness, stress, stomach weakness, tumors

Use for cats: yes

Applications

Gastrointestinal system: Maitake mushroom supports microbiome diversity after antibiotic usage, which is key for systemic recovery.

Heart: Maitake supports the cardiac system by increasing circulation and strengthening the cardiac muscle, bringing down blood pressure and helping to regulate blood flow.

Lymphatic system: Increases circulation, which is key for lymphatic drainage and supporting the liver. Mix maitake with turkey tail to help dogs with lipomas. Combined, they help with heat and stagnation in the liver and help with detoxification of fat soluble toxins.

Preparation and Dosing Schedule

	Extra-Small Dog	Small Dog	Medium Dog	Large Dog	Extra-Large Dog
Extracted dried powder	¹⁄₁₆ teaspoon	⅛ teaspoon	¼ teaspoon	½ teaspoon	¾ teaspoon
Glycerite	0.5 ml per every 10 pounds of your dog's body weight, given before feeding				
Decoction	¼ teaspoon	½ teaspoon	1–2 teaspoons	1–2 tablespoons	3–6 tablespoons

Potential Concerns

Herb-drug interactions: blood thinners, diabetes medications

Cautions: none known

◣ Poria (*Poria cocos, Wolfiporia extensa*)

Family: Polyporaceae

Part used: sclerotium

Energetics: neutral to cool, dry

Energetic patterns indicating its use: warm to hot energetics, cool energetics, dampness

Long-term use: yes

Actions: antiallergy, anticancer, anti-inflammatory, antifungal, antioxidant, antiparasitic, antiseptic, anti-tumor, antiviral, diuretic, immune modulator, sedative, synergistic, tonic

Constituents: beta-glucan, caprylic acid, enzymes, fatty acids, fiber, lauric acid, pachymaran, heteropolysaccharides, polysaccharides, sterols, triterpenes, undecanoic acid

Nutrients: calcium, copper, iron, magnesium, manganese, niacin, protein, vitamin B2, zinc

Cofactors: antibiotic use, anxiety, biting paws, cancer, candida, colitis, dementia, dermatitis, diarrhea, digestive upset, digestive weakness, dizziness, edema, food sensitivities, gastritis, heart palpitations, heart weakness, hyperpigmentation, immune weakness, incontinence, interdigital cysts, insomnia, kidney inflammation and weakness, leaky gut, lymphatic stagnation, melanoma, nausea, nervous conditions, paw edema and swelling, restlessness, ringworm, skin tumors, spleen weakness, stress, swellings, vomiting, worms, yeast

Use for cats: yes

Applications

Gastrointestinal system: Bringing down inflammation in the gut is key to healing your dog's gut lining and decreasing permeability and food sensitivities. Poria mushroom helps decrease inflammation, increase digestive secretions, and improve immune function in the gut.

Lymphatic system: Lymphatic stimulation and flow is a key component to your dog's health. Poria is a stimulant that supports lymphatic circulation, which makes it a great addition to any successful lipoma protocol.

Paws: Poria mushroom is an effective, systemic anti-inflammatory with an affinity toward the extremities and paws. It is great for licking, biting, and swellings affecting your dog's feet, including interdigital cysts.

Preparation and Dosing Schedule

	Extra-Small Dog	Small Dog	Medium Dog	Large Dog	Extra-Large Dog
Extracted dried powder	1/16 teaspoon	1/8 teaspoon	1/4 teaspoon	1/2 teaspoon	3/4 teaspoon
Glycerite	0.5 ml per every 10 pounds of your dog's body weight, given before feeding				

Potential Concerns

Herb-drug interactions: sedatives, benzodiazepines
Cautions: none known

⚑ Reishi (*Ganoderma lucidum*)

Family: Ganodermataceae
Energetics: slightly warm, damp (but dry long term)
Energetic patterns indicating its use: cold, coolness, dampness, relaxation
Parts used: fruiting body and mycelium
Long-term use: yes
Actions: adaptogen, antibacterial, antifungal, antihistamine, antioxidant, antiviral, astringent, bitter, hepatodetoxifier, hepatoprotective, immune modulator
Constituents: amino acids, beta-glucan, beta-lactone, glucuronoglucan, ergone, ganoderans, ganoderenic acid, ling zhi-8, polysaccharides, triterpenes

Nutrients: calcium, copper, germanium, iron, manganese, riboflavin, vitamins B_2 and C, zinc

Cofactors: acid reflux, adrenal depletion, allergies, arthritis, asthma, autoimmune disease, bronchitis, deficiency, early aging, high blood pressure, high blood sugar, high liver enzymes, histamine excess, immune weakness, insomnia, kidney coldness, kidney weakness, lethargy, lipomas, liver weakness, low vagal tone, lung afflictions, lung weakness, mast cell tumor, muscle spasm, nerve pain, pathogens, restlessness, respiratory imbalance, stress, sympathetic excess, unbalanced hormones (in unspayed females), UTIs, warts

Use for cats: yes

Applications

Heart: Helps increase circulation and lower blood pressure. Improves overall heart function. Through its influence on the autonomic nervous system, it can help the heartbeat more quickly return to a normal rate after a sympathetic episode.

Immune: Reishi helps build and modulate the immune system, reducing autoimmune excess, reactivity, and systemic inflammation. It helps balance hormones, mitigate autoimmune conditions, and calm the nervous system, relieving tension.

Kidneys: Decreases inflammation; detoxifies and strengthens kidney tissues.

Liver: Reishi increases glutathione production, which reduces inflammatory oxidation. It helps lower liver enzymes and balances hormones, histamine, food sensitivities, and "allergic" reactions. This helps with conditions like leaky gut, lipomas, and gastrointestinal distress.

Lungs: Helps stop coughing and increases a dog's ability to absorb oxygen. In chronic lung conditions, it helps reduce and calm spasm, strengthen lung capacity, and modulate the immune system helping improve overall lung health.

Nervous System: Reishi addresses the parasympathetic nervous system and helps keep it balanced so that organs can function properly; especially helpful for liver detoxification.

Preparation and Dosing Schedule

	Extra-Small Dog	Small Dog	Medium Dog	Large Dog	Extra-Large Dog
Extracted dried powder	1/16 teaspoon	1/8 teaspoon	1/4 teaspoon	1/2 teaspoon	3/4 teaspoon
Glycerite	6–8 drops	10–15 drops	15–20 drops	20–30 drops	30–60 drops
Decoction	1 teaspoon	1 tablespoon	1/4 cup	1/2 cup	1 cup

. . . .

Tip! Reishi mushroom is bitter, and many dogs don't enjoy the taste. Give it as a glycerite, in capsules, or mixed with food.

. . . .

Potential Concerns
Herb-drug interactions: anticoagulants, antiplatelet drugs
Cautions: Can be drying long-term.

🌿 Tremella (*Tremella fuciformis*)
Family: Tremellaceae
Part used: fruiting body
Energetics: neutral to cool and damp
Energetic patterns indicating its use: warm to hot energetics, dryness, tension
Long-term use: yes
Actions: antiaging, anti-inflammatory, antioxidant, antitumor, hepatoprotective, immune modulator, mild laxative, neuroprotective, vulnerary; stimulates the production of SOD (superoxide dismutase) in the brain and liver
Constituents: beta-glucan, ergosterol, ergosta-5,7-dien-3ß-ol, ergosta-7-en-3ß-ol, fatty acids, flavonoids, galactose, glycoprotein, glycuronic acid, lauric acid, linoleic acid, mannose, myristic acid, oleic acid, palmitic acid, palmitoleic acid, pentadecanoic acid, phosphatidylethanolamine, phosphatidylcholine, phosphatidyl glycerol, phosphatidylserine, phosphatidylinositol, polysaccharides, stearic acid, tridecanoic acid, undecanoic acid, xylose

Nutrients: calcium, copper, fiber, folate, iron, magnesium, potassium, protein, vitamins (B_1, B_2, B_6, D), zinc

Cofactors: acid reflux, arthritis, asthma, bladder stones, chronic lung conditions, cognitive decline, dementia, dermatitis, dry cough, dry skin, dryness, constipation, kidney dryness, gastrointestinal heat, heat in the lungs, heart weakness, high blood sugar, high cholesterol, high triglycerides, inflammation, leaky gut, low circulation, low white/red blood cells, lung inflammation, musculoskeletal weakness, nervousness, trauma, stress, stiffness, ulcers, urinary tract infection, x-rays

Use for cats: yes

Applications

Gastrointestinal system: Tremella mushroom is a demulcent that adds mucilage to the entire gastrointestinal tract. It can help protect and heal your dog's gut lining and decrease intestinal permeability, which helps decrease food sensitivities, itching, and scratching.

Kidneys: You can mix tremella and reishi mushroom if your dog has a urinary tract infection. Tremella will soothe the tract and bring down irritation while it works with reishi to help modulate the immune system and stregthen and balance the renal system.

Musculoskeletal system: Dryness is one of the tissue states that can aggravate arthritis and especially painful, stiff joints that crack. Tremella adds moisture to your dog's musculoskeletal system, helping improve mobility.

Preparation and Dosing Schedule

	Extra-Small Dog	Small Dog	Medium Dog	Large Dog	Extra-Large Dog
Extracted dried powder	1/16 teaspoon	1/8 teaspoon	1/4 teaspoon	1/2 teaspoon	3/4 teaspoon
Glycerite	0.5 ml per every 10 pounds of your dog's body weight, given before feeding				
Decoction	1/4 teaspoon	1/2 teaspoon	1–2 teaspoons	1–2 tablespoons	3–6 tablespoons

Potential Concerns

Herb-drug interactions: none known

Cautions: not for damp conditions

✕ Turkey Tail (*Trametes versicolor*)

Family: Polyporaceae

Energetics: neutral, dry

Energetic patterns indicating its use: warm and cool energetics, dampness

Parts used: fruiting body and mycelium

Long-term use: yes

Actions: antibacterial, antihistamine, anti-inflammatory, antimicrobial, antioxidant, antitumor, antiviral, immune modulator

Constituents: beta-glucan, beta-sitosterol, cerevisterol, ergosterol, ergosta-7, fungisterol, lipids, polysaccharides, polysaccharide-K, sterols, polysaccharide peptide, triterpenoids

Nutrients: protein, selenium, vitamins B_3 and D

Cofactors: allergies, antibiotic use, arthritis, asthma, autoimmune diseases, cancer, candida overgrowth, chemotherapy, coughing, fatty liver, high histamine levels, itchiness, leaky gut, lipomas, low immune function, lung weakness, mast cell tumor, papillomas, poor appetite, radiation exposure, scratching, surgery, tumors, UTIs, warts, weakness

Use for cats: yes

Applications

Gastrointestinal system: In the gut, turkey tail modulates the immune system, helps clear dampness, and reduces symptoms of leaky gut, diarrhea, high histamine levels, and food sensitivities. It acts as a prebiotic, helping to balance the microbiome. Turkey tail is high in polysaccharides that support the gut mucosa, which can help heal leaky gut.

Liver: Turkey tails are a good source of antioxidants, which can reduce overall oxidation in the body and relieve the load on the liver. It also reduces liver enzymes, helping support healthy phase 1 and phase 2 detoxification pathways. This process makes them anticancer and antitumor, helping decrease lipoma formation and preventing new lipomas. I recommend turkey tail mushrooms as part of an overall lipoma reduction program; you need higher dosages of this mushroom for this purpose.

Preparation and Dosing Schedule

	Extra-Small Dog	Small Dog	Medium Dog	Large Dog	Extra-Large Dog
Extracted dried powder	¹⁄₁₆ teaspoon	⅛ teaspoon	¼ teaspoon	½ teaspoon	¾ teaspoon
Glycerite	0.5 ml per every 10 pounds of your dog's body weight, given before feeding				
Decoction	1 teaspoon	1 tablespoon	¼ cup	½ cup	1 cup

Potential Concerns

Herb-drug interactions: none known

Cautions: Can cause digestive upset in some dogs. If this happens, give with more food, decrease the dosage, or discontinue.

Phytoembryonics

Below are monographs of the phytoembryonic herbal remedies that I find most useful. As far as energetics goes, these remedies are more flexible and balancing. All of them can be used acutely. These types of remedies are at the forefront of research-based herbal medicine; their language and use continue to unfold.

For the purpose of clarity and comparison in the monographs below, phytoembryonic pertains to the mother tincture of the buds, young tissues, seeds, barks and rootlets of a plant. Gemmotherapy refers to the diluted mother tincture to a D1 (1:200) homeopathic potency. In commerce, both of these remedies belong under the blanket term "gemmotherapy."

For dosing, start out administering once daily, work slowly up to suggested dosage. See how your dog does with one dose, then you can add a second daily dose. For maximum results, mix remedies with water for taste and syringe into the mouth. You can also drip on a treat or put in food.

🌥 Beech (*Fagus sylvatica*)

Energetics: slightly warm to neutral, dry

Energetic patterns indicating its use: cool to warm energetics, dampness

Part used: bud

Long-term use: yes

Actions: antibacterial, anti-inflammatory, antihistamine, antioxidant, antiviral, antiyeast

Constituents: amino acids (alanine, cysteine, glutamine), betulin, epicatechin, coumaric acid, flavanone, glutathione, glycosides, hydroxyproline, hydroxybenzoic acid, para-cymene and cis-ocimene, polysaccharides, propolis, sabinene, salicortin, tannins, and vanillin.

Nutrients: barium, calcium, choline, gold, iron, manganese, magnesium, nickel, potassium, sodium, vitamins (C, D, E), zinc

Cofactors: antibiotics use, candida overgrowth, chronic viral infections, *E. coli* infections, emotional sensitivity, feline AIDS, food sensitivities, grief, gut sensitivity, high histamine levels, high uric acid levels, kidney weakness, leaky gut, liver weakness, low enzyme production, low IgA levels, low immune function, low immunoglobulin levels, low kidney function, UTIs, yeast overgrowth

Use for cats: yes; use gemmotherapy

Dosing Schedule

	Extra-Small Dog	Small Dog	Medium Dog	Large Dog	Extra-Large Dog
Phytoembryonic	I drop	2 drops	3 drops	4 drops	5 drops
Gemmotherapy	4 drops	8 drops	9 drops	12 drops	15 drops

Potential Concerns

Herb-drug interactions: none
Cautions: none

⚐ Black Currant (*Ribes nigrum*)

Energetics: warm and dry; can be used acutely or topically for all energetic patterns

Energetic patterns indicating its use: cool to cold energetics, dampness

Part used: bud

Long-term use: yes

Actions: adaptogenic, antiaging, anti-allergy, anti-anemic, antihistamine, anti-inflammatory, antimicrobial, antioxidant, anti-thrombotic, blood detoxifier, chemoprotective, COX-2 inhibitor, diuretic, natural cortisone

Constituents: amino acids (glutamine, proine, serine, threonine, valine) citric acid, citronellol, flavonoids, gamma-linolenic-acid, limonene, linalool, linoleic acid, lutein, pectin, polyphenols, quercetin, terpinene

Nutrients: biotin, boron, calcium, chromium, copper, iron, manganese, magnesium, niacin, nickel, phosphorus, potassium, quercetin, selenium, silicon, silver, sodium, sulfur, thiamine, vitamins (B_1, B_2, B_3, B_{12}, C, E), zinc

Cofactors: Addison's disease, allergies, allergy to pharmaceuticals, anaphylactic shock, ankylosing spondylitis, antibiotics recovery, anxiety, arthritis, asthma, autoimmune diseases, broken bones, burns, CCL tears, chronic pancreatitis, conjunctivitis, dry eyes, dryness, ear-nose-throat conditions, flea allergy, gastritis, heartworm, high blood pressure, high cholesterol, hives, inflammation, inflamed joints, inflamed ligaments and tendons, inflamed mucous membranes, itchiness, itchiness due to detoxification, kennel cough, lethargy, low adrenal function, low immunity, low pituitary function, mast cell tumor, osteoporosis, poor appetite, poor circulation, rabies vaccine, restlessness, steroid damage, vaccine damage, worms

Use for cats: yes

Dosing Schedule

	Extra-Small Dog	Small Dog	Medium Dog	Large Dog	Extra-Large Dog
Phytoembryonic	1 drop	2 drops	3 drops	4 drops	5 drops
Gemmotherapy	4 drops	8 drops	9 drops	12 drops	15 drops

Potential Concerns

Herb-drug interactions: steroids

Cautions: Avoid use in dogs that have seizures, as it's stimulating. Avoid in cases of high cortisol levels.

✄ Bramble (*Rubus fruticosus*)

Energetics: cool and slightly dry

Energetic patterns indicating its use: warm to hot energetics

Part used: young shoot

Long-term use: yes

Actions: analgesic, antibacterial, anti-inflammatory, antioxidant, antisclerotic, astringent, balancing, hemostatic

Constituents: anthocyanin, arbutin, ascorbic acid, beta-amyrin, beta-carotene, carotenoids, chlorogenic acid, cyanidin-3-glucoside, ellagic acid, ferulic acid, lutein, hydroquinone, lactic acid, malic acid, neochlorogenic acid, quercetin, stigmasterol, succinic acid, tannin, urosilic acid, zeaxanthin

Nutrients: calcium, copper, inositol, iron, magnesium, manganese, nickel, phosphorus, selenium, tin, vitamin B-complex and C, zinc

Cofactors: ankylosing spondyloarthritis, arthritic pain, arthritis, decalcification, diarrhea, endometriosis, fibromyalgia, food sensitivities, gastritis, gastrointestinal weakness, general pain, geriatric raw feeding, joint pain, knee pain, loose stool, lung inflammation, lung weakness, mouth inflammation, musculoskeletal weakness, osteoporosis, spinal weakness, stomatitis, uterine conditions

Use for cats: no

Dosing Schedule

	Extra-Small Dog	Small Dog	Medium Dog	Large Dog	Extra-Large Dog
Phytoembryonic	1 drop	2 drops	3 drops	4 drops	5 drops
Gemmotherapy	3–4 drops	4–6 drops	6–8 drops	8–10 drops	10–15 drops

Potential Concerns

Herb-drug interactions: none
Cautions: none

⚔ Cowberry (*Vaccinium vitis-idaea*)

Energetics: warm and slightly dry
Energetic patterns indicating its use: cool to cold energetics
Part used: young shoot
Long-term use: yes
Actions: antibacterial, anti-inflammatory, antioxidant, antispasmodic
Constituents: arbutin, ascorbic acid, avicularin, benzoic acid, beta-carotene, neochlorogenic, caffeic acid, chlorogenic acid, cinnamic acid, carbohydrate ester, citric acid, cyanidin, epicatechin, ericolin, fructose,

glucose, hyperoside, isoquercitrin, kaempferol, lycopene, malic acid, organogermanium, pectin, phytoestrogen, quercetin, salidroside, tyrosol, zeaxanthin

Nutrients: calcium, copper, chromium, boron, iron, magnesium, manganese, phosphorus, potassium, selenium, silicon, sodium, sulphur, titanium, vitamins C and K, zinc

Cofactors: antibiotics use, arthritis, bladder infections, bladder inflammation, bladder stones, bladder toxicity, chronic constipation, constipation, diarrhea from antibiotics use, female osteoporosis (helps calcium absorption in the gut), food sensitivities, *Helicobacter pylori* infection, IBD, incontinence from being spayed, inflammation, interstitial cystitis, irregular menstrual cycle, leaky gut, low ocular circulation, lung spasm, mucosa damage, nephritis, oxalate and calcium stones, parvo, parvo vaccine, periodontal disease, poor eyesight, poor night vision, pyometra, rapid transit of food through the colon, spleen weakness, thyroid adenoma, UTIs

Use for cats: yes; use gemmotherapy

Dosing Schedule

	Extra-Small Dog	Small Dog	Medium Dog	Large Dog	Extra-Large Dog
Phytoembryonic	1 drop	2 drops	3 drops	4 drops	5 drops
Gemmotherapy	3–4 drops	4–6 drops	6–8 drops	8–10 drops	10–15 drops

Potential Concerns

Herb-drug interactions: none

Cautions: avoid in estrogen-positive cancers

⚕ Fig (*Ficus carica*)

Energetics: neutral

Energetic patterns indicating its use: relaxation and excessive tension (balancing)

Part used: bud

Long-term use: yes

Actions: antibacterial, antiemetic, antifungal, anti-inflammatory, antimicrobial, antioxidant, antiviral, autoimmune, hepatoprotective

Constituents: amino acids (alanine, arginine, cystine, glycine, histidine, isoleucine, leucine, lysine, methionine, phenylalanine, serine, threonine, tyrosine, valine), ascorbic acid, aspartic acid, bergapten, beta-amyrin, beta-carotene, beta-sitosterol, caffeic acid, citric acid, cystine, ferulic acid, fiber, ficin, fructose, fumaric acid, glucose, glutamic acid, guaia-zulene, kaempferol, linoleic acid, lipase, lupeol, lutein, malic acid, muci-lage, myristic acid, oleic acid, palmitic acid, pectin, psoralen, quercetin, quinic acid, rutin, stearic acid, stigmasterol, succinic acid, sucrose, tryp-tophan, xanthotoxin, xanthotoxol, xylose

Nutrients: calcium, copper, barium, boron, magnesium, phosphorus, potas-sium, vitamins (B_1, B_2, B_3, B_5, B_6, C, E), zinc

Cofactors: acid reflux, anxiety, autoimmune diseases, burping, congested liver, damaged mucous membranes, diarrhea, digestive insufficiency, digestive upset, emotional reactivity, endocrine disorders, esophageal disorders, excessive gas, enzyme insufficiency, IBD, IBS, inflammation, leaky gut, low vagal tone, megaesophagus, microbiome damage, motion sickness, nervous pooping, nervous stomach, obsessive behavior, parvo, parvo vaccination, poor appetite, rabies vaccination with aggression, restlessness, stress, sympathetic excess, vomiting

Use for cats: yes; use gemmotherapy

Dosing Schedule

	Extra-Small Dog	Small Dog	Medium Dog	Large Dog	Extra-Large Dog
Phytoembryonic	1–2 drops	2–3 drops	3–4 drops	4–5 drops	4–8 drops
Gemmotherapy	3 drops	6 drops	8 drops	10 drops	15 drops

Potential Concerns

Herb-drug interactions: none

Cautions: If your dog experiences any stomach upset, cut back on the dosage.

⚞ Heather (*Calluna vulgaris*)

Energetics: neutral

Energetic patterns indicating its use: dampness

Part used: young shoot

Long-term use: yes

Actions: antibacterial, anti-inflammatory, anticancer, antioxidant, antitumor, antiseptic, antiviral, diuretic

Constituents: apigenin, arbutasa, arbutin, anthocyanidins, caffeic acid derivatives, chlorogenic acid, coumarins, citric acid, escopoletol, esculetol, flavonoids, friedelin, fumaric acid, glucosides, hydroquinones, hydroxycinnamic acid, isoquercetrin, kaempferol, luteolin, methylarbutin, organic acids, phenolic acids, phenols and their glycosides, proanthocyanidins, quercetin, rutin, steroids, tannins, taraxasterol and taraxerone, triterpenes, terpenoids

Nutrients: vitamins C and E

Cofactors: arthritis, autoimmune diseases, bladder cancer, bladder gravel, bladder weakness, bleeding gums, CCL tears, fear, cystitis, gallbladder weakness, gastrointestinal inflammation, gum inflammation, incontinence (not hormone related), joint pain, kidney disease, kidney stones, kidney weakness, leaky gut, mammary tumors, obesity, poor microbiome health, rheumatoid arthritis, sensitivity to noises, trauma, tumors, UTIs, warts, weak joints, weak teeth

Use for cats: yes

Dosing Schedule

	Extra-Small Dog	Small Dog	Medium Dog	Large Dog	Extra-Large Dog
Phytoembryonic	1 drop	2 drops	3 drops	4 drops	5 drops
Gemmotherapy	2–3 drops	4–6 drops	6–8 drops	8–10 drops	10–15 drops

Potential Concerns

Herb-drug interactions: none

Cautions: none

⚹ Horsetail (*Equisetum arvense*)

Energetics: neutral, slightly damp

Energetic patterns indicating its use: dryness, relaxation

Part used: young shoot

Long-term use: yes
Actions: antispasmodic, diuretic, hemostatic
Constituents: aconitic acid, ascorbic acid, beta-carotene, beta-sitosterol, caffeic acid, campesterol, cholesterol, equicetrin, equistetolic acid, ferulic acid, fiber, flavonoids, florigen, gallic acid, isofucosterol, isoquercitrin, isoquercitroside, kaempferol, linoleic acid, luteolin, malic acid, methylsulfonylmethane (msm), naringenin, nicotine, oleic acid, palustrine alkaloid, palustrinine alkaloid, paba, saponins, silicic acid, silicates, tannins, tannic acid, thiaminase, vanillic acid
Nutrients: calcium, copper, iron, magnesium, manganese, phosphorus, potassium, selenium, silica, tin, vitamins (B_2, B_2, B_3, C), zinc
Cofactors: anal fissures, anal growths, bleeding, bone loss, bone loss in the mouth, brittle nails, broken bones, bronchitis, burping, CCL tears, conjunctivitis, cystitis, damaged cartilage, edema, enlarged prostate, gout, hair loss, hairline fractures, hot spots, incontinence (all types), incontinence in puppies and young dogs, irritable bladder, leaky gut, low calcium levels, musculoskeletal weakness, nose bleeds, skin growths, stomatitis, UTIs, weak connective tissues, weak teeth
Note: Horsetail phytoembryonic is collagen-stimulating and a calcium stabilizer.
Use for cats: yes

Dosing Schedule

	Extra-Small Dog	Small Dog	Medium Dog	Large Dog	Extra-Large Dog
Phytoembryonic	1 drop	2 drops	3 drops	4 drops	5 drops

Potential Concerns

Herb-drug interactions: digitalis, digoxin, lithium
Cautions: The phytoembryonic remedy provides a lower risk of thiamine deficiency compared to mature horsetail, but some risk still exists. Signs of low thiamine include dragging of extremities, difficulty walking, decline of muscle coordination, confusion, and dementia. Don't use in high doses or for longer than 3 months. Don't mix with hawthorn. Horsetail is a diuretic and can cause excessive potassium loss.

⚹ Mountain Pine (*Pinus montana*)

Energetics: neutral to cool, slightly damp

Energetic patterns indicating its use: tension

Part used: bud

Long-term use: yes

Actions: analgesic, anti-allergic, antibacterial, antihistamine, anti-inflammatory, antioxidant, antipyretic, antiseptic, antispasmodic, antitumor, and antiviral

Constituents: adenine, alpha-carotene, alpha-phellandrene, alpha-pinene, alpha-terpinene, anisaldehyde, ascorbic acid, beta-carotene, beta-myrcene, beta-phellandrene, beta-pinene, beta-sitosterol, borneol, bornyl-acetate, butyric acid, campesterol, camphene, capric acid, caryophyllene, chamazulene, citral, d-limonene, dehydroabietane, dehydroabietic acid, delta-3-carene, delta-cadinene, dihydroquercetin, dipentene, epicatechin, estragole, eugenol-methyl-ether, enzogenol, fructose, furfural, germanium, limonene, lutein, phenol, pinitol, pinocembrin, pinosylvin, protocatechuic acid, epicatechin, quercetin, quinic acid, sabinene, shikimic acid, sucrose, tannin, terpineol, testosterone, vanillic acid, xylose

Nutrients: choline, copper, iron, magnesium, manganese, potassium, silicon, vitamin C

Cofactors: broken bones, CCL tears, high cholesterol, high histamine levels, high levels of heavy metals, high toxic load, hip dysplasia, hip and knee deformities, IBS, kidney weakness, liver weakness, low sperm motility, low testosterone levels, low vagal tone, mast cell cancer, muscle twitching, musculoskeletal damage (cartilage, ligaments, tendons, and bones), slow lymph drainage, spinal weakness, sympathetic excess

Note: Mountain pine phytoembryonic is a strong anti-inflammatory and pain reliever.

Use for cats: yes

Dosing Schedule

	Extra-Small Dog	Small Dog	Medium Dog	Large Dog	Extra-Large Dog
Phytoembryonic	1–2 drops	2–3 drops	3–6 drops	4–8 drops	6–12 drops
Gemmotherapy	4 drops	6 drops	8 drops	12 drops	12–15 drops

Potential Concerns

Herb-drug interactions: Vetprofen

Cautions: Can be stimulating and can affect sleep in some dogs (and people). Don't give within 2 hours of bedtime.

🌿 Olive (*Olea europaea*)

Energetics: neutral to warm, slightly dry

Energetic patterns indicating its use: dampness

Part used: bud

Long-term use: yes

Actions: antibacterial, antiestrogenic, antisclerotic, antimicrobial, antiviral, anti-yeast

Constituent: alpha-tocopherol, antiestrogenic (acetoside), apigenin, beta-carotene, beta-sitosterol, caffeic acid, calcium, catechin, cinchonine alkaloid, esculetin, esculin, estrone estrogenic, fiber, fructose, glucose, kaempferol, linoleic acid, luteolin, mannitol, myristic acid, oleanolic acid, oleic acid, oleocanthal, oleuropein, palmitic acid, pectin, protocatechuic acid, quercetin, rutin, squalene, stearic acid, tannins

Nutrients: boron, calcium, choline, copper, estrone, fiber, iron, phosphorus, magnesium, manganese, phosphorus, potassium, silicon, sodium, vitamin E

Cofactors: artery deposits bacterial overgrowth, bladder infections, colon inflammation, constipation, fear, heartworm, *Helicobacter pylori* infection, high cholesterol, high nitric oxide, high triglycerides, IBD, leaky gut, Lyme and its co-infections (all types), necrotic tissue, parasitic overgrowth, poor circulation, senility, severe infection, tachycardia, worms, yeast overgrowth

Use for cats: yes

Dosing Schedule

	Extra-Small Dog	Small Dog	Medium Dog	Large Dog	Extra-Large Dog
Phytoembryonic	1–2 drops	2–3 drops	3–5 drops	4–7 drops	6–8 drops
Gemmotherapy	1–4 drops	3–6 drops	4–8 drops	6–12 drops	8–15 drops

Potential Concerns
Herb-drug interactions: none
Cautions: none
Note: Phytoembryonic olive can be used together with an herbal olive leaf remedy. If use of an herbal olive leaf remedy causes nausea or vomiting, use the phytoembryonic alone.

⚔ Walnut (*Juglans regia*)

Energetics: neutral to cool, slightly damp
Energetic patterns indicating its use: warm energetics, dryness, balancing
Part used: bud
Long-term use: yes
Actions: antibiotic, antifungal, anti-inflammatory, anti-infectious, antimycobacterial, antiparasitic, antiviral, prebiotic, probiotic
Constituents: amino acids (arginine, adenosine), alpha-tocopherol, ascorbic acid, avicularin, beta-carotene, beta-sitosterol, campesterol, delta-tocopherol, ellagic acid, fiber, gamma lactones, gamma-tocopherol, juglandin, juglandic acid, juglone, alpha-hydrojuglone, glycoside beta-hydrojuglone, bisjuglone, trijuglone, polyunsaturated fatty acids, alpha linolenic acid, methyl palmitate, lutein, melatonin, molybdenum, myricetin, myricitrin, oleic acid, palmitic acid, polyamines, polyphenols, progesterone, quercetin, serotonin, stearic acid, sterols, stigmasterol, zeaxanthin
Nutrients: boron, chlorine, chromium, copper, gold, iodine, iron, beta-sitosterol, boron, chlorine, chromium, copper, gold, iodine, iron, magnesium, manganese, nickel, phosphorus, potassium, selenium, sodium, vitamins C and E, zinc
Cofactors: antibiotics use, arthritis, bacterial infections, bronchitis, candidiasis, chronic pancreatitis, chronic UTI, collapsed trachea, constipation, dry skin conditions, excessive gas, gastrointestinal distress, giardiasis, hypothyroidism, inflammatory skin conditions, leaky gut, low immune function, painful diarrhea, poor absorption, poor assimilation, streptococcus or staphylococcus infections, imbalanced microbiome, yeast infection
Use for cats: yes

Dosing Schedule

	Extra-Small Dog	Small Dog	Medium Dog	Large Dog	Extra-Large Dog
Phytoembryonic	1 diluted drop	1–2 drops	2–3 drops	3 drops	4 drops
Gemmotherapy	1–2 drops	3–4 drops	5–6 drops	7–8 drops	9–10 drops

Potential Concerns

Herb-drug interactions: none

Cautions: Can cause yeast die-off reactions if given at too high a dosage too soon; if symptoms occur, give every other day. Avoid in horses.

⚲ Willow (*Salix alba*)

Energetics: neutral, dry

Energetic patterns indicating its use: dampness

Part used: bud

Long-term use: yes

Actions: analgesic, anticoagulant (*mild*), anti-inflammatory, antiseptic, astringent, diuretic, inflammation modulating, pain reliever, sedative, and tonic

Constituent: apigenin, ascorbic-acid, beta-carotene, catechin, cellulose, cyanidin, fiber, fragilin, gallic acid, glucomannan, glucose, isoquercitrin, isosalicin, isosalipurposide, lignin, quercetin, rutin, salicin, salicortin, salicoylsalicin, salidroside, saligenin, salipurposide, starch, tannin, tremulacin, triandrin, xylose

Nutrients: chromium, iron, magnesium, manganese, phosphorus, potassium, selenium, thallium, zinc

Cofactors: acne, anal tumors, antibiotics use, arthritis, back-end weakness, candidiasis, colon cancer, dandruff, dry growths, early aging, fungal infections, hair loss, heart weakness, high blood pressure, high levels of heavy metals, IBD, joint weakness, localized inflammation, low immune function, low testosterone levels, lymphatic stagnation, mammary cancer, osteoarthritis, pain, pathogenic overgrowth in the gut, poor circulation, rough paw pads, SIBO, stomach cancer, systemic inflammation, tension, upper respiratory infections, warts, yeast infection

Use for cats: no

Dosing Schedule

	Extra-Small Dog	Small Dog	Medium Dog	Large Dog	Extra-Large Dog
Phytoembryonic	1–2 drops	2–3 drops	3–4 drops	4–5 drops	5–6 drops
Gemmotherapy	4 drops	6 drops	8 drops	8–10 drops	10–12 drops

Potential Concerns

Herb-drug interactions: anti-inflammatories, aspirin, clopidogrel, heparin, methotrexate, metoclopramide, pentoxifylline, phenytoin, potassium-sparing diuretics, probenecid, seizure medications, spironolactone, spironolactone, sulfonamide drugs, ticlopidine, valproate, warfarin

Cautions: Do not use in dogs with an aspirin allergy, bleeding disorder, kidney disease, or gout. Do not use together with ginkgo.

Flower Essences

I love flower essences for their ability to calm the nervous system and adjust a dog's emotional center. Below are some of my favorite flower essences that I use in my practice. I suggest giving a couple drops of flower essence in the mouth or on the ears twice daily for 8–12 weeks. You can mix flower essences, combining two to six essences.

Agrimony: for skin eruptions, stoicism, restlessness at night, pacing, grief, chewing of feet and sometimes entire body, attachment to abuser, high histamine levels, leaky gut

Aspen: to inspire courage and inner peace; for sleeplessness, nightmares, fear of the unknown, thunderstorms, fireworks, vet visits, car rides, low hum sounds, anxiety

Beech: for yeast infections, allergies, territorial feelings, high histamine levels, leaky gut; to support confidence and getting along with others

Bleeding heart: for grief or loss of a friend, caregiver, or littermate

Boneset: for low immune function, severe trauma, broken bones, surgery recovery, low vitality, grief

Borage: for grief, loss, trauma, lethargy, dryness, anxiety, leaky gut

Bougainvillea: for general stress, lung weakness, grief; good for female dogs

Centaury: for weakness, nervous exhaustion, debility, energetic cold, sympathetic excess, anxiety, worms

Comfrey: for trauma, deep trauma, rescue dogs coming from extreme situations, nervous system disorders, anxiety, grief, leaky gut

Crab apple: for cleansing and detoxifying; for poop eating, anal gland infections, mange, dogs prone to fleas, unexpected peeing or pooping, surgery recovery, vet visits, obsessive grooming, itchiness, sores and wounds, abandonment, constipation, nerve support, skin odor, skin conditions, antibiotics damage, incontinence, bladder stones; as a preventive prior to boarding

Easter lily: for female reproductive conditions in spayed and unspayed females and in breeding females; for incontinence and lipomas

Fireweed: for shock, trauma, lethargy, low vitality, change of family, fear of males, recovery from chronic illness, bladder stones, nervous system support, lung conditions; useful for working dogs

Gorse: for hopelessness, trauma, loss grief, despair

Impatiens: for gastrointestinal issues, itchiness and scratching, hair-trigger emotional responses, anxiety, restlessness, pain, aversion to touch; useful during training

Mimulus: for general fear, kidney weakness, anxiety

Nasturtium: for hyperactivity, excessive barking, spleen weakness, low immune function; useful for dogs that are hard to train

Oak: for lingering illness, major illness, trauma, stoicism, muscle twitching, weak musculature, incontinence

Olive: for allergies, Lyme disease and coinfections, seizure support, adrenal fatigue, viral infection support, lung conditions, grief, gastritis; useful for geriatric dogs and working dogs

Pine: useful for dogs that are new to a family, rescue dogs, dogs who take on the stress of their owners, dogs who are sensitive to strong emotion and yelling, for grief

Red chestnut: for kidney weakness, anxiety, worry, inability to be alone, separation anxiety

Rescue Remedy: for fear, fright, anxiety, panic, nausea

Rock rose: for fright, panic, need to escape, trauma, uneasiness, leaky gut

Star of Bethlehem: for trauma, shock, abuse, gastritis; useful in situations with extreme temperatures

Tomato: for fear and anxiety, fear of loud noises, debility, weakness, anxiety; promotes agility; useful for working dogs

Vervain: for restlessness, nervous disorders, excessive barking, hyperactivity, grief, high histamine levels

Vine: for dogs that are dominant, forceful, territorial; for stones

Walnut: for environmental and food allergies and sensitivities, worms, antibiotics damage, high histamine levels, gastritis

White chestnut: for OCD behaviors, training issues, chewing, scratching, insomnia, seasonal allergies, restlessness, lung weakness

APPENDIX 1
Herbal Actions

You don't need to be an expert in chemistry to be successful in herbalism, but you do need to know how herbs and their constituents affect the body and its systems. Most herbs have multiple actions in the body, and working with all of them, in addition to plant chemistry and constituents, can be overwhelming. Don't fret. You'll pick things up as you get more familiar with using herbs to help your dog. They'll become increasingly familiar when you start using herbal actions in context. For example, one action of German chamomile (*Matricaria chamomilla*) is that it is antispasmodic. That simply means it relieves tension in smooth muscle tissue. In context, that means it's useful for relaxing the digestive tract. It's also a carminative, meaning that it reduces gas, and it's a bitter, helping to stimulate the production of digestive enzymes.

Once you begin to understand herbal actions, you'll begin to understand plant language. In canine herbalism, some actions are more important than others. Let's go over a few.

Adaptogens: help your dog adapt to both internal and external stress. Adaptogens work with the whole body and strengthen the vital force by supporting the body's elimination systems, improving the processes of digestion, glandular and immune function, and tissue renewal.

Alteratives: gradually restore systemic function by purifying the blood, increasing elimination, and assisting with nutrient assimilation. They have a strong influence on major organs like the liver, intestines, skin, and kidneys. Some alteratives you might recognize are burdock root, nettles, and plantain.

Analgesics: help reduce internal or external pain through their influence on the nervous and digestive systems. Some popular analgesics include skullcap, passionflower, and St. John's wort.

Antacids: decrease stomach acid and can help with digestion. Three antacid examples are fennel, marshmallow, and slippery elm.

Antibacterials: can be used internally and externally, inhibiting the growth of bacteria. Popular examples include goldenseal root, Oregon grape root, and usnea.

Anticatarrhals: like dandelion and goldenrod decrease mucus buildup. Mucus helps the body eliminate foreign invaders and infections; it's one way the body says, "Hey, something is wrong here." Anticatarrhals thin mucus through constituents called saponins, astringents, tannins, and volatile oils.

Antidiarrheals: shrink tissues and soothe the bowels. My favorites for acute diarrhea are blackberry leaf and plantain.

Antiemetics: reduce nausea and help prevent vomiting. They help settle digestion and relax the digestive muscles. Fennel and ginger are popular examples.

Antifungal: herbs help minimize internal and external fungi. Examples include calendula and pau d'arco.

Antihistamines: work against the body's histamine response. Herbal antihistamines are gentle and nonsedating. They help alleviate allergic-type reactions like seasonal allergies and food sensitivities. Two examples are nettles and turmeric.

Anti-inflammatories: decrease inflammation. Herbal anti-inflammatories support the natural healing process rather than suppressing it; they modulate the inflammatory response. Turmeric and rose hips are two anti-inflammatories I recommend for systemic inflammation. The constituents most involved in aiding the inflammation response are mucilage, resins, saponins, flavonoids, volatile oils, salicylates, and essential fatty acids.

Antimicrobials: are a class of herbs that include antibiotics, antifungals, antiparasitics, antiseptics, and antivirals. They can be used internally or on the skin. Calendula, chamomile, goldenseal, Oregon grape root, sage, St. John's wort, and yarrow are all canine-safe antimicrobials.

Antiseptics: reduce pathogens and clean the blood. Burdock root and echinacea are good examples.

Antispasmodics: relieve and prevent spasms by relaxing smooth muscle tissue. Many of these herbs relieve tension through emotional and physical pathways. Alkaloids, salicylates, and volatile oils aid in these actions. Popular herbal antispasmodics include chamomile and skullcap.

Astringents: help reduce fluids and tighten blood vessels, mucous membranes, and tissues; their tannin content is often responsible for this astringency. They can have a slight constipating effect when taken internally and are best administered in small amounts. Examples include agrimony, elecampane, goldenrod, plantain, and yarrow.

Bitters: are so called due to their bitter flavor, which stimulates the production of digestive juices and supports the whole digestive process. They can have a laxative and diuretic effect in the body. Bitter herbs include chamomile, dandelion, and Oregon grape root.

Carminatives: help the stomach relax and encourage the elimination of gas from the digestive tract, thus supporting the digestive process. They have high levels of volatile oils. Carminative herbs include chamomile and fennel.

Demulcents: have a high mucilage content. Mucilage is a watery, gelatinous substance rich in polysaccharides. Thanks to their mucilage, demulcents soothe and protect internal tissues and provide relief from irritation of the mucous membranes. Demulcent examples include marshmallow root, mullein leaf, and slippery elm.

Digestives: work with the stomach and digestive system, helping normalize their function. Examples are chamomile, fennel, and meadowsweet.

Diuretics: are the go-to for removing fluid from the body. They work with the kidneys, liver, and vascular system to increase secretions and urination. A few diuretic examples include cleavers, dandelion leaf, and parsley.

Expectorants: thin and loosen mucus from the respiratory tract. A few examples include elecampane, fennel, and mullein.

Hemostatics: (styptics) stop bleeding. Yarrow is one of the best examples of a good hemostatic since it stops bleeding and pain; others include mullein and plantain.

Immune modulators: change the way your dog's immune system responds according to what the body needs. They have a more sustained response compared to stimulants.

Immune stimulants: increase your dog's immune function and support its components to fight off disease and/or pathogens.

Laxatives: move the stool body. Herbal laxatives vary in strength; some are more stimulating, while others add moisture. Examples include cleavers and marshmallow root.

Nervines: calm, tone, and strengthen the nervous system. They can be relaxing, like milky oats, or stimulating, like rosemary.

Nutritives: provide nutrition: proteins, carbohydrates, fats, vitamins, minerals, and micronutrients. Nutritive herbs can be safely consumed in large quantities. Examples are nettles and milky oats.

Stimulants: denote action or an increase in some part of your dog's physiological makeup or ecosystem.

Tonics: strengthen the whole body, a system, or specific organs. They have a normalizing effect on the body and, in many cases, provide micronutrients. I love to use them for seasonal healing. A few dog-friendly tonics are burdock, chamomile, dandelion, and nettles.

Trophorestoratives: give deep, systemic support with their restorative action on the health of the dog-as-ecosystem. Some have an affinity to a specific system. For example, there are many nervous system trophorestoratives.

Vulneraries: promote wound healing. They include burdock, calendula, chickweed, cleavers, and plantain.

🍃

Adaptogens, bitters, demulcents, and nervines are actions that require further explanation and a deeper understanding. They are frequently used in canine herbalism and often misunderstood.

Adaptogens

Adaptogens help your dog's body deal with everyday stressors. It's critical to think holistically and energetically before taking strong adaptogens. I find they work best for autoimmune disorders, deficiency, cancer, insomnia, long-term stress, nervous disorders, thyroid imbalances, and some types of sympathetic excess. Many adaptogenic herbs have short and long-term effects, especially on cortisol levels. Be cautious of herbs labeled as adaptogenic, even if their marketing labels them safe for long-term use. Labeling isn't always accurate, and it tends to display an allopathic perspective of the plant, disregarding the plant (and patient!) as an individual. Paul Bergner, director of the North American Institute of Medical Herbalism, observes, "The term adaptogen is not well defined by science outside of tonic effects, it ignores the possible consequences of overstimulation, of masking effects, [of] rebound effects after use or abuse, and [it] promotes overgeneralization both in contemporary herbal literature and in scientific writings on the concept."[1]

Adaptogens can have a dark side, and without proper use, they can cause harm and severe side effects. Using energetics is key to picking the appropriate adaptogens but looking at the entire dog-as-ecosystem is the most important aspect. It's critical that you address the root cause of stress and imbalance. Adaptogens aren't one-size-fits-all for stress and fatigue. They aren't recommended for acute conditions or high levels of dampness and stagnation. Addressing deficiency is the main tenet of adaptogens. Once a dog returns to normal functioning, adaptogens should be discontinued as they can easily overstimulate.

I once had client with a highly stressed-out dog who was peeing and marking in the house. He had been on ashwagandha for more than six months. We discontinued the ashwagandha, and the peeing immediately stopped.

One example of an often-misused adaptogen is schisandra berry. I've seen it recommended for dogs with sympathetic excess, meaning they can't shut off their sympathetic nervous system, which controls fight or flight. Schisandra is an adaptogen, but it is stimulating, and unlike other adaptogens, it isn't well indicated for dogs with sympathetic excess because it can activate the sympathetic system and increase heart rate, blood pressure, and urination. Many times it will have the opposite effect of what's intended.

Adaptogens can also energize the body; cordyceps is one example. This may help dogs who are cool to cold and deficient. But it is *not* what the body needs if it's hot and overstimulated.

When thinking about adding an adaptogen to your dog's health regimen, ask yourself the following questions: What is your reason for using an adaptogen? What's the root cause of your dog's stress? Is it lifestyle, food, the gut, the nervous system? Is it your stress? Trauma? Liver stagnation? When did it start happening?

Some practitioners mistake tonics for adaptogens. In the vast world of herbalism, tonic and adaptogenic actions can overlap, and distinguishing between them gets confusing depending on how someone learns about them. I recommend working directly with the plants to fully understand their range of influence.

When looking at adaptogens there are herbs that are widely known and accepted in this action category, but there are also herbs that have a more mild adaptogenic effect on a dog's stress response.

Popular adaptogens: American ginseng, ashwagandha, cordyceps mushroom, devils club, Siberian ginseng (eleuthero), licorice, reishi mushroom, rhodiola, and schizandra berry

Mild adaptogens: burdock, chaga, cleavers, dandelion, milky oats, and nettle seed

Bitters

Bitter herbs have an affinity for the gastrointestinal tract and the entire liver system. They predominantly affect digestive function, helping to balance insufficiency and tone digestive function. Your dog has bitter receptors throughout their body, including the gut but also the lungs, heart, and vasculature. In the gut, bitters trigger receptors to activate the production and release of hydrochloric acid, bile, and digestive enzymes. This builds your dog's digestive fire, enabling food to be thoroughly broken down. In the long term bitters are drying, but in the short term they increase fluids in the digestive tract, aiding digestion and protecting mucous membranes.

Energetically, most bitters are cooling. They bring energy (and fluids) from the head down toward the core and heart center and then out through the elimination organs.

Dogs who belch in your face (yuck), burp, and have excessive gas can benefit from bitters. But not all digestive problems need bitters.

Administering bitters when they're not well indicated works against the dog-as-ecosystem. And consideration of energetics is important. If bitters were indicated for a cold dog, they likely wouldn't be beneficial if administered on their own. However, you could mix warming herbs like ginger with the bitters, balancing them energetically so the dog can tolerate and benefit from the herbs.

Bitters have other properties too. When well indicated, bitters can help stimulate appetite, regulate blood sugar, and help heal the gut wall, increasing nutrient assimilation. They can have a systemic effect because they cleanse the blood, balance the liver-skin connection, and stimulate lymphatic drainage, depending on the herb. Bitters can regulate dogs in sympathetic excess by activating the vagus nerve, which modulates not only the digestive process but also the parasympathetic nervous system. I like using flower essences from bitter plants like blessed thistle, burdock, milk thistle, gentian, and skullcap to help calm notoriously hyperactive dogs.

Some bitters shouldn't be used long-term. Avoid using them for dogs that are pregnant or have ulcers, kidney and gallbladder stones, gastro-esophageal reflux disease (GERD), or acid reflux.

Strong bitters: aloe vera, blue vervain, gentian, goldenseal, Oregon grape root, turmeric, yellow dock root

Mild bitters: angelica, artichoke, blessed thistle, burdock root, calendula, Ceylon cinnamon, chamomile, dandelion, ginger, milk thistle, peppermint, reishi mushroom, skullcap, St. John's wort, wood betony, yarrow

Demulcents

Demulcents are sweet, full of moisture, cooling, and nourishing, with lots of carbohydrates and starch. They help remedy deficiency and dryness. They have an affinity for the digestive, musculoskeletal, respiratory, urinary tract, and reproductive systems, but they act on the entire organism. I use demulcents for inflammation, dried-out tissues, acid reflux, and constipation.

Dogs with dryness, anxiety, and excess nervous energy can benefit from demulcents, as can dogs with poor appetite, excessive thirst, dry oral mucosa, constipation, weakness in the lower back, and dryness-related arthritis. Dryness depletes a dog's secretions, drying tissues, including surfaces, junctions, and membranes. Excess dryness degrades the dog-as-ecosystem because mucous membranes protect against bacteria overgrowth, pathogens, respiratory pollutants, urinary inflammation, infection, and oversensitivity. When the mucous membranes are dried out, the body loses their protection—everywhere. Everything is connected.

Demulcents have a lot of mucilaginous polysaccharides. Dissolve slippery elm in warm water and you'll better understand what mucilage is. Water is vital for extracting the mucilaginous polysaccharides, so, when giving a demulcent to your dog, use an infusion. A tincture won't work well for this purpose. If your dog is finicky, you could also administer a demulcent herb as a powder added to food or as a capsule.

Popular demulcents: aloe vera, couch grass, licorice, marshmallow root, mullein leaf, plantain, red clover, slippery elm, Solomon's seal, tremella mushroom, violet

Diuretics

Simply put, diuretics encourage your dog to pee more. They support your dog's kidneys, benefiting the urinary system, eliminating wastes, and supporting the entire inner cleansing process. Diuretics help eliminate metabolic wastes, toxins, and products of inflammation. Diuretics' elimination action is crucial in musculoskeletal conditions, as waste products and toxins are the root cause of many inflammatory problems, including arthritis. Diuretic herbs relieve swollen joints, draining fluids from the extracellular space (the interstitial fluid) and moving it toward the kidneys for elimination.

Kidneys filter excess fluid in blood; to do this, they need a certain biochemical balance in place, including a proper sodium-to-potassium ratio. Sodium and potassium salts are electrolytes, and they are involved in many body processes, like regulation of blood pressure, nerve impulse transmission, and muscle contraction. When dogs ingest too much sodium, they can lose their electrolyte balance. Many commercial dog foods, particularly the canned foods, have high sodium levels; they use sodium as a preservative and to enhance the flavor. Diuretic herbs promote salt and water excretion. By helping release sodium from the body, they can benefit many dogs on commercial food diets.

Diuretic herbs should be used only when well indicated and not for extended periods, as they can dry out your dog's constitution. A possible adverse effect of diuretic herbs is an increased risk of hypokalemia and a lower-than-normal potassium level. If your dog is taking glucosamine, you may need to increase the dosage, as diuretics may reduce its effectiveness.

Popular diuretics: ashwagandha, burdock root, chamomile, chickweed, cleavers, couch grass, dandelion, goldenrod, hawthorn, juniper berry, marshmallow, uva-ursi, violet, yarrow

Nervines

Nervines act on your dog's central nervous system. The central nervous system governs functions across the body, so nervine herbs express many kinds of therapeutic activity. Remember, everything is connected. Your dog's nervous system should be considered in any health and healing regimen. Nervines can calm and sedate dogs with hyperactivity or anxiety and restore a sense of well-being in a depressed dog. They can be effective in reducing stress associated with chronic pain.

The two main types of nervines are tonic and relaxant. You'll find more information on each one inside the monograph section of this book.

Tonic Nervines

Nervine tonics strengthen and restore tissues directly. If your dog has damaged nerve tissue, whether from pathological causes or physical trauma, nervine tonics can help with stress while also aiding in healing. Nervine tonics include herbs known as trophorestoratives. These herbs have a general affinity toward a particular organ or system, bringing it to balance and slowly restoring function.

Popular tonic nervines: ashwagandha, chamomile, lion's mane mushroom, milky oats, skullcap, and St. John's wort.

Relaxant Nervines

Nervine relaxants have sedating and calming activity. They're helpful if your dog struggles with anxiety, stress, restlessness, hyperactivity, and insomnia or needs behavior modification. Relaxants should be used only when well indicated. Look at the cofactors for each relaxing nervine herb and consider which system they have an affinity for, as they have a direct action on specific organ systems and many are not interchangeable.

Popular relaxant nervines: chamomile, lemon balm, passionflower, and skullcap

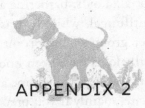

APPENDIX 2
Herbal Constituents

Metabolites are compounds formed through an organism's metabolism. For a plant, primary metabolites are compounds used to maintain growth and structure; they include lipids, protein, and starches, among others. Secondary metabolites make up a plant's communication system and help guard against the outside world. Scientists think that secondary metabolites are responsible for plants' actions in animals and humans.

The following is a list of important herbal constituents. Learning about them can help you know a plant as an individual and better understand its effect on your dog's body.

Alcohol: is found in plants as a constituent of volatile oils (defined below). An example of a plant alcohol is menthol, a constituent of peppermint. Other forms of alcohol can be found in the fatty acids and waxes that coat plant leaves.

Alkaloids: are a powerful and highly medicinal group of secondary metabolites. They include compounds responsible for the poisonous, hallucinogenic, and bitter effects of plants. Alkaloids are mainly extracted by alcohol, rather than water, and dissipate with heat. Vinegar, too, can extract alkaloids and tends to magnify their effects. Not all alkaloids are toxic; small amounts can help heal the digestive system, nerves, liver, and lungs, as well as other parts of the body. Alkaloids are nitrogen-rich, with their potency varying from herb to herb. Generally, plants with a high alkaloid content need to be used cautiously. Of the thirteen alkaloid classifications, one group, the isoquinolines group, includes two important alkaloids: berberine and hydrastine. Berberine is antibacterial and antifungal, while hydrastine is antiseptic as well as hemostatic. Another group of important alkaloids is the pyrrolizidines. Pyrrolizidine alkaloids have been known to cause liver disease in mammals. Plants containing pyrrolizidine alkaloids, such as comfrey, need to be used with care, mainly if you prepare them via an alcoholic extraction.

Carbohydrates: include glucose, starch, and fructose. They give plants energy and structure and help produce cooling mucilages like those found in slippery elm bark and marshmallow root.

Chlorophyll: a powerful constituent, transforms sunshine into energy and nutrition. Chlorophyll is an antiseptic that supports the entire digestive tract and vital organs like the liver.

Coumarins: are antimicrobial and antispasmodic and help clot blood. Herbs with high levels of coumarins, like cinnamon, can have negative interactions with pharmaceuticals and should be used with care.

Carotenoids: are pigmented antioxidants. They're found in red, white, and yellow veggies and herbs like St. John's wort and yarrow.

Flavonoids: reduce inflammation and positively affect liver detoxification through their interaction with oxidation. They can be antispasmodic, increase circulation, and improve kidney function. Flavonoids can be extracted by both water and alcohol. Violet and yarrow are examples of herbs high in flavonoids.

Glycosides: are a group of sugar constituents. Some are toxic; some are nontoxic. They can be extracted by both water and alcohol.

Lignans: repair liver cells, protect the body from toxins, and have antioxidant action. Milk thistle is a popular example of an herb rich in lignans.

Mucilages: are mostly water-soluble, gelatinous polysaccharides. Polysaccharides are nutritive and stimulate the immune system. Plants produce mucilage for the hydration and storage of liquids. Because of their gel-like consistency, they protect mucous membranes from irritation. They're cooling, nourishing for the body, and sweet in taste.

Phenols: are secondary metabolites that can relieve pain but also can be toxic. One beneficial phenol that most people are familiar with is salicin. You may know it as the popular drug aspirin, but originally salicin was discovered in white willow bark.

Resins: are thick, sticky, and often antifungal. Myrrh is a popular resin, and you can find resins in plants like calendula.

Saponins: are glycosides usually found in anti-inflammatory herbs, and they form the building blocks of other compounds. Saponins are soluble in water and alcohol. They can help emulsify fat molecules both internally and externally. Saponins can disrupt endocrine function and increase gut permeability; however, many herbs with high levels of saponins have other constituents that modulate the saponins' effects, exemplifying the benefits of whole-plant medicine. At high dosages, saponins can cause side effects like diarrhea, nausea, and vomiting. Alfalfa is an example of an herb with saponins.

Sterols: have a similar structure to cholesterol and come from a plant's cell walls. They support heart health, reduce harmful cholesterol, and aid circulation. Natural examples include astragalus, mushrooms, calendula, and elecampane.

Terpenes: are a group of secondary metabolites made up of carbon and hydrogen. They're the constituents that deter highly aromatic insects due to their volatile oil content. Terpenes can be both toxic and nontoxic. Burdock, lemon balm, and rosemary are all terpene-rich herbs.

Tannins: tone and astringe tissues while protecting the digestive system and skin from irritation. Tannins can be extracted in water, alcohol, and glycerin. Both meadowsweet and mullein are high in tannins.

Volatile oils: are abundant in aromatic plants. They are usually stimulating, antiseptic, and anti-inflammatory. They can irritate internal and external tissues and cross the blood-brain barrier when ingested. Volatile oils evaporate quickly, so herbs high in volatile oils must be protected against oxidation. Herbs with volatile oils profiled in this book include mullein, parsley, and passionflower.

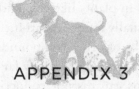

APPENDIX 3
Vitamins and Minerals

Vitamins

Vitamins are categorized according to whether they are water-soluble or fat-soluble. Water-soluble vitamins are not stored within the body except in small amounts. Any extra is excreted through a dog's kidneys. Thanks to this process, water-soluble vitamins are not likely to reach toxic levels, though it's still possible if an excessive amount is administered. Since these vitamins aren't stored in the body, it's essential for a dog to consume adequate amounts through the diet and, if necessary, supplementation.

Fat-soluble vitamins are stored in cells called lymphocytes. Since they're not quickly absorbed and/or excreted, over-supplementation is something to be mindful of when administering fat-soluble vitamins to your dog. Too much of a vitamin over time causes vitamin excess, which leads to toxic symptoms. Fat-soluble vitamins in their synthetic form can accumulate in the fatty tissues and cause signs of toxicity.

Water-Soluble Vitamins
Vitamin B₁ (Thiamine)
Synthetics: thiamine hydrochloride, thiamine mononitrate
Benefits: Energy and carbohydrate metabolism, assists in blood formation and improves circulation, critical for muscle tone, helps produce ATP, strengthens immunity and decreases stress, essential for hydrochloric acid production, helps prevent allergies and food sensitivities. Thiamine antagonist is sugar.

Food sources: brown rice, chicken, eggs, liver, mushrooms, mussels, organ meats, pork, peas, raw cow milk, raw goat milk

Deficiency symptoms: anorexia, confusion, digestive conditions, enlarged heart, muscle weakness

Toxicity symptoms: Thiamine is nontoxic, but you don't want to overdo it.

Vitamin B₂

Synthetics: riboflavin

Benefits: Needed for the formation of red blood cells and antibodies. Helps combat free radicals, prevent cataracts, and prevent tongue and mouth inflammation as well as cracks in corners of the mouth. A coenzyme for the metabolic process of turning carbohydrates, fats, and proteins into energy.

Food sources: avocados, broccoli, dulse, egg yolks, fish, nuts, poultry, raw cheese, raw cow milk, raw goat milk, raw yogurt (plain), rice bran, spinach, watercress, whole grains

Deficiency symptoms: bloodshot eyes, itchy eyes, light sensitivity, mouth inflammation, stomatitis

Toxicity symptoms: appetite loss, constipation, diarrhea, muscle tremors, seizures

Vitamin B₃ (Niacin)

Synthetics: nicotinic acid

Benefits: Supports nervous system and brain function, helps maintain healthy skin, clears heat from the stomach, aids in proper digestion, helps lower cholesterol, strengthens the spleen. A coenzyme for NAD (nicotinamide adenine dinucleotide), which increases circulation.

Food sources: avocado, beef liver, broccoli, carrots, chicken eggs, organ meats, mackerel, mushroom, peas, potatoes, raw cow milk, raw goat milk, rice bran, salmon (wild), sardines

Deficiency symptoms: anxiety, bad breath, dementia, darkening of tongue, lethargy, mouth sores, poor appetite, tendency toward agitation

Toxicity symptoms: Toxicity is rare but can cause liver inflammation

Vitamin B₄ (Choline)

Synthetic: choline bitartrate, choline chloride

Benefits: A coenzyme for metabolism; prevents excessive fat from accumulating in the liver. Can be converted from tryptophan in a healthy body. Manufactures neurotransmitters and aids in nerve and brain health. An important component of DNA and RNA

Food sources: chard, chicken, cod, collard greens, egg yolks, kale, liver, raw cow milk, raw goat milk, red meat, romaine lettuce, salmon (wild-caught), summer squash, turmeric

Deficiency symptoms: Deficiency is rare.

Toxicity symptoms: diarrhea, lethargy, loss of appetite, seizures, tremors, vomiting

Vitamin B₅ (Pantothenic Acid)

Synthetic: calcium d-pantothenate

Benefits: Aids adrenal glands' cortisol response to stress, helps create red blood cells and sex hormones, helps heal wounds (including leaky gut), decreases systemic inflammation, helps relieve stress, clears heat, supports the spleen. A critical component of coenzyme A (CoA); essential for fat, carbohydrate, and protein metabolism.

Whole Food versus Synthetic Vitamins

Most commercial diets, including many freeze-dried and dehydrated brands, are balanced with synthetic vitamins and minerals. Synthetic vitamins are harder for the body to absorb and assimilate than natural vitamins. A dog's body, like a human's body, has vitamin receptors throughout. There is some question as to whether these receptors recognize synthetic vitamins as vitamins or whether the synthetic versions contribute to clogging these receptors and not allowing the natural form of the vitamins to be metabolized. A good example of this is folic acid, the synthetic form of folate. Folic acid binds to a dog's receptors and blocks natural folate, degrading liver detoxification processes.

There are other potential dangers associated with synthetic vitamin isolates. Some are not recognized by the body or are recognized as toxins and circulate in the body without being absorbed. As is the case with herbs, when possible, we want the whole natural vitamin, not an isolate or lab-produced facsimile of it.

Note: Dogs are individuals, of course; some can tolerate synthetics or whole-food vitamins, while others can't.

Food sources: avocados, blackstrap molasses, broccoli, brown rice, cabbage, eggs, kale, legumes, mushrooms, nutritional yeast, organ meats, raw cow milk, raw goat milk

Deficiency symptoms: Deficiency is rare but can cause early graying, gastrointestinal distress, heart conditions, and lethargy.

Toxicity symptoms: acid reflux, diarrhea, early graying, edema, joint pain, nausea

Vitamin B₆ (Pyridoxine)

Synthetic: pyridoxine hydrochloride

Benefits: Aids the manufacturing of neurotransmitters and serotonin, supports more than a hundred enzymes, supports red blood cell production, needed for vitamin B_{12} absorption, supports immunity, helps assimilation of fats and proteins, protects the nervous system, supports kidney function

Food sources: alfalfa, artichokes, avocados, bananas, chlorella, eggs, dark leafy greens, fish, meat, moringa, phytoplankton, raw cow milk, raw goat milk, sardines, spirulina

Deficiency symptoms: cracking of lips, lethargy, low immune function, nervousness, seizures, skin rashes (scaly)

Toxicity symptoms: constipation, diarrhea, lethargy, loss of appetite, muscle tremors

Vitamin B₇ (Biotin)

Synthetic: d-biotin

Benefits: Helps break down carbohydrates, fats, and proteins; helps regulate cellular communication; promotes healthy skin and coat

Food sources: almonds, avocados, egg yolks, fish, nuts, organ meats, raw cow milk, raw goat milk, sweet potatoes, walnut oil

Deficiency symptoms: brittle nails, crusty skin conditions, thinning hair

Toxicity symptoms: diarrhea, vomiting

Vitamin B₉ (Folate)

Synthetic: folic acid, pteroylglutamic acid

Benefits: Needed for proper methylation and for vitamin B_{12} absorption and utilization; essential for red blood cell formation; maintains healthy homocysteine levels; supports nervous system function.

Food sources: anchovies, asparagus, cauliflower, beets, broccoli, broccoli sprouts, Brussel sprouts, eggs, lentils, liver, mussels, phytoplankton, raw cow milk, raw goat milk, romaine lettuce, sardines, seaweed, spinach, sweet potatoes (note that cooking foods depletes their folate content)

Deficiency symptoms: dementia, diarrhea, lethargy, mouth sores, muscle weakness, neurological conditions, weight loss

Toxicity symptoms: agitation, diarrhea, gastrointestinal upset, insomnia, nausea, seizures, vomiting

---

A Note on Folic Acid

There are many supplements that contain folic acid. It is NOT the same as natural folate and has a different chemical structure that makes it "highly absorbable," easily leading to too much folic acid absorption. Your dog's body can only convert so much synthetic folic acid into folate. The rest of it remains unconverted in your dog's blood. Why is this important to know? Unconverted folic acid can bind to folate receptors and compete with usable natural folate, disrupting a process called methylation, a process responsible for healthy immune function, cell growth, and genetic expression. Make sure your dog is not getting an abundance of synthetic folic acid in their food, supplements, and treats. For example, if folic acid is on your dog's food label, make sure they are not getting it anywhere else.

Vitamin B_{12}

Synthetic: cyanocobalamin, hydroxocobalamin (prescription version)

Benefits: Helps protect DNA and brain cells; helps regulate healthy gene function; responsible for neurotransmitter production; supports nerve function and red blood cell. Healthy levels of vitamin B_{12} are dependent on healthy gut flora and proper levels of intrinsic factor.

Food sources: clams, eggs, fish, nutritional yeast, organ meats, poultry, raw cow milk, raw goat milk

Deficiency symptoms: anxiety, chronic diarrhea, cognitive impairment, gait impairment, gastrointestinal distress, incontinence, lethargy, muscle weakness, poor appetite, poor vision, shortness of breath

Toxicity symptoms: diarrhea, fatigue, nausea, and vomiting

Vitamin C

Synthetic: ascorbic acid

Benefits: A building block for connective tissues, cartilage, bones, blood vessels, and teeth. Aids in utilization of carnitine, production of collagen, and absorption of folic acid. Supports healthy histamine response and immune function.

Food sources: amla berries, bell peppers, black currants, broccoli, Brussel sprouts, camu camu berries, cantaloupe, cauliflower, citrus, kale, kiwis, peas, pineapples, potatoes, pumpkin, raw cow milk, raw goat milk, rose hips, spinach, spleen, strawberries

Deficiency symptoms: allergy-like reactions, bad breath, bloody gums, dull coat, low immune function, musculoskeletal weakness, slow wound healing, weak or loose teeth, weakness

Toxicity symptoms: toxicity is low in dogs; look for signs of diarrhea or nausea with high dosages

Note: look for non-GMO sources. Be aware if you are supplementing calcium, vitamin B_{12}, vitamin E, or zinc, they can decrease C levels. Whole food sources are best as they contain balanced nutrients and bioavailable sources.

Fat-Soluble Vitamins

Vitamin A (Beta-carotene, Retinol, Retinal)

Synthetics: vitamin A acetate and vitamin A palmitate

Benefits: Vital for many important functions of the body. Protects against free radicals and supports the liver. Important for growth, vision, healthy bones, and blood. Retinol is a form of vitamin A that comes from animal sources.

Food sources: *retinol*—butter, cod liver oil, egg yolks, fish, liver, organ meats, raw cow milk, raw goat milk, shellfish; *beta-carotene*—broccoli, most dark leafy greens, orange and yellow fruits and vegetables, raw cow milk, raw goat milk

Deficiency symptoms: bone fractures, crusty skin conditions, dry coat, hair loss, poor appetite, poor vision, seizures, vomiting, wasting

Toxicity symptoms: diarrhea, excessive thirst, lethargy, seizures, vomiting, weight loss

Note: Dogs with hypothyroidism can have difficulty converting vitamin A in the intestines.

Vitamins D₂ and D₃ (Cholecalciferol)

Synthetics: ergocalciferol (D₂), calcitriol, calcipotriene, doxercalciferol

Benefits: Supports the nervous system, immune function, cardiac function, and musculoskeletal formation; aids in the absorption of calcium and phosphorus. Offers cancer support/prevention.

Food sources: beef liver, cod liver and its oil (only use oil if you are testing vitamin D levels), mackerel, raw cow milk, raw goat milk, salmon (wild-caught), sardines

Deficiency symptoms: cancer, drooling, dull eyes, hair loss, insomnia, lameness, lethargy, lymphoma, musculoskeletal issues, viral infections

Toxicity symptoms: diarrhea, excessive thirst, musculoskeletal issues, vomiting, wasting

Note: Test your dog's vitamin D levels yearly, along with other vitamin levels. Don't supplement this vitamin unless tests show that your dog is deficient. Vitamin D₃ comes from animal sources and D₂ from plant sources like mushrooms. When providing whole food vitamin D sources, high levels are uncommon. Make sure to give D with K for proper absorption.

Vitamin E (RRR-alpha-tocopherol, d-alpha-tocopherol)

Synthetic: rac-alpha-tocopherol, dl-alpha-tocopherol, vitamin E acetate, vitamin E succinate

Benefits: Anticancer; a powerful antioxidant; essential to the formation and function of cell membranes; helps prevent oxidation and protect dogs from air pollutants; reduces blood lipids; supports structure and function of smooth muscles; supports immune health

Food sources: almonds, asparagus, avocados, beet greens, bell peppers, butter (grass-fed), collard greens, egg yolks, mangoes, pumpkin, raw cow milk, raw goat milk

Deficiency symptoms: aggression or changes in behavior, chronic skin conditions, low immune function, neurological conditions, poor vision, retinopathy, uncontrolled body movements, weight loss

Toxicity symptoms: diarrhea, lethargy, muscle weakness, nausea, shaking, vomiting

Minerals

Minerals are naturally occurring inorganic (not made by living organisms) substances that are essential to healthy cells and balanced bodily functions. Without minerals, your dog's body couldn't utilize hormones and enzymes, maintain blood pressure, manufacture neurochemicals like serotonin, or have properly functioning systems and structures.

Macro Minerals

Calcium

Benefits: Supports bone growth and function and affects neurological and hormone function. Requires magnesium for complete function.

Food sources: broccoli, chicken eggs and necks, kelp, phytoplankton, raw bones, raw cow milk, raw goat milk, spinach, turkey necks

Deficiency symptoms: bone disorders, decreased growth, hyperparathyroidism, lameness

Toxicity symptoms: irregular heartbeat, itchiness, kidney dysfunction, nausea, severe bone and joint abnormalities, vomiting

Magnesium

Benefits: Essential for cellular oxidation, heart health, and function of enzymes (along with calcium). Supports hydrochloric acid production, carbohydrate and fat metabolism, bone structure, muscle contraction, and brain-muscle function.

Food sources: almonds, collard greens, green beans, kelp, mackerel, phytoplankton, raw cow milk, raw goat milk, sardines, sea vegetables, seeds (hemp, pumpkin, sunflower), spinach, Swiss chard, wheatgrass

Deficiency symptoms: cardiac arrhythmia, hypomagnesemia, muscle pain, muscle tremors, spasms, stiffness

Toxicity symptoms: diarrhea and gas, gastrointestinal spasm, nausea

Note: Calcium, potassium, and sodium are all dependent on magnesium. Low levels of magnesium can result is low functioning of these other minerals, especially potassium, and sodium. Antibiotics use can deplete magnesium.

Phosphorus

Benefits: Plays a major role in energy production and metabolism, protein synthesis, cell membrane formation, and fatty acid production. Required for proper function of B vitamins.

Food sources: beans, beef, chicken, herring, mackerel, muscle and organ meats, phytoplankton, pork, raw cow milk, raw goat milk, turkey

Deficiency symptoms: Deficiency is rare but can cause bone conditions, poor appetite, poor coat, and skin conditions.

Toxicity symptoms: high calcium levels and deposits, kidney damage, weak bones

Note: Everything is connected. Phosphorus and calcium form and maintain the health of bones (including teeth). This relationship is responsible for heart function, cellular reproduction, and other metabolic functions.

Potassium

Benefits: An electrolyte; helps maintain acid balance and supports cardiac function, cellular function, muscle contraction, and nerve function.

Food sources: bananas, beef, beet greens, dried apricots, herring, kelp, mushrooms, peas, phytoplankton, pork, raw cow milk, raw goat milk, salmon, spinach, squash, sweet potatoes, Swiss chard

Deficiency symptoms: cardiac arrhythmia, deficiency, diarrhea, excessive urination, gas, hypokalemia, lethargy, muscle paralysis, muscle weakness, poor appetite, poor growth, restlessness

Toxicity symptoms: nausea, shortness of breath, vomiting

Note: Antibiotics deplete potassium.

Sodium Chloride

Benefits: An electrolyte; helps maintain acid balance and supports the nervous system and muscle contractions. Also helps maintain fluid levels in the dog-as-ecosystem. Is involved in the production of hydrochloric acid in the stomach.

Food sources: eggs, herring, kale, kelp, mackerel, raw cow milk, raw goat milk

Deficiency symptoms: dehydration, dry skin, hair loss, heart conditions, kidney disease, lethargy, muscle weakness, poor growth

Toxicity symptoms: diarrhea, edema, heart rate issues, high blood pressure, low calcium levels, nausea, restlessness, seizures

. . . .

Tip! Potassium and sodium can be affected in typical Addison's disease. You'll see high potassium levels with lowered sodium and a decline in cortisol.

. . . .

Sulfur

Benefits: Supports the skin, phase II liver detoxification, the immune system, and healthy serotonin and dopamine levels. Helps keep the balance between beneficial and pathogenic bacteria in the gut.

Food sources: asparagus, beans, broccoli, eggs, fish, grains, molasses, muscle meat, raw cow milk, raw goat milk

Deficiency symptoms: allergies, fur discoloration, skin conditions

Toxicity symptoms: allergies, constipation, diarrhea, gas, gastrointestinal inflammation, lethargy, nausea, nosebleeds

Note: Dogs eating too much folic acid (synthetic) instead of folate (natural) can have problems with sulfur buildup if they consume too much sulfur through their diet or supplements.

Micro Minerals

Micro or trace minerals are essential for cellular health and all bodily functions. Your dog must get these from outside sources in "trace" amounts. These micronutrients help your dog's body utilize macronutrients like calcium, magnesium, and vitamin D.

Boron

Benefits: Helps calcium and magnesium with bone formation and maintenance. Supports healthy immune function, endocrine function, and the entire musculoskeletal system.

Food sources: apples, avocados, beans, brewer's yeast, broccoli, peaches, pears, peanut butter, potatoes, raw cow milk, raw goat milk, turkey, shellfish

Deficiency symptoms: diarrhea, dry skin, gastrointestinal upset, nausea, vomiting

Toxicity symptoms: arthritis, bone conditions, bone weakness, mineral imbalances (calcium, magnesium, phosphorus)

Cobalt

Benefits: Helps a dog absorb iron by aiding in the production of red blood cells. A part of vitamin B_{12}; affects total metabolic function. Supports antiviral and antibiotic protection. Helps balance thyroid function.

Food sources: apricots, beets, cabbage, fish, meat, nuts, raw cow milk (trace), raw goat milk (trace), shellfish; also any good source of vitamin B_{12}

Deficiency symptoms: anemia, B_{12} malfunction, lethargy, low intrinsic factor levels, low immune function

Toxicity symptoms: cardiac and endocrine malfunction, cognitive issues, enlarged thyroid, excessive concentration of red blood cells in the blood, tremors

Copper

Benefits: Helps the body absorb iron; prevents anemia; supports the nervous, musculoskeletal, and immune systems.

Food sources: grains, leafy greens, mollusks, organ meats, raw cow milk (trace), raw goat milk (trace), shiitake mushrooms, spirulina

Deficiency symptoms: anemia, bone conditions, coat discoloration, enzyme deficiency, lethargy, low immune function, musculoskeletal weakness, tendon and ligament weakness

Toxicity symptoms: anemia, bloody urine, diarrhea, kidney and liver disease, poor appetite

Fluoride

Benefits: Aids tooth and bone development.

Food sources: oatmeal, potatoes, raw cow milk (trace), raw goat milk (trace), spinach

Deficiency symptoms: dental weakness and deformities

Toxicity symptoms: arthritis, bone deformities, bone weakness, cancer, kidney and liver damage

Note: Fluoride is a naturally occurring trace mineral that most dogs get enough or too much of by drinking unfiltered fluorinated water. Never supplement fluoride. If needed, a homeopathic cell salt of fluoride (6X or 12X) can be given.

Iodine

Benefits: Important for metabolic function and endocrine health, especially thyroid health.

Food sources: cod, dairy, eggs, kelp, raw cow milk, raw goat milk, seaweed, shrimp

Deficiency symptoms: anxiety, constipation, dry skin, hair loss, lethargy, muscle weakness, sensitivity to cold

Toxicity symptoms: diarrhea, hyperthyroidism, nausea, vomiting

Note: Use care if you are supplementing iodine. Natural sources are best for this trace mineral (but avoid tuna as a source; it is high in mercury).

Iron

Benefits: Helps the body produce red blood cells, hemoglobin, and myoglobin. Helps bring oxygen to the organs and musculoskeletal system. (Hemoglobin carries oxygen to your dog's cells, and myoglobin carries it to your dog's muscles.)

Food sources: beans, broccoli, cabbage, leafy greens, liver, meat, nuts, peas, pumpkin seeds, raw cow milk, raw goat milk

Deficiency symptoms: anemia, brittle nails, dry coat, lethargy, growth issues

Toxicity symptoms: anorexia, diarrhea, mineral deficiencies (copper, manganese, zinc)

Manganese

Benefits: Helps with musculoskeletal formation, including cartilage. Works with iodine for thyroid hormone production. This is an underappreciated mineral; it contributes to amino acid metabolism, antioxidant protection, blood clotting, bone health, carbohydrate metabolism, cartilage formation and health, cognition, collagen production, enzyme activation, iron absorption, mitochondria health, and nervous system health.

Food sources: beans, berries, brown rice, chickpeas, lentils, mussels, peas, pineapples, raw cow milk, raw goat milk, spinach, sweet potatoes

Deficiency symptoms: abnormal carbohydrate metabolism, bone conditions, impaired growth, lameness, musculoskeletal conditions, seizures

Toxicity symptoms: facial spasms, iron deficiency, severe neurological conditions, tremors

Molybdenum

Benefits: Supports cellular health, metabolizes nitrogen, and balances copper, uric acid, and sulfur. Responsible for enzyme function, including sulfite oxidase and xanthine oxidase, which are integral to the body's detoxification process. Helps break down toxins in the body.

Food sources: bananas, beef, brown rice, chicken, dairy, eggs, grains, leafy greens, potatoes

Deficiency symptoms: toxic sulfur levels, low uric acid levels, risk of esophageal cancer

Toxicity symptoms: anemia, improper growth, kidney failure, low metabolic copper levels, seizures, stunted growth

Selenium

Benefits: Supports the immune system, helps prevent premature aging by being an antioxidant superpower, helps prevent cancer and inflammation, and protects DNA from oxidative damage.

Food sources: bananas, Brazil nuts, brown rice, cashews, eggs, fish, mushrooms, oats, raw cow milk, raw goat milk, spinach, sunflower seeds

Deficiency symptoms: early graying, hair loss, lethargy, muscle cramping, poor appetite, sympathetic excess, weak immune system

Toxicity symptoms: brittle nails, cancer, diarrhea, heart failure, kidney failure, nausea, restlessness

Silicon

Benefits: Helps the body heal and is integral for healthy skin and nails; supports musculoskeletal health, including cartilage formation, and strengthens the immune system.

Food sources: bananas, brown rice, green beans, nuts, oats, organ meats, raw cow milk, raw goat milk, shellfish, spinach

Deficiency symptoms: artery hardening, brittle nails, dry skin and coat, hair loss, heart disease, joint issues, low stomach acid, weak teeth

Toxicity symptoms: Toxicity is rare, as silicon is excreted in the urine.

Note: Silicon levels naturally decline as a dog ages.

Zinc

Benefits: Helps the body utilize copper, calcium, phosphorus, vitamin A, and B vitamins. Supports enzymatic and antibody functions. Contributes to antiviral protection, immune function, liver function, protection against heavy metals, protein metabolism, and white blood cell proliferation.

Food sources: almonds, beans, beef, chicken, eggs, green beans, kale, lamb, legumes, liver, oats, oysters, pork, potatoes, pumpkin seeds, raw cow milk, raw goat milk, shiitake mushrooms, squash

Deficiency symptoms: coat discoloration, diarrhea, dry coat, hair loss, impaired immune function, skin issues, infertility, poor appetite

Toxicity symptoms: low nutrient absorption, diarrhea, nausea, poor appetite, stomach damage, vomiting

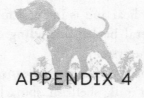

APPENDIX 4
Supplements

Activated charcoal: is absorbent and binding. It binds toxins to its surface area so that they can be eliminated from the body. Activated charcoal works well to eliminate most but not all toxins; it works best when given at the time of toxin ingestion. *Dosage:* Give 1 gram for every 5 pounds of your dog's body weight, mixed with warm water. (Single dose at time of toxin ingestion or as soon after as possible.)

Apple cider vinegar: is warming, balances pH, helps keep candida populations in check, supports heart health, and helps balance the microbiome. *Dosage:* 1/4 teaspoon for extra-small dogs; 1/2 teaspoon for small dogs; 1 teaspoon for medium dogs; 2 teaspoons for large dogs; 1 tablespoon for extra-large dogs. Once daily.

Betaine hydrochloride: helps the body restore a healthy level of stomach acid and absorb proteins. It increases digestive strength, pancreatic activity, and bile production. Caution: Avoid using betaine with NSAIDs. This supplement is usually part of a formula.

Black seed or black cumin seed (*Nigella sativa*): is a warm remedy, high in antioxidants. It is antibacterial, anti-inflammatory, antiparasitic, and hepatoprotective. It supports cognition, immune health and promotes longevity. *Freshly ground seed dosage:* 1/8 teaspoon for extra-small dogs; 1/4 teaspoon for small dogs; 1/2 teaspoon for medium dogs; 1 teaspoon for large dogs; 1 1/2 teaspoons for extra-large dogs. Once daily. If using the seed oil, halve the doses recommended here.

Bromelain: is an enzyme found in pineapple that helps the body break down proteins and improves assimilation. It also helps reduce swelling and inflammation and has an affinity for the joints, ears, nose, and throat. Caution: Some dogs are sensitive to bromelain, usually resulting in itchiness, nausea, and vomiting. *Dosage:* 25 mg for every 15 pounds of your dog's body weight, twice daily with food.

Butyric acid: is a short-chain fatty acid that supports the colon through the microbiome. It's produced naturally by beneficial microbes and helps prevent leaky gut by strengthening the gut lining and decreasing inflammation. As a supplement, it is usually part of a formula, but it can be used alone as sodium butyrate. *Dosage:* 1/16 teaspoon for extra-small dogs; 1/8 teaspoon for small dogs; 1/4 teaspoon for medium dogs; 1/2 teaspoon for large dogs; 1 teaspoon for extra-large dogs. Give in the morning, once daily.

CBD (cannabidiol): is an extract of cannabis that is slightly warming with systemic benefits including relief from inflammation, seizures, pain, and anxiety. As a plant, cannabis is drying; it can be less drying when mixed with certain base oils. Make sure to use a full-spectrum, organic oil specifically formulated for dogs. *Dosage*: will vary depending on the situation. Most CBD comes in bottles containing 150 mg for extra-small dogs, 300 mg for small dogs, 600 mg for medium to large dogs and 1000 mg for extra-large dogs. Give as needed and read dosing directions on the bottle.

Chlorella: is a type of freshwater algae that has high levels of chlorophyll, B vitamins, amino acids, folate, and vitamin C. It decreases EMF damage, cleanses the blood, binds heavy metals, aids nutrient assimilation, and eliminates toxins. *Dosage:* 1/16 teaspoon for extra-small dogs; 1/8 teaspoon for small dogs; 1/4 teaspoon for medium dogs; 1/2 teaspoon for large dogs; 1 teaspoon for extra-large dogs. Give twice daily.

Coenzyme Q10: helps protect the body against radiation and supports the immune system. It helps prevent oxidative stress, supports heart health, and deters early aging. Make sure you source this substance from non-GMO sources. *Dosage:* 1 mg per pound of your dog's body weight, once daily.

Colostrum: is warm and nourishes the digestive system, soothes allergies, and provides growth factors. It helps with leaky gut treatment by supporting the repair of the gut lining. It also supports a healthy immune system, decreases food sensitivities, and increases IgA and beneficial bacteria. Choose ethically produced grass-fed and grass-finished sources. *Dosage:* 1/8 teaspoon for every 10 pounds of your dog's body weight, once daily.

Cranberries: are cool and contain manganese, quercetin, and vitamins C, E, and K1, as well as antioxidants, fiber, quercetin, D-mannose, anthocyanin, and proanthocyanidins. They help liver oxidation and support kidney and bladder health. *Dosage:* 150 milligrams for extra-small dogs; 200–300 milligrams for small dogs; 400 milligrams for medium dogs; 500–600 milligrams for large dogs; 700-800 milligrams for extra-large dogs. Once daily.

Digestive enzymes: support digestion and assimilation and therefore most other systems and structures in the body. They can be an especially important supplement for dogs that are fed kibble or cooked, freeze-dried, or dehydrated foods, which due to their processing often have low levels of enzymes. Digestive enzymes also help break up biofilm in the digestive tract and should be a part of all yeast/candida removal protocols (for this purpose, feed your dog the enzymes 3 hours after meals in broth). Note: If digestive enzymes make your dog itch, switch enzymes or use a lower dose. Purchase dog-specific enzymes. Start at a quarter of the manufacturer's recommended dose and work slowly up to the recommended dosage

D-mannose: is a unique simple sugar that keeps harmful bacteria from sticking to a dog's gut wall. *Dosage:* 1 gram of powder for every 20 pounds of your dog's weight daily.

Green-lipped mussels: are from New Zealand. They are warming and anti-inflammatory and a good alternative to NSAIDs for dogs with osteoarthritis and joint pain. *Dosage:* A good starting dose is 150 mg for every 10 pounds of your dog's body weight, twice daily. Make sure the supplement you're giving is at least 6 percent fat to ensure its absorption.

Green tea (decaffeinated): is slightly cool, highly antioxidant, and anti-inflammatory. It has anticancer properties and supports brain and immune function. Never give your dog caffeine; it can make them sick. *Dosage:* Give in tea form only and in the same dosages used for a standard infusion: 1/8 cup for an extra-small dog; 1/4 cup for a small dog; 1/2 cup for a medium dog; 3/4–1 cup for a large dog, and 1 1/2–2 cups for an extra-large dog. Administer twice daily.

Humic and fulvic acids: help balance the microbiome, provide trace minerals, fight the effects of glyphosate, and decrease candida populations. *Dosage:* Give 2 or 3 drops per day in food or liquid. If using a powdered supplement, consult the dosage instructions on the package, but start at a lower dose than what is suggested.

Honey (raw): is good for wound care, coughs, immune support, digestive issues, allergies, food sensitivities, liver detoxification, and systemic inflammation. Manuka honey, in particular, is specifically antibacterial and can be used internally and externally. *Dosage:* 1/8 teaspoon for extra-small dogs; 1/4 teaspoon for small dogs; 1/2 teaspoon for medium dogs; 3/4 teaspoon for large dogs; 1 teaspoon for extra-large dogs. Once daily.

Hyaluronic acid: helps create synovial fluid for joints. It's best used in a formula because too much can cause diarrhea, loss of appetite, and nausea.

Larch arabinogalactan: is a polysaccharide-rich prebiotic plant fiber. It supports a healthy microbiome and immune system, while tightening gut junctions. *Dosage:* 1/2 teaspoon for every 5 pounds of your dog's body weight, twice daily.

L-glutamine: is an amino acid that helps repair and support the gut lining by supporting cellular energy. It's antiviral and antibacterial and reduces immune cascade cycles. *Dosage:* L-glutamine is usually found in a formula for dogs, but the general dosage is 150 mg for every 10 pounds of your dog's body weight, once daily.

MCT oil: is medium-chain triglycerides usually sourced from coconuts. MCT oil supports the brain, gut, skin, and coat and is used in treatments for seizures and allergies. *Dosage:* 1/4 teaspoon for every 5 pounds of your dog's body weight, once daily.

Monolaurin: is sourced from coconuts. It helps break down and decreases biofilm due to its high lauricidin content. *Dosage:* 1/16 teaspoon for extra-small dogs; 1/8 teaspoon for small dogs; 1/4 teaspoon for medium dogs; 1/2 teaspoon for large dogs; 3/4 teaspoon for extra-large dogs. Once daily.

MSM (methylsulfonylmethane): provides sulfur, which is responsible for healthy DNA formation and repairs damaged cells. It also helps keep cellular membranes flexible, and it is integral to collagen formation. It supports your dog's immune, musculoskeletal, and nervous systems. *Dosage:* when needed, give 100 mg for every 5 pounds, once daily.

N-acetylcysteine: commonly known as NAC, helps clear the body of heavy metals and other toxins and breaks down biofilm in the intestines. *Dosage:* 1/16 teaspoon for extra-small dogs; 1/8 teaspoon for small dogs; 1/4 teaspoon for medium dogs; 1/2 teaspoon for large dogs; 3/4 teaspoon for extra-large dogs. Once daily.

PEA (palmitoylethanolamide): is an anti-inflammatory fatty acid used to treat arthritis, osteoarthritis, allergies, urinary tract infections, nerve pain, and other inflammatory conditions. *Dosage:* 1/16 teaspoon for extra-small dogs; 1/8 teaspoon for small dogs; 1/4 teaspoon for medium dogs; 1/2 teaspoon for large dogs; 1 teaspoon for extra-large dogs. Once daily. Like turmeric, PEA is absorbed better with a small amount of fat.

Phytoplankton: is a super-green, containing everything needed for life. It is a wee food packed with antioxidants, amino acids, carotenoids, chlorophyll, DHA, EPA, essential fatty acids, fiber, minerals, protein, vitamins, and trace minerals. As a supplement, phytoplankton increases mobility, strengthens digestion and liver detoxification, supports mitochondria and overall cellular function, and lowers anxiety. *Dosage:* 1/32 teaspoon (small pinch) for extra-small dogs; 1/16 teaspoon for small dogs; 1/8 teaspoon for medium dogs; 1/2 teaspoon for large dogs; 3/4 teaspoon for extra-large dogs. Once daily.

Propolis: is a bee product with high levels of antioxidants and polyphenols. It's antibacterial, anticancer, antifungal, antiviral, and immunoprotective. It is also extremely astringent, so mix it with something palatable or use it in a formula. Caution: Do not give propolis to dogs that are allergic to beestings. *Dosage:* 1/16 teaspoon for extra-small dogs; 1/8 teaspoon for small dogs; 1/4 teaspoon for medium dogs; 1/2 teaspoon for large dogs; 1 teaspoon for extra-large dogs. Once daily. Unless you are using it in a protocol under the supervision of a holistic vet or herbalist, limit its use to 2 weeks at a time, with a 3-week break between cycles, due to its antibacterial properties.

Quercetin: is a natural antihistamine that doesn't negatively affect stomach acid. It helps decrease gastrointestinal inflammation and heal leaky gut. It is also antipathogenic and supports beneficial bacteria in the large intestine and lungs. *Dosage:* 25 mg for every 5 pounds of your dog's body weight, twice daily.

Saccharomyces boulardii: is a probiotic yeast that helps control candida populations and reestablish balance in the microbiome. It's a powerhouse player in increasing glycocalyx and IgA production, allowing beneficial bacteria to grow and populate the gut. It helps reduce candida populations and keep candida inside the digestive tract and out of the bloodstream. *Dosage:* 1/16 teaspoon for extra-small dogs; 1/8 teaspoon for small dogs; 1/4 teaspoon for medium dogs; 1/2 teaspoon for large dogs; 1 teaspoon for extra-large dogs. Once daily. Start at one-quarter dose and work your way up slowly.

Sea vegetables: are high in trace minerals, enzymes, and protein, among other beneficial compounds. They have anti-inflammatory and anticancer effects, and they work to remove heavy metals from the body and support heart health, thyroid function, healthy teeth, and digestion. Sea vegetables include brown seaweed, kelp, dulse, kombu, nori, wakame. *Dosage:* 1/16 teaspoon for extra-small dogs; 1/8 teaspoon for small dogs; 1/4 teaspoon for medium dogs; 1/2 teaspoon for large dogs; 1 teaspoon for extra-large dogs. Once daily.

Spirulina: is a type of blue-green algae that is extremely nutritive, with high levels of vitamins, minerals, and trace minerals, along with other beneficial compounds. It helps slow yeast overgrowth and prevent recurring infections, protect cell membranes and the microbiome, resolve food sensitivities, and detoxify heavy metal accumulation. Quality is a huge issue with spirulina, so be sure to obtain it from trusted suppliers who test for mycrocystins, a liver toxin found in some blue-green algae, especially those grown in open ponds. *Dosage:* 1/16 teaspoon for every 5 pounds of your dog's body weight, once daily.

Zeolite: is a mineral that, as a supplement, helps absorb toxins, supports cellular function, and increases assimilation and elimination. Like bentonite clay, zeolite is negatively charged, which is how it binds toxins, but it doesn't interfere with nutrient absorption like clay does. *Dosage:* 1/8 teaspoon in olive oil or MCT oil for every 5 pounds of your dog's body weight, once daily. Or, if you are using a nanotized liquid, 1 drop for every 10 pounds of your dog's body weight. Look for clinoptilolite zeolite.

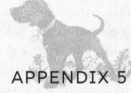

Food Energetics

Energetics is a system of patterns, and it's a guide. Is it always correct? No. No system of healing is 100 percent correct because, again, dogs are individuals. However, energetics is the best way I've found to address my dog's individuality. It helps me choose foods, herbs, supplements, and formulas that support my dog's health and longevity.

Below, I've listed the energetics of common ingredients in foods and supplements, including those used in popular pre-mixed formulas. At the end of the chapter I've also provided the energetics for herbs not included in the monographs in this book. When you consult these lists, remember that energetics is a range, and a particular food's energetics may depend on how it was grown (organic or not, for example) and how it interacts with a dog's energetics. A food that is warm can express a range of warmth, a food that is neutral can be slightly warm or slightly cool, and so on.

General Guidelines

1. Generally speaking, a healthy dog does best when fed foods that range from neutral to the opposite of the dog's natural energetics. In other words, if your dog is warm, feed foods that are neutral to cool. Feed a cold dog foods that run from neutral to warm.
2. If your dog is healthy, you can give foods in opposition to the above guideline as part of a rotating diet or as a snack. For example, if you have a naturally warm dog, you could give them cooked salmon (a warming food) as a rotation or treat a few times a month.

3. Ear-test any food, supplement, or remedy that you suspect may be energetically inappropriate for your dog; see page 150.

4. If a particular food seems to fall slightly out of your dog's range, the seasons could affect their tolerance. For example, a warm dog who is unable to tolerate chicken in the summer may do fine with it in the winter.

5. Treat acute conditions first, then chronic conditions. That means you may need to administer energetically inappropriate remedies for a short period (1 to 2 weeks) to treat an acute health condition. That's okay.

6. Probiotics tend to be neutral.

7. Amino acids and additives tend to be neutral. For example, N-acetylcysteine (NAC) is neutral.

8. If your dog is warm and has any imbalance, avoid digestive enzymes containing bromelain.

9. Avoid rabbit with dogs that are excessively dry or anxious and nervous.

10. Some of my observations differ from the energetics lists you may find online. My assessments come from my experience of these substances in my practice. Many of the lists you'll find online come from traditional Chinese medicine and were created at a time when factory farming didn't exist, animals were less stressed, vegetables were grown organically, soils were healthier, water was much cleaner, and food was simpler.

11. Energetic range can also depend on the types of feed meat animals are consuming. For example, cows have warmer energetics when they are fed poor diets. A cow fed native grasses will have cooler energetics than a cow fed monoculture grasses and/or genetically modified corn and candy derivatives.

12. You may read that a protein is warming or cooling—but in comparison to what? For example, many TCM lists say beef is warming. Yes, it is when compared to cooler meats like white fish, duck, and rabbit. But beef is cooler than lamb/mutton, venison, goat, chicken, and turkey. Use the lists below as a guide. Animal-based proteins come from living, breathing beings with their own set of energetic ranges—and, as humans, our knowledge is limited.

13. Conventional produce is warmer than organic produce.

Meat

Anchovies / neutral / damp

Beaver / hot / dry

Beef / neutral to cool / dry

Beef heart / neutral to cool / dry

Beef tripe / neutral / slightly dry

Bison / cool / slightly damp

Bovine colostrum / warm / neutral

Calamari / cool / damp

Camel / warm / damp

Catfish / warm / dry

Cow milk (raw) / neutral to cool / warm / slightly damp

Cow milk (pasteurized) / warm / damp

Chicken / warm / dry

Chicken eggs / neutral / slightly damp

Clams / warm / dry

Codfish / cool / damp

Crab / warm / dry

Cricket / cool / dry

Duck / cool / damp

Duck eggs / neutral / damp

Elk / neutral to warm / dry

Frog / warm / dry

Emu / warm / damp

Goat / warm / drying to slightly damp

Green-lipped mussel / warm / dry to slightly damp

Guinea fowl / neutral / slightly dry

Halibut / cool / damp

Herring / neutral / damp

Kangaroo / warm to hot / dry

Lake trout (non-farmed) / cool / dry

Lamb / hot / slightly damp

Lobster / hot / dry

Mackerel / neutral to cool / damp

Ostrich / warm / dry

Oyster / warm / damp

Partridge / cool / damp

Pheasant / cool / dry

Pigeon / cool / dry

Pollock / cool / damp

Pork / cool to cold / damp

Quail /neutral / neutral to damp

Rabbit / neutral to cool / dry

Salmon / warm / damp

Sardines / neutral / damp

Scallops / warm / dry

Shrimp / warm / dry

Sole / cool / dry

Squirrel / warm / damp

Tilapia: Avoid due to toxicity concerns.

Tuna / slightly warm / dry

Turkey / neutral to slightly warm / damp

Venison / hot / dry

Wild boar / cool / damp

Grains and Legumes

Amaranth / warm / dry

Barley / warm / dry

Black rice / neutral / damp

Brown rice / cool / damp

Buckwheat / warm / dry
Chickpeas / neutral / dry
Kamut / warm / dry
Lentils / cool / dry
Millet / warm / damp
Oats / cool / dry
Peas / neutral / damp
Quinoa / warm / dry
Rice bran / cool / dry

Rye / warm / dry
Sorghum / cool / slightly damp
Spelt / cool / dry
Wheat (organic) / neutral damp
Wheat bran / neutral / damp
Wheat germ / neutral / damp
White rice / warm / dry
Wild rice / cool / dry

Vegetables and Fruits

Açaí berries / warm / dry
Acorn squash / neutral / damp
Adzuki beans / cool / dry
Apples / neutral / damp
Apricots / cool / damp
Artichokes / neutral / damp
Arugula / slightly warm / dry
Asparagus / cool / dry
Avocados / neutral / damp
Bananas / warm / damp
Barley grass / neutral / dry
Beets / cool / dry
Black beans / cool / dry
Blackberries / cool / damp
Black currants / warm / damp
Blueberries / cool / dry
Bok choy / cool / damp
Boysenberries / cool / damp
Broccoli / cool / damp
Broccoli sprouts / cool / damp
Brussels sprouts / neutral / dry
Butternut squash / neutral / dry
Cabbage / warm / damp
Cactus pears / warm / damp
Cantaloupe / cool / damp

Carrots / neutral / dry
Cauliflower / cool / damp
Celery / cold / dry
Chard / cool / damp
Cherry / neutral / dry
Chinese cabbage / warm / slightly
  drying
Clementines / warm / dry
Coconut / neutral / damp
Collard greens / warm / slightly
  damp
Corn (sweet) / warm / dry
Cranberries / cool / dry
Cucumbers / cold / damp
Eggplant / warm / damp
Fennel bulb/ warm / dry
Garlic / warm / dry
Green beans / cool / dry
Hearts of palm / warm / damp
Honeydew melon / cool / damp
Kale / warm / dry
Kidney beans / warm / damp
Kiwi / warm / damp
Kohlrabi / warm / dry
Kumquats / cool / damp

Lemons / warm / dry

Lettuce / cold / slightly drying

Lima beans / cool / damp

Limes / cool / dry

Lingonberries / neutral / damp

Loganberries / cool / damp

Mangoes / neutral / damp

Marionberrries / warm / dry

Mustard greens / warm / dry

Navy beans / neutral / damp

Olives / neutral / slightly damp

Oranges / warm / dry

Papayas / cool / damp

Parsnips / cool / dry

Passion fruit / cool / damp

Peaches / cold / damp

Pears / slightly warm / dry

Peas / neutral / dry

Pineapple / warm / damp

Pink peppercorns / warm / dry

Pinto beans / cool / dry

Plums / cool / damp

Pomegranates / neutral / slightly dry

Potatoes (cooked) / neutral / damp

Pumpkin / neutral to cool / dry

Radish / cool but pungent / dry

Raspberries / cool / damp

Romaine lettuce / cool / slightly drying/balancing

Rutabagas / hot / dry

Snow peas / cool / dry

Soybean (organic) / neutral / damp

Spaghetti squash / cool / dry

Spinach / warm / slightly dry

Strawberries / slightly warm / damp

String beans / cool / dry

Summer squash (yellow) / warm / dry

Sweet potatoes / neutral / dry

Tangerines / warm / dry

Tomatoes / neutral / damp

Turnips and turnip greens / warm / dry

Watercress / neutral to warm / dry

Watermelon / cold / damp

Winter squash / cool / dry

Yams / cool / dry

Zucchini / slightly warm / damp

Mushrooms

Agarikon / warm / dry

Artist's conk / cool / dry

Chaga / neutral to cool / dry

Chanterelle / neutral / damp

Cordyceps / slightly hot / dry

Cremini / neutral / damp

Lion's mane / neutral to cool / damp

Maitake / cool / damp

Oyster / slightly warm / dry

Poria / neutral / dry

Portobello / neutral / damp

Reishi / slightly warm / dry

Shiitake / warm / dry

Tremella / neutral to cool / damp

Turkey tail / neutral / dry

Oils, Nuts, and Seeds

Ahi oil / neutral / damp

Almond oil / warm / damp

Almonds / warm / slightly damp

Avocado oil / cool / damp

Brazil nuts / neutral / damp

Calamari (squid) oil / cool / damp

Canola oil: Avoid.

Cashews / cool / damp

CBD oil / slightly warm / slightly drying

Chia seed / neutral / damp

Coconut oil / neutral / slightly damp

Corn oil: Avoid.

Flaxseed oil / neutral / damp

Flaxseeds / neutral / damp

Green-lipped mussel oil / warm / damp

Hemp seed oil / slightly warm / damp

Hemp seeds / slightly warm / damp

Olive oil / neutral / slightly damp

Peanuts / neutral / damp

Pistachio nuts / warm / dry

Pumpkin seed oil / cool / damp

Pumpkin seeds / cool / damp

Rapeseed oil: Avoid.

Rice bran oil / cool / damp

Safflower oil / warm / damp

Salmon oil / warm / damp

Sesame seed oil / cool / dry

Sesame seeds / cool / dry

Soybean oil: Avoid.

Sunflower seed oil / warm / damp

Sunflower seeds / warm / dry

Tahini / cool / slightly damp

Walnuts / cool / damp

Walnut oil / cool / slightly damp

Other Common Dog Supplement/Food Ingredients

Algae-derived calcium / neutral / damp

Aloe vera / cool / damp

Apple cider vinegar / warm / dry

Astaxanthin / warm / dry

Bee pollen / neutral / balancing

Bee propolis / warm / dry

Bentonite clay / neutral / dry

Brewer's yeast / warm / damp

Broccoli sprout powder / cool / damp

Bromelain / warm / neutral

Brown rice syrup / cool / damp

Chlorella / cool / slightly damp

Deer antler / warm / dry

Glycerin / neutral / damp

Green tea / slightly cool / dry

Honey / neutral / damp

Papain / cool / damp

Phytoplankton / neutral / dry

Psyllium / cool / damp

Seaweed / neutral / slightly dry

Spirulina / slightly warm / damp

Tapioca / neutral / damp

Vanilla / warm / dry

Herbs Not Found in This Book

American ginseng (*Panax quinquefolius*) / cool / damp

Andrographis (*Andrographis paniculata*) / cool / dry

Bacopa (*Bacopa monnieri*) / cool / dry / balancing

Barberry (*Berberis vulgaris, aristate*) / cool / dry

Bayberry (*Myrica cerifera*) / slightly warm / dry

Basil (*Ocimum basilicum*) / warm / dry

Black pepper (*Piper nigrum*) / warm / dry

Black walnut (*Juglans nigra, regia*) / slightly cool / dry

Bladderwrack (*Fucus vesiculosus*) / cool / damp

Bilberry (*Vaccinium myrtillus*) / cool / dry / balancing

Blessed thistle (*Cnicus benedictus*) / cool / dry

Blue flag iris (*Iris versicolor*) / cool / dry

Blue vervain (*Verbena hastata*) / cool / dry

Boneset (*Eupatorium perfoliatum*) / cool / dry

Borage (*Borago officinalis*) / cool / damp

Bugleweed (*Lycopus virginicus*) / cool / dry

Bupleurum (*Bupleurum chinense, scorzoneraefolium*) / cool / dry

California poppy (*Eschscholzia californica*) / cool / slightly damp

Cardamom (*Eletteria cardamomum*) / warm / dry

Catnip (*Nepeta cataria*) / cool to slightly warm

Cat's claw (*Uncaria tomentosa*) / cool / dry

Ceylon cinnamon (*Cinnamomum verum*) / warm / dry

Chaste berry (*Vitex agnus-castus*) / warm / dry

Cilantro (*Coriandrum sativum*) / cool / damp

Clove (*Eugenia caryophyllata*) / warm / dry (use caution)

Coltsfoot (*Tussilago farfara*) / cool / damp

Comfrey (*Symphytum officinale*) / cool / damp (use caution)

Corn silk (*Zea mays*) / neutral / slightly dry / balancing

Cramp bark (*Viburnum opulus*) / cool / dry

Devil's claw (*Harpagophytum procumbens*) / cool / dry

Dill (*Anethum graveolens*) / warm / dry

Dulce (*Palmaria palmata*) / cool / damp

Elder (*Sambucus canadensis, nigra*) / cool / dry

Elderberry (*Sambucus canadensis, nigra*) / cool / damp

Eleuthero (*Eleutherococcus senticosus*) / slightly warm / balancing

Eyebright (*Euphrasia officinalis*) / cool / dry

Fenugreek seed (*Trigonella foenum-graecum*) / warm / dry

Feverfew (*Tanacetum parthenium*) / cool / dry

Flaxseed (*Linum usitatissimum*) / cool / damp

Frankincense (*Boswellia serrata*) / warm / dry

Gentian (*Gentiana lutea*) / cold / dry

Ginkgo (*Ginkgo biloba*) / neutral / slightly dry

Ginseng (*Panax ginseng*) / warm / damp

Grindelia (*Grindelia* spp.) / warm /dry

Hibiscus (*Hibiscus rosa-sinensis*) / cool / dry

Holy basil (*Ocimum sanctum*) / cool / dry

Horehound (*Marrubium vulgare*) / cool / dry

Horse chestnut (*Aesculus hippocastanum*) / cool / dry

Horsetail (*Equisetum arvense*) / cool / dry

Hydrangea (*Hydrangea arborescens*) / cool / dry

Irish moss (*Chondrus crispus*) / cool / damp

Japanese knotweed (*Reynoutria japonica*) / cool / slightly dry

Kelp (*Laminaria* spp.) / neutral / damp

Kudzu (*Pueraria lobata, thunbergiana*) / cool / damp / balancing

Lavender (*Lavandula officinalis, angustifolia*) / slightly warm / dry

Lemongrass (*Cymbopogon citratus*) / cool / dry

Linden (*Tilia* spp.) / slightly warm / damp

Lobelia (*Lobelia inflata*) / slightly warm / slightly dry (use caution)

Maca (*Lepidium meyenii*) / warm / slightly damp

Marjoram (*Origanum majorana*) / warm / dry

Motherwort (*Leonurus cardiaca*) / cool / dry

Moringa leaf (*Moringa oleifera*) / warm / damp

Myrrh (*Commiphora* spp.) / warm / dry

Neem (*Azadirachta indica*) / cool / dry

Oak (*Quercus* spp.) / warm / dry

Oregano (*Origanum vulgare*) / warm / dry

Osha (*Ligusticum porteri*) / warm / dry

Papaya leaf (*Carica papaya*) / cool / dry

Paprika (*Capsicum annuum*) / warm / dry

Peppermint (*Mentha piperita*) / cool / dry

Pipsissewa (*Chimaphila umbellata*) / cool / dry

Pleurisy root (*Asclepias tuberosa*) / cool / damp

Prickly ash (*Zanthoxylum Americanum*) / warm / dry

Pulsatilla (*Pulsatilla vulgaris*) / cool / dry

Red raspberry (*Rubus idaeus*) / cool / dry

Red root (*Ceanothus americanus*) / neutral / dry

Rehmannia (*Rehmannia glutinosa*) / cool / neutral / balancing

Rhodiola (*Rhodiola rosea*) / cool / dry

Saffron (*Crocus sativus*) / warm / dry

Sage (*Salva officinalis*) / warm / dry

Saw palmetto (*Sabal serrulata*) / warm / damp

Self-heal (*Prunus vulgaris*) / cool / slightly dry

Schisandra (*Schisandra chinensis*) / neutral / balancing

Shatavari (*Asparagus racemosus*) / cool / balancing

Shepherd's purse (*Capsella bursa-pastoris*) / warm / dry

Teasel (*Dipsacus asper*) / cool / dry

Thyme (*Thymus vulgaris*) / warm / dry

Valerian (*Valeriana officinalis*) / warm / slightly dry

Wheatgrass (*Triticum aestivum*) / cool / slightly dry

Willow (*Salix* spp.) / cool / slightly dry

Wormwood (*Artemisia absinthium*) / cool / dry

Yerba mansa (*Anemopsis californica*) / warm / dry

Yucca (*Yucca glauca*) / cool / damp

Glossary

adrenal glands: two small endocrine glands located above the kidneys; they produce hormones that regulate many bodily systems, including the fight-or-flight response

adrenaline: a hormone produced by the adrenal glands, especially during times of fear, anger, or stress, that is responsible for the fight-or-flight response

astringent: acting to bind together or constrict

energetics: the energetic properties of an herb as it acts on the body; the energetic qualities of a condition or imbalance; or the energetics of a person or animal

enteric nervous system: the network of neurons covering the gastrointestinal tract; sometimes called the intrinsic nervous system

glyphosate: a broad-spectrum herbicide linked to cancer and dysfunction of the microbiome

histamine: a chemical released by the immune system as part of a signaling system for local immune responses, among other functions; it can contribute to food sensitivities and allergic responses

holism: the view that everything is connected and cannot function when divided into separate parts

interstitial fluid: the fluid between cells, which helps oxygenate cells and eliminate wastes; a vital component of the lymphatic system; also called matrix

intrinsic factor: a protein that allows the gastrointestinal tract to absorb vitamin B_{12}

mechanistic view: seeing living beings as if they were machines, a view that lacks empathy

menstruum: a solvent used in the preparation of an herb

meridians: pathways of energy flow in traditional Chinese medicine

myelin sheath: a protective and conductive layer that forms around nerves; when the sheath is damaged, electrical impulses (which serve as messages between the brain and body) slow down

oxalate stone: the most common type of kidney and bladder stone in dogs; made of calcium and oxalate

oxidation: a chemical reaction that takes place when a substance comes into contact with oxygen; in the body, oxidation is a normal process employed to fight pathogens and reduce the risk of infection, among other functions

oxidative stress: a condition of excessive oxidation caused by free radicals (atoms with an unpaired electron) reacting with oxygen in the body, which has a negative effect on many organs and systems in body, including the liver

oxytocin: a hormone that relieves stress

peristalsis: the process that moves food from the mouth to the anus

pH: a scale measuring the relative acidity or alkalinity of a substance

portal vein: a major blood vessel that delivers blood from the gallbladder, pancreas, spleen, and gastrointestinal tract to the liver

sepsis: a life-threatening bacterial infection in the bloodstream

SIBO: small intestinal bacterial overgrowth is a condition in which an overgrowth of bacteria in the small intestine causes gastrointestinal upset

solvent: a liquid substance that can dissolve other substances, turning them into a solution

synergy: a condition in which a combination of elements produces an effect greater than the sum of the elements acting on their own

thyroxine: a hormone produced by the thyroid

tone: continuous tension within tissues; think of low tone as flabby and high tone as strong and tight—and sometimes too tight

toxic burden: the volume of toxins in the body

vagus nerve: the dominant nerve that controls parasympathetic (rest, relaxation, digestion, immune function) activity

vital force: innate energy or spirit that animates living creatures; the energy that leaves or stops when an organism dies

wildcrafting: procuring plants from their natural habitats for use as food or medicines; foraging

Notes and References

Chapter 1. Holistic Canine Herbalism

1. Antonia Demas, "Celebrating Ancient Green Thoughts on Food and Health," Food Studies Institute website, n.d.
2. J. L. Casanova and L. Abel, "The Genetic Theory of Infectious Diseases: A Brief History and Selected Illustrations." *Annual Review of Genomics and Human Genetics* 14 (2013): 215–43.
3. S. P. Wiertsema, J. van Bergenhenegouwen, J. Garssen, and L. M. J. Knippels, "The Interplay between the Gut Microbiome and the Immune System in the Context of Infectious Diseases throughout Life and the Role of Nutrition in Optimizing Treatment Strategies," *Nutrients* 13, no. 3 (2021): 886.
4. M. C. Horzinek, "Vaccine Use and Disease Prevalence in Dogs and Cats." *Veterinary Microbiology* 117, no. 1 (2006): 2–8.
5. Megan Pond, "Adjuvants in Vaccines," Weston A. Price Foundation website, August 3, 2015.
6. E. C. Rosenow, "Experimental Studies on the Etiology of Encephalitis: Report of Findings in One Case," *JAMA* 79, no. 6 (1922): 443–48.
7. R. Lee, R. E. Seidel, and M. E. Winter, "The Rife Microscope, or 'Facts and Their Fate,'" Lee Foundation for Nutritional Research reprint 47, 1950 (orig. pub. 1944).
8. Ronald Hamowy, "The Early Development of Medical Licensing Laws in the United States 1875–1900," *Journal of Libertarian Studies* 3, no. 1 (1979): 73–119.
9. Eric Schewe, "How Did Big Pharma Get Big?" *JSTOR Daily*, March 19, 2017; R. L. Sur and P. Dahm, "History of Evidence-Based Medicine," *Indian Journal of Urology* 27, no. 4 (2011): 487–89.
10. T. J. Smith and B. H. Ashar, "Iron Deficiency Anemia Due to High-Dose Turmeric," *Cureus* 11, no. 1 (2019): e3858.
11. E. Williamson, "Synergy and Other Interactions in Phytomedicines," *Phytomedicine*, 8, no. 5 (2001): 401–9.
12. U. Bingel, L. Colloca, and L. Vase, "Mechanisms and Clinical Implications of the

Placebo Effect: Is There a Potential for the Elderly? A Mini-Review," *Gerontology* 57, no. 4 (2011): 354–63.

13. S. Rawat and S. Meena, "Publish or Perish: Where Are We Heading?" *Journal of Research in Medical Sciences* 19, no. 2 (2014): 87–89.

14. Jalees Rehman, "Can the Source of Funding for Medical Research Affect the Results?" *Scientific American* blog post, September 23, 2012.

15. M. Valentino and P. Pavlica, "Medical Ethics," *Journal of Ultrasound* 19 (2016): 73–76; Shaoni Bhattacharya, "Research Funded by Drug Companies Is 'Biased,'" New Scientist website, May 30, 2003.

16. B. Capps, "Can a Good Tree Bring Forth Evil Fruit? The Funding of Medical Research by Industry," *British Medical Bulletin* 118, no. 1 (2016): 5–15; Michelle Llamas, "Big Pharma's Role in Clinical Trials," Drugwatch website, April 24, 2015.

17. Michael F. Dahlstrom, "The Narrative Truth about Scientific Misinformation," *PNAS* 118, no. 15 (2021).

18. Susanne Tabert, "What Are Alkaloids in Plants & How to Extract Them," blog post, Mountain Rose Herbs website, January 11, 2023.

19. Demas, "Celebrating Ancient Green Thoughts on Food and Health."

20. Marc Bekoff, "Dogs Mirror Our Stress and We Know More about How and Why," blog post, Psychology Today website, June 8, 2019.

21. K. Uvnas-Moberg and M. Petersson, "Oxytocin, ein Vermittler von Antistress, Wohlbefinden, Sozialer Interaktion, Wachstum und Heilung" [Oxytocin, a mediator of anti-stress, well-being, social interaction, growth and healing], *Zeitschrift für Psychosomatische Medizin und Psychotherapie* 51, no. 1 (2005): 57–80.

22. Clara Wilson, Kerry Campbell, Zachary Petzel, and Catherine Reeve, "Dogs Can Discriminate between Human Baseline and Psychological Stress Condition Odours," *PLOS One* 17, no. 9 (2022): e0274143; Stanley Coren, "Do Humans Serve as a 'Safe Haven' for Stressed Dogs," blog post, Psychology Today website, March 20, 2013.

23. Rollin McCraty, *Science of the Heart: Exploring the Role of the Heart in Human Performance*, vol. 2 (HeartMath Institute, 2015).

24. Jessica Morales, "The Heart's Electromagnetic Field Is Your Superpower," blog post, Psychology Today website, November 29, 2020.

25. Temple Grandin, *The Autistic Brain: Thinking across the Spectrum* (Houghton Mifflin, 2013); Judith Orloff, MD, *Emotional Freedom: Liberate Yourself from Negative Emotions and Transform Your Life* (Random House, 2009).

26. A. Madison and J. K. Kiecolt-Glaser, "Stress, Depression, Diet, and the Gut Microbiota: Human-Bacteria Interactions at the Core of Psychoneuroimmunology and Nutrition," *Current Opinion in Behavioral Science* 28 (2019): 105–10.

27. Judith Orloff, MD, "The Power of an Animal's Unconditional Love," blog post, Psychology Today website, November 21, 2011.

Chapter 2. Food as Medicine

1. Ethan Shaw, "Animals That Are Carnivores," Sciencing website, August 19, 2018.

2. Judy Morgan, DVM, "20 Harmful Ingredients Found in Pet Food," blog post, Naturally Healthy Pets website, September 6, 2018.

3. Barbara Royal, DVM, "Understanding Pet Digestion," Innovative Veterinary Care website, April 12, 2018.

4. Ecology Center, "Pets Beware: Toxic Chemicals in Pet Food Cans—Press Release," EcoCenter.org website, June 29, 2017.

5. K. Leverett, R. Manjarín, E. Laird, D. Valtierra, T. M. Santiago-Rodriguez, R. Donadelli, and G. Perez-Camargo, "Fresh Food Consumption Increases Microbiome Diversity and Promotes Changes in Bacteria Composition on the Skin of Pet Dogs Compared to Dry Foods," *Animals* (Basel), 12, no. 15 (2022): 1881.

6. Steve Brown, "What You Should Know about Nutrition and Recipe Basics: An Intro to Homemade Pet Food with Renowned Formulator Steve Brown & Dr. Susan Recker," *The Inside Scoop Live* podcast, with Rodney Habib and Dr. Karen Becker of Planet Paws, July 2, 2023.

7. Peter Dobias, DVM, "Complete Guide to Natural Dental Care for Dogs," Peter Dobias website, accessed July 30, 2024.

8. G. Ianiro, S. Pecere, V. Giorgio, A. Gasbarrini, and G. Cammarota, "Digestive Enzyme Supplementation in Gastrointestinal Diseases," *Current Drug Metabolism* 17, no. 2 (2016): 187–93.

9. Y. Poitelon, A. M. Kopec, and S. Belin, "Myelin Fat Facts: An Overview of Lipids and Fatty Acid Metabolism," *Cells* 9, no. 4 (2020): 812.

10. Billy Hoekman, personal correspondence with the author via email, June 1, 2024.

11. Melissa Nohr, "Top 3 Healthy Fats & Which Fats To NEVER Eat," DrJockers website, n.d.

12. Burton Moomaw, "How Cold Food and Drink Affect Digestion," Burton Moomaw Acupuncture website, April 20, 2021.

13. E. E. Bray, Z. Zheng, M. K. Tolbert, B. M. McCoy, Dog Aging Project Consortium, M. Kaeberlein, and K. F. Kerr, "Once-Daily Feeding Is Associated with Better Health in Companion Dogs: Results from the Dog Aging Project," *GeroScience* 44, no. 3 (2022): 1779–90.

14. M. Razzoli, C. Pearson, S. Crow, and A. Bartolomucci, "Stress, Overeating, and Obesity: Insights from Human Studies and Preclinical Models," *Neuroscience & Biobehavioral Reviews* 76, part A (2017): 154–62.

15. L. Medalie, N. T. Baker, M. E. Shoda, W. W. Stone, M. T. Meyer, E. G. Stets, and M. Wilson, "Influence of Land Use and Region on Glyphosate and

Aminomethylphosphonic Acid in Streams in the USA," *Science of the Total Environment* 707 (2020): 136008.

16. Ryan Felton, "What's Really In Your Bottled Water," Consumer Reports website, September 24 2020.

Chapter 3. Canine Energetics

1. Paul Pitchford, *Healing with Whole Foods: Asian Traditions and Modern Nutrition* (North Atlantic Books, 2002), 309.

2. Pitchford, *Healing with Whole Foods,* 314–16.

3. Pitchford, *Healing with Whole Foods,* 312–13.

4. Pitchford, *Healing with Whole Foods,* 311–12.

5. Pitchford, *Healing with Whole Foods,* 313–14.

6. Pitchford, *Healing with Whole Foods,* 310–11.

7. Matthew Wood, *The Practice of Traditional Western Herbalism: Basic Doctrine, Energetics and Classification* (North Atlantic Books, 2004), 47.

8. Sajah Popham, Materia Medica Monthly, Herbal Foundations, Energetics, Temperature, Hot/Cold Polarity, video course materials, from the School of Evolutionary Herbalism, 2014–2015.

9. Wood, *The Practice of Traditional Western Herbalism,* 47.

10. Wood, *The Practice of Traditional Western Herbalism,* 50

11. Popham, Materia Medica Monthly course materials.

12. Wood, *The Practice of Traditional Western Herbalism,* 50.

13. J. R. Sheehan, C. Sadlier, and B. O'Brien, "Bacterial Endotoxins and Exotoxins in Intensive Care Medicine," *BJA Education* 22, no. 6 (2022): 224–30.

14. Cheryl Schwartz, DVM, *Four Paws, Five Directions: A Guide to Chinese Medicine for Cats and Dogs* (Celestial Arts, 1996), 271.

15. Matthew Wood and Sajah Popham, notes from Herbal Medicine Course, School of Evolutionary Herbalism, Oregon, September 29–30, October 20–21, November 3–4, December 1–2, 2018, and February 16–17, March 9–10, 2019.

16. Wood, *The Practice of Traditional Western Herbalism,* 48–49.

17. Wood, *The Practice of Traditional Western Herbalism,* 48–49.

18. Wood and Popham, notes from Herbal Medicine Course.

19. Schwartz, *Four Paws, Five Directions,* 271.

20. Wood, *The Practice of Traditional Western Herbalism,* 56–58.

21. Sajah Popham, Materia Medica Monthly, Herbal Foundations, Energetics, Tone, Relaxant-Tonic Polarity, video course materials, from the School of Evolutionary Herbalism, 2014–2015.

22. Randy Kidd, DVM, *Dr. Kidd's Guide to Herbal Dog Care* (Storey Publishing, 2000), 142.

23. Sajah Popham, Materia Medica Monthly, Herbal Foundations, Energetics, Moisture, Damp-Dry Polarity, video course materials, from the School of Evolutionary Herbalism, 2014–2016.

24. Wood, *The Practice of Traditional Western Herbalism*, 53–56.

25. Wood, *The Practice of Traditional Western Herbalism*, 47–48.

Chapter 4. Everything Is Connected

1. Kara E. Hannibal and Mark D. Bishop, "Chronic Stress, Cortisol Dysfunction, and Pain: A Psychoneuroendocrine Rationale for Stress Management in Pain Rehabilitation," *Physical Therapy* 94, no. 12 (2014): 1816–25.

2. M. Katayama, T. Kubo, K. Mogi, K. Ikeda, M. Nagasawa, and T. Kikusui, "Heart Rate Variability Predicts the Emotional State in Dogs," *Behavioural Processes* 128 (2016): 108–12.

3. A. Arruda, C. Mesquita, R. Couto, V. Sousa, and C. Mendonça, "Dogs Barking and Babies Crying: The Effect of Environmental Noise on Physiological State and Cognitive Performance," *Noise & Health* 25, no. 119 (2023): 247–56.

4. M. Carabotti, A. Scirocco, M. A. Maselli, and C. Severi, "The Gut-Brain Axis: Interactions between Enteric Microbiota, Central and Enteric Nervous Systems," *Annals of Gastroenterology* 28, no. 2 (2015): 203–9.

5. Guido Masé, "Guido Masé on Bitters: The Gym for Your Digestion," blog post, Urban Moonshine website, n.d.

6. Y. Han, B. Wang, H. Gao, C. He, R. Hua, C. Liang, S. Zhang, Y. Wang, S. Xin, and J. Xu, "Vagus Nerve and Underlying Impact on the Gut Microbiota-Brain Axis in Behavior and Neurodegenerative Diseases," *Journal of Inflammation Research* 15 (2022): 6213–30.

7. Jane A. Foster, Linda Rinaman, and John F. Cryan, "Stress & the Gut-Brain Axis: Regulation by the Microbiome," *Neurobiology of Stress* 7 (2017): 124–36.

8. H. M. Al-Awami, A. Raja, and M. P. Soos. "Physiology, Gastric Intrinsic Factor." StatPearls, July 17, 2023.

9. Jim McDonald, "Fight, Flight, Freak, & Freeze: Understanding Sympathetic Stress," in *Herbal Clinician V: Energetics, Herbal Actions & Further Therapeutics*, ed. Jesse Wolf Hardin and Kiva Rose Hardin (independently published, 2020).

10. Masé, "Guido Masé on Bitters."

11. P. Harkins, E. Burke, C. Swales, and A. Silman, "'All Disease Begins in the Gut'— the Role of the Intestinal Microbiome in Ankylosing Spondylitis," *Rheumatology Advances in Practice* 5, no. 3 (2021): rkab063.

12. Jim McDonald, "Surviving Sinusitis & Other Catarrhal Catastrophes," in *Herbal Clinician IV: Herbal Treatments for Lungs, Liver, Heart, Kidneys & Bladder*, ed. Jesse Wolf Hardin and Kiva Rose Hardin (independently published, 2020), 275.

13. R. Uauy, P. Peirano, D. Hoffman, P. Mena, D. Birch, and E. Birch, "Role of Essential Fatty Acids in the Function of the Developing Nervous System," *Lipids* 31, suppl. (1996): S167–76.

14. P. Hemarajata and J. Versalovic, "Effects of Probiotics on Gut Microbiota: Mechanisms of Intestinal Immunomodulation and Neuromodulation," *Therapeutic Advances in Gastroenterology* 6, no. 1 (2013): 39–51.

15. P. S. Mortimer and S. G. Rockson, "New Developments in Clinical Aspects of Lymphatic Disease," *Journal of Clinical Investigation* 124, no. 3 (2014): 915–21.

16. Betsy Costilo-Miller, "The Language of Lymph," in *Herbal Clinician III: Inflammation, Immune, Structural & Gut Therapeutics* (independently published, 2020), 88.

17. Matthew Wood, "Lymph Immune System—Part I," in *Herbal Clinician III: Inflammation, Immune, Structural & Gut Therapeutics* (independently published, 2020), 32–41.

18. J. I. Park, S. W. Cho, J. H. Kang, and T. E. Park, "Intestinal Peyer's Patches: Structure, Function, and In Vitro Modeling," *Tissue Engineering and Regenerative Medicine* 20, no. 3 (2023): 341–53.

19. Cheryl Schwartz, DVM, *Four Paws, Five Directions: A Guide to Chinese Medicine for Cats and Dogs* (Celestial Arts, 1996), 243–44.

20. Y. Zhang and X. M. Fang, "Hepatocardiac or Cardiohepatic Interaction: From Traditional Chinese Medicine to Western Medicine," *Evidence-Based Complementary and Alternative Medicine* 2021: 6655335.

21. Patricia Jordan, DVM, "A Vet's Guide to Elevated Liver Enzymes in Dogs," Dogs Naturally website, October 2022.

22. David Jockers, "8 Proven Ways to Improve Your Detoxification System," DrJockers website, n.d.

23. Karen A Moriello, DVM, "Structure of the Skin in Dogs," *Merck Veterinary Manual* (online), June 2018.

24. Dana Ullman, "Don't Confuse Real Healing with Suppression of the Disease," blog post, *Huffington Post,* November 17, 2011.

25. Jean Dodds, DVM, and Diana R. Laverdure, *The Canine Thyroid Epidemic: Answers You Need for Your Dog* (Dogwise Publishing, 2011).

26. Peter Dobias, DVM, "Natural Approach to Treating Skin Infections, Allergies and Hot Spots," Dr. Dobias Natural Healing website, n.d.

27. R. H. Hunt, M. Camilleri, S. E. Crowe, E. M. El-Omar, J. G. Fox, et al., "The Stomach in Health and Disease," *Gut* 64, no. 10 (2015): 1650–68.

28. Dan Richardson, "The Dog Digestive System," blog post, Vetericyn website, September 10, 2019.

29. Al-Awami, Raja, and Soos, "Physiology, Gastric Intrinsic Factor."

30. R. H. Patel and S. S. Mohiuddin, "Biochemistry, Histamine," StatPearls, May 1, 2023.

31. H. T. Debas and S. H. Carvajal, "Vagal Regulation of Acid Secretion and Gastrin Release," *Yale Journal of Biology and Medicine* 67, no. 3–4 (1994): 145–51.

32. A. R. Ballegaard and K. L. Bøgh, "Intestinal Protein Uptake and IgE-Mediated Food Allergy," *Food Research International* 163 (2023): 112150.

33. J. R. Rapin and N. Wiernsperger, "Possible Links between Intestinal Permeability and Food Processing: A Potential Therapeutic Niche for Glutamine," *Clinics* (São Paulo) 65, no. 6 (2010): 635–43.

34. D. A. Fritsch, M. I. Jackson, S. M. Wernimont, G. K. Feld, D. V. Badri, J. J. Brejda, C. Y. Cochrane, and K. L. Gross, "Adding a Polyphenol-Rich Fiber Bundle to Food Impacts the Gastrointestinal Microbiome and Metabolome in Dogs," *Frontiers in Veterinary Science* 9 (2023): 1039032.

35. I. Trefflich, H. U. Marschall, R. D. Giuseppe, M. Ståhlman, A. Michalsen, A. Lampen, K. Abraham, and C. Weikert, "Associations between Dietary Patterns and Bile Acids: Results from a Cross-Sectional Study in Vegans and Omnivores," *Nutrients* 12, no. 1 (2019): 47.

36. J. M. Ridlon, D. J. Kang, P. B. Hylemon, and J. S. Bajaj, "Bile Acids and the Gut Microbiome," *Current Opinions in Gastroenterology* 30, no. 3 (2014): 332–28.

37. S. Waniek, R. di Giuseppe, T. Esatbeyoglu, I. Ratjen, J. Enderle, G. Jacobs, U. Nöthlings, M. Koch, S. Schlesinger, G. Rimbach, and W. Lieb, "Association of Circulating Vitamin E (α- and γ-Tocopherol) Levels with Gallstone Disease," *Nutrients* 10, no. 2 (2018): 133.

38. E. Mondo, G. Marliani, P. A. Accorsi, M. Cocchi, and A. Di Leone, "Role of Gut Microbiota in Dog and Cat's Health and Diseases," *Open Veterinary Journal* 9, no. 3 (2019): 253–58.

39. A. Madison and J. K. Kiecolt-Glaser, "Stress, Depression, Diet, and the Gut Microbiota: Human-Bacteria Interactions at the Core of Psychoneuroimmunology and Nutrition," *Current Opinion in Behavioral Science* 28 (2019): 105–10.

40. Rachel Pilla and Jan Suchodolski, "The Role of the Canine Gut Microbiome and Metabolome in Health and Gastrointestinal Disease," *Frontiers in Veterinary Science* 6 (2020).

41. G. P. Donaldson, M. S. Ladinsky, K. B. Yu, J. G. Sanders, B. B. Yoo, et al., "Gut Microbiota Utilize Immunoglobulin A for Mucosal Colonization," *Science* 360, no. 6390 (2018): 795–800.

42. A. Qamar, S. Aboudola, M. Warny, P. Michetti, C. Pothoulakis, J. T. LaMont, and C. P. Kelly, "*Saccharomyces boulardii* Stimulates Intestinal Immunoglobulin A Immune Response to Clostridium difficile Toxin A in Mice," *Infection and Immunity* 69, no. 4 (2001): 2762–65.

43. Y. Koga, "Microbiota in the Stomach and Application of Probiotics to Gastroduodenal Diseases," *World Journal of Gastroenterology* 28, no. 47 (2022): 6702–15.

44. E. Rinninella, P. Raoul, M. Cintoni, F. Franceschi, G. A. D. Miggiano, A. Gasbarrini, and M. C. Mele, "What Is the Healthy Gut Microbiota Composition? A Changing Ecosystem across Age, Environment, Diet, and Diseases," *Microorganisms* 7, no. 1 (2019): 14.

45. A. Piccolo, G. Celano, and P. Conte, "Adsorption of Glyphosate by Humic Substances," *Journal of Agricultural and Food Chemistry* 44, no. 8 (1996): 2442–46; Deby Hamilton, MD, "Humic Acid: The Power of Detox and Immune Support All in One," *Research Review* 12 (2018).

46. Jillian Levy, "7 Fulvic Acid Benefits & Uses: Improve Gut, Skin & Brain Health," Dr. Axe website, September 3, 2019.

47. Schwartz, *Four Paws, Five Directions,* 225.

48. Jessica Morales, "The Heart's Electromagnetic Field Is Your Superpower," blog post, Psychology Today website, November 29, 2020.

49. Schwartz, *Four Paws, Five Directions,* 225–27.

50. Karuna Meda, "The Heart's 'Little Brain,'" *Thomas Jefferson University Research Magazine* 3, no. 1, article 13 (2022).

51. B. Y. Nguyen, A. Ruiz-Velasco, T. Bui, L. Collins, X. Wang, and W. Liu, "Mitochondrial Function in the Heart: The Insight into Mechanisms and Therapeutic Potentials," *British Journal of Pharmacology* 176, no. 22 (2019): 4302–18.

52. Zhang and Fang, "Hepatocardiac or Cardiohepatic Interaction."

53. Pip Waller, *Holistic Anatomy: An Integrative Guide to the Human Body* (North Atlantic Books, 2010), 135–43.

54. Malcolm Weir, DVM, and Sonya G. Gordon, DVM, "Home Breathing Rate Evaluation," VCA Animal Hospitals website, n.d.

55. E. R. Lillehoj and K. C. Kim, "Airway Mucus: Its Components and Function," *Archives of Pharmacal Research* 25, no. 6 (2002): 770–80.

56. Schwartz, *Four Paws, Five Directions,* 209–10.

57. Josie Beug, DVM, TCVM, email exchange, February 3, 2023.

58. Schwartz, *Four Paws, Five Directions,* 211–24.

59. Schwartz, *Four Paws, Five Directions,* 209.

60. Rodney Habib and Karen Shaw Becker, DVM, *The Forever Dog, Surprising New Science to Help Your Canine Companion Live Younger, Healthier & Longer* (Harper Wave, 2021), 377.

61. Cheshire Pet, "Urine Test," Cheshire Pet website, n.d.

62. Schwartz, *Four Paws, Five Directions,* 290–92.

63. B. Schoener and J. Borger, "Erythropoietin Stimulating Agents," StatPearls, March 11, 2023.

64. Waller, *Holistic Anatomy*, 183–90.

65. Peter Dobias, DVM, "Holistic Approach to Kidney Disease Treatment," Dr. Dobias Natural Healing website, n.d.

66. Gregory F. Grauer, "Reassessment of 'Normal' Values in Dogs and Cats with Chronic Kidney Disease," International Renal Interest Society website, n.d.

67. S. Gueye, S. M. Seck, Y. Kane, P. O. Tosi, S. Dahri, et al., "La néphrite de Lyme chez l'homme: Bases physiopathologiques et spectre lésionnel rénal" [Lyme nephritis in humans: Physio-pathological bases and spectrum of kidney lesions], *Néphrologie & Thérapeutique* 15, no. 3 (2019): 127–35.

68. J. Kim, J. Lee, K. N. Kim, K. H. Oh, C. Ahn, J. Lee, D. Kang, and S. K. Park, "Association between Dietary Mineral Intake and Chronic Kidney Disease: The Health Examinees (HEXA) Study," *International Journal of Environmental Research and Public Health* 15, no. 6 (2018): 1070.

Chapter 5. Remedies

1. Tina Wismer, DVM, "Ethanol Toxicosis: A Review," *Today's Veterinary Practice*, March/April 2017.

2. T. G. O. Achufusi and R. K. Patel, "Milk Thistle," StatPearls, September 12, 2022.

3. A. Shah, Y. Wang, and F. E. Wondisford, "Differential Metabolism of Glycerol Based on Oral versus Intravenous Administration in Humans," *Metabolites* 12, no. 10 (2022): 890.

4. Swanie Simon, herbalist, personal interview with the author via email, 2017.

5. Y. Wu, Y. Zhang, G. Xie, A. Zhao, X. Pan, et al., "The Metabolic Responses to Aerial Diffusion of Essential Oils," *PLoS One* 7, no. 9 (2012): e44830.

6. Dee Blanco, DVM, personal interview with the author via phone, 2017.

7. Robert Tisserand, "Proof of Safety: Challenges Facing Essential Oil Therapy" (paper presented at the 2007 AIA Conference in Denver, Colorado).

8. N. J. Sadgrove, G. F. Padilla-González, O. Leuner, I. Melnikovova, and E. Fernandez-Cusimamani, "Pharmacology of Natural Volatiles and Essential Oils in Food, Therapy, and Disease Prophylaxis," *Frontiers in Pharmacology* 12 (2021): 740302.

9. Patrice de Bonneval and Cathy Skipper, *Aromatic Medicine: Integrating Essential Oils into Herbal Practice* (Editions des Savoirs Naturels, 2013), 47.

10. Anja Rothe, "The Dirt on Hydrosols," Fat of the Land Apothecary website, Spring 2022.

11. Josh Axe, "Sandalwood Essential Oil Benefits for the Brain & Body," Dr. Axe webite, March 3, 2023.

12. United Plant Savers, "Your Essential Oils Might Be at Risk," United Plant Savers website, n.d.

13. Andrea Barra, "Factors Affecting Chemical Variability of Essential Oils: A Review of Recent Developments," *Natural Product Communications* 4, no. 8 (2008): 1147–54.

14. F. Capetti, A. Marengo, C. Cagliero, E. Liberto, C. Bicchi, P. Rubiolo, and B. Sgorbini, "Adulteration of Essential Oils: A Multitask Issue for Quality Control. Three Case Studies: *Lavandula angustifolia* Mill., *Citrus limon* (L.) Osbeck and *Melaleuca alternifolia* (Maiden & Betche) Cheel.," *Molecules* 26, no. 18 (2021): 5610.

15. Elisabeth Anderson and Jinpeng Li, "Essential Oils—An Overview," Michigan State University Center for Research on Ingredient Safety website, August 17, 2020.

16. Matthew Wood, *Vitalism, The History of Herbalism, Homeopathy, and Flower Essences* (North Atlantic Books, 2000), 185–94.

17. Jeffrey R. Cram, "A Psychological and Metaphysical Study of Dr. Edward Bach's Flower Essence Stress Formula," *Subtle Energies & Energy Medicine Journal Archives* 11, no. 1 (2000).

18. Marcello Nicoletti and Fernando Piterà di Clima, *Gemmotherapy, and the Scientific Foundations of a Modern Meristemotherapy* (Cambridge Scholars Publishing, 2020), 23.

19. Max Tetau, MD, *Gemmotherapy: A Clinical Guide* (Editions Similla, 2010); Stephen Blake, DVM, *Gemmotherapy for Our Animal Friends* (independently published, 2011), 19–21.

Chapter 6. Planning Herbal Protocols

1. Rajneesh Kumar Sharma, "Arndt Schultz Law and Its Applications in Homeopathy," Homeobook website, June 4, 2012.

2. Notes from a lecture given by Matthew Wood, "Introduction to the Simple & Mysterious in Herbal Medicine," Radiance Herbs and Gifts, Olympia, Washington, November 2016.

Chapter 7. Herbal Applications

1. C. P. Haworth, "Low Stomach Acid—Everything You Need to Know," Functional Gut Clinic website, June 28, 2022.

2. S. Pucci and C. Incorvaia, "Allergy as an Organ and a Systemic Disease," *Clinical and Experimental Immunology* 153, suppl. 1 (2008): 1–2.

3. Peter Dobias, DVM, "Holistic and Natural Approach to Treating Diarrhea in Dogs," blog post, Dr. Dobias Natural Healing website, accessed May 15, 2024.

4. K. Farzam, S. Sabir, and M. C. O'Rourke, "Antihistamines," StatPearls, July 10, 2023.

5. A. M. Fardous and A. R. Heydari, "Uncovering the Hidden Dangers and Molecular Mechanisms of Excess Folate: A Narrative Review," *Nutrients* 15, no. 21 (2023): 4699.

6. Conor Brady, "Anal Glands in Dogs," Dogs First website, May 5, 2016.

7. Rania Golakner, DVM, "Metronidazole," VCA Hospitals website, n.d.

8. Rodney Habib and Karen Shaw Becker, DVM, *The Forever Dog, Surprising New Science to Help Your Canine Companion Live Younger, Healthier & Longer* (Harper Wave, 2021), 171.

9. A. Caneschi, A. Bardhi, A. Barbarossa, and A. Zaghini, "The Use of Antibiotics and Antimicrobial Resistance in Veterinary Medicine, a Complex Phenomenon: A Narrative Review," *Antibiotics* (Basel), 12, no. 3 (2023): 487.

10. V. T. Pham, S. Dold, A. Rehman, J. K. Bird, and R. E. Steinert, "Vitamins, the Gut Microbiome and Gastrointestinal Health in Humans," *Nutrition Research* 95 (2021): 35–53.

11. Alena Pribyl, "The Effects of Antibiotics on the Gut Microbiome," Microba website, November 28, 2018.

12. Sophie Fessi, "What Happens to the Gut Microbiome after Taking Antibiotics," *The Scientist,* May 5, 2022.

13. T. De Campos, J. C. Assef, and S. Rasslan, "Questions about the Use of Antibiotics in Acute Pancreatitis," *World Journal of Emergency Surgery* 1 (2006): 20.

14. R. G. Xiong, D. D. Zhou, S. X. Wu, S. Y. Huang, A. Saimaiti, Z. J. Yang, A. Shang, C. N. Zhao, R. Y. Gan, and H. B. Li, "Health Benefits and Side Effects of Short-Chain Fatty Acids," *Foods* 11, no. 18 (2022): 2863.

15. Amy Myers, "Why Soil-Based Probiotics Are Best for SIBO," Amy Myers, MD, website, accessed July 10, 2024.

16. M. Cavalheiro and M. C. Teixeira, "*Candida* Biofilms: Threats, Challenges, and Promising Strategies," *Frontiers in Medicine* 5 (2018).

17. Habib and Becker, *The Forever Dog,* 171.

18. B. Medeiros-Fonseca, A. I. Faustino-Rocha, R. Medeiros, P. A. Oliveira, and R. M. Gil da Costa, "Canine and Feline Papillomaviruses: An Update," *Frontiers in Veterinary Science* 10 (2023): 1174673.

19. John Munday and Susan Shaw, "Skin Cutaneous Papilloma in Dogs," Vetflexion website, 2016.

20. A. C. C. C. Branco, F. S. Y. Yoshikawa, A. J. Pietrobon, and M. N. Sato, "Role of Histamine in Modulating the Immune Response and Inflammation," *Mediators of Inflammation* (2018): 9524075.

21. E. B. Thangam, E. A. Jemima, H. Singh, M. S. Baig, M. Khan, C. B. Mathias,

M. K. Church, and R. Saluja. "The Role of Histamine and Histamine Receptors in Mast Cell-Mediated Allergy and Inflammation: The Hunt for New Therapeutic Targets," *Frontiers in Immunology* 9 (2018): 1873.

22. Lauren Deville, MD, "Methylation Defects," Dr. Lauren Deville website, September 23, 2023.

23. J. Talkington and S. P. Nickell, "*Borrelia burgdorferi* Spirochetes Induce Mast Cell Activation and Cytokine Release," *Infection and Immunity* 67, no. 3 (1999): 1107–15.

24. Chris Kresser, "What You Should Know about Histamine Intolerance," Chris Kresser website, June 26, 2019.

25. S.-H. Kim, D.-E. Park, H.-S. Lee, H.-R. Kang, and S.-H. Cho, "Chronic Low Dose Chlorine Exposure Aggravates Allergic Inflammation and Airway Hyperresponsiveness and Activates Inflammasome Pathway," *PLoS ONE* 9, no. 9 (2014): e106861; Karen Thomas, "The Health Dangers and Histamine Triggers of Chlorine," *Naturally Recovering Autism* podcast, episode 128, June 2, 2021.

26. S. Sánchez-Pérez, O. Comas-Basté, A. Duelo, M. T. Veciana-Nogués, M. Berlanga, M. L. Latorre-Moratalla, and M. C. Vidal-Carou, "Intestinal Dysbiosis in Patients with Histamine Intolerance," *Nutrients* 14, no. 9 (2022): 1774.

27. Conor Brady, *Feeding Dogs: Dry or Raw? The Science behind the Debate* (Farrow Road Publishing, 2020), 219–26.

28. Jonathan Leake, "Killer Liver Disease on Rise Due to Overeating," *The Times* (London), May 3, 2015.

29. J. H. Chang, C. R. Vogt, G. Y. Sun, and A. Y. Sun, "Effects of Acute Administration of Chlorinated Water on Liver Lipids," *Lipids* 16, no. 5 (1981): 336–40.

30. I. Gambino, F. Bagordo, T. Grassi, A. Panico, and O. De Donno, "Occurrence of Microplastics in Tap and Bottled Water: Current Knowledge," *International Journal of Environmental Research and Public Health* 19, no. 9 (2022): 5283.

31. Mia DiFelice and Ben Murray, "5 Reasons to Rein In The Bottled Water Industry," Food and Water Watch website, November 10, 2023.

32. Hannah Hickey, "Scented Laundry Products Emit Hazardous Chemicals through Dryer Vents," University of Washington News website, August 24, 2011.

33. Jennifer L. Weinberg, MD, "An Integrative Medicine Approach to Lipomas," Rupa Health website, October 11, 2023.

34. Karen Beltran, Rita Wadeea, and Karen L. Herbst, "Infections Preceding the Development of Dercum Disease," *IDCases* 19 (2020): e00682.

35. Jean Dodds, DVM, "Glyphosate and Your Companion Pets," Hemopet website, January 13, 2020.

36. Deby Hamilton, MD, "Humic Acid: The Power of Detox and Immune Support All in One," *Research Review* 12 (2018).

37. Charles Turlington, "Phases of Healing Following Surgery," Solstice Wellness website, n.d.

Chapter 8. Plant and Fungi Monographs

The monographs are a collaboration of my experience in my clinical practice and the works cited here.

General References

Garran, Thomas Avery, *Western Herbs according to Traditional Chinese Medicine: A Practitioner's Guide* (Healing Arts Press, 2008).

Holmes, Peter, *The Energetics of Western Herbs: A Materia Medica Integrating Western and Chinese Herbal Therapeutics* (Snow Lotus Press, 2007).

Sinadinos, Christa, *The Essential Guide to Western Botanical Medicine* (self-published, 2022).

Skenderi, Gazmend, *Herbal Vade Mecum* (Herbacy Press, 2003).

Tilford, Greg, and Mary L. Wulff, *Herbs for Pets: The Natural Way to Enhance Your Pet's Life*, 2nd ed. (Bowtie Press, 2009).

Wood, Matthew, *The Earthwise Herbal,* vol. 1, *A Complete Guide to Old World Medicinal Plants* (North Atlantic Books, 2008), and vol. 2, *A Complete Guide to New World Medicinal Plants* (North Atlantic Books, 2009).

Agrimony

Cascardi, Laura, "Agrimony Materia Medica," monograph on the Hawthorn Tree website, n.d.

Paluch, Z., L. Biriczová, G. Pallag, E. Carvalheiro Marques, N. Vargová, and E. Kmoníčková, "The therapeutic effects of *Agrimonia eupatoria* L.," *Physiological Research* 69, suppl. 4 (2020): S555–71.

Popham, Sajah, "Agrimony: The Tense but Relaxed Remedy," School of Evolutionary Herbalism website, August 16, 2023.

Wood, *The Earthwise Herbal,* vol. 1, 54–60.

Alfalfa

British Herbal Pharmacopoeia (British Herbal Medicine Association, 1996).

Sinadinos, *The Essential Guide to Western Botanical Medicine,* 1.

Skenderi, *Herbal Vade Mecum,* 8.

Tilford, Greg, and Mary L. Wulff-Tilford, *Herbs for Pets: The Natural Way to Enhance Your Pet's Life* (Bowtie Press, 1999), 66–68.

Wood, *The Earthwise Herbal,* vol. 1, 338–41.

Aloe

National Center for Complementary and Integrative Health (NCCIH), "Aloe Vera," NCCIH website, August 2020.

Sinadinos, *The Essential Guide to Western Botanical Medicine,* 4–8.

Skenderi, *Herbal Vade Mecum,* 10.

Tilford, Greg, and Mary L. Wulff-Tilford, *Herbs for Pets: The Natural Way to Enhance Your Pet's Life* (Bowtie Press, 1999), 69–70.

Angelica

Brinker, F., *Herb Contraindications and Drug Interactions,* 3rd ed. (Eclectic Medical Publications, 2001).

British Herbal Pharmacopoeia (British Herbal Medical Association, 1983).

Garran, *Western Herbs according to Traditional Chinese Medicine,* 121–22.

Hoffmann, David, *Medical Herbalism* (Healing Arts Press, 2003), 427.

Holmes, *The Energetics of Western Herbs,* 383.

Johnson, Talitha, "Angelica," monograph on the HerbRally website, n.d.

Mills, S., and K. Bone, *Principles and Practice of Phytotherapy* (Churchill Livingstone, 2000).

Sinadinos, *The Essential Guide to Western Botanical Medicine,* 16–19.

Skenderi, *Herbal Vade Mecum,* 13.

Wood, *The Earthwise Herbal,* vol. 1, 91–98.

Artichoke

Sinadinos, *The Essential Guide to Western Botanical Medicine,* 34–37.

Skenderi, *Herbal Vade Mecum,* 19.

Wood, *The Earthwise Herbal,* vol. 1, 54–60.

Ashwagandha

The Ayurvedic Pharmacopoeia of India, part 1, vol. 1 (Government of India, Ministry of Health and Family Welfare, Department of Indian Systems of Medicine & Homoeopathy, 1978).

Popham, Sajah, "Ashwagandha Materia Medica," Materia Medica Monthly course materials (volume 34), from the School of Evolutionary Herbalism, 2019.

Sinadinos, *The Essential Guide to Western Botanical Medicine,* 38–40.

Skenderi, *Herbal Vade Mecum,* 23.

Thompson, Krystal, "Ashwagandha (*Withania somnifera*)," monograph on the HerbRally website, n.d.

Upton, R., ed., "Ashwagandha Root *Withania somnifera*: Analytical, Quality Control, and Therapeutic Monograph," part of the American Herbal Pharmacopoeia and Therapeutic Compendium (American Herbal Pharmacopoeia, April 2000).

Astragalus

Bensky, D., and A. Gamble, *Chinese Herbal Medicine: Materia Medica* (Eastland Press, 1986).

Brinker, F., *Herb Contraindications and Drug Interactions*, 4th ed. (Eclectic Medical Publications, 2010).

Holmes, *The Energetics of Western Herbs*, 256.

Sinadinos, *The Essential Guide to Western Botanical Medicine*, 45–48.

Thompson, Krystal, "Astragalus Monograph," monograph on the HerbRally website, n.d.

Tierra, Lesley, *Healing with the Herbs of Life* (Crown, 2003), 51–52.

Tilford and Wulff, *Herbs for Pets*, 56–58.

Bee Balm

Crow, T. M., *Native Plants, Native Healing: Traditional Muskogee Way* (Native Voices, 2001).

Doyle, Ashley, "*Monarda fistulosa menthafolia*—A Student Monograph," the Forager's Path School of Botanical Studies website, November 19, 2019.

Johnson, Jackie, "Benefits of Bee Balm: Mondarda fistulosa and M. didyma," Herbal Academy website, July 28, 2015.

Rosethorn, Kiva, "Honeyed Spice of the Canyons," Enchanter's Green website, n.d.

Skenderi, *Herbal Vade Mecum*, 39.

Wood, *The Earthwise Herbal*, vol. 2, 240–42.

Blackberry

Grieve, Maud, "Blackberry," in *A Modern Herbal* (1931), posted in a hypertext edition on the Botanical.com website.

Holmes, *The Energetics of Western Herbs*, 808.

Sinadinos, *The Essential Guide to Western Botanical Medicine*, 68–72.

Wood, *The Earthwise Herbal*, vol. 2, 309–12.

Zia-Ul-Haq, M., M. Riaz, V. De Feo, H. Z. Jaafar, and M. Moga, "Rubus fruticosus L.: Constituents, Biological Activities and Health Related Uses," *Molecules* 19, no. 8 (2014): 10998–1029.

Burdock

Garran, *Western Herbs according to Traditional Chinese Medicine*, 69–71.

Kress, Henriette, "Herb of the Week: Burdock," blog post, Henriette's Herbal Homepage, February 26, 2012.

Holmes, *The Energetics of Western Herbs,* 696.

Miller, Betsy Costilo, "Burdock," in *Herbal Allies & Plant Profiles: A Practitioner's Guide to Essential Medicinal Herbs,* vol. 2 of *Materia Medica,* ed. Jesse Wolf Hardin and Kiva Rose Hardin (Plant Healer Magazine, 2020), 92.

Sinadinos, *The Essential Guide to Western Botanical Medicine,* 87–90.

Tierra, Michael, "Dandelion, Burdock, and Cancer," blog post, East West School of Planetary Herbology website, accessed January 22, 2016.

Tilford and Wulff, *Herbs for Pets,* 67–69.

Wood, *The Earthwise Herbal,* vol. 1, 103–7.

Calendula

Holmes, *The Energetics of Western Herbs,* 611.

Kidd, Randy, DVM, *Dr. Kidd's Guide to Herbal Dog Care* (Storey Publishing, 2000), 155.

Levy, Juliette de Bairacli, *The Complete Herbal Handbook for Farm and Stable* (Farrar, Straus and Giroux, 1991).

Popham, Sajah, "Calendula Materia Medica," Materia Medica Monthly course materials (volume 1), from the School of Evolutionary Herbalism, 2017.

Sinadinos, *The Essential Guide to Western Botanical Medicine,* 97–100.

Tilford and Wulff, *Herbs for Pets,* 70–72.

Wood, *The Earthwise Herbal,* vol. 1, 154–59.

Cayenne

Sinadinos, *The Essential Guide to Western Botanical Medicine,* 119–21.

Wood, *The Earthwise Herbal,* vol. 2, 93–97.

Chamomile

Garran, *Western Herbs according to Traditional Chinese Medicine,* 209–11.

Levy, Juliette de Bairacli, *The Complete Herbal Handbook for the Dog and Cat* (Faber and Faber, 1955), 182.

Sinadinos, *The Essential Guide to Western Botanical Medicine,* 124-127

Skenderi, *Herbal Vade Mecum,* 91.

Tilford and Wulff, *Herbs for Pets,* 76–78.

Wood, *The Earthwise Herbal,* vol. 1, 177–82.

Chickweed

Levy, Juliette de Bairacli, *The Complete Herbal Handbook for the Dog and Cat* (Faber and Faber, 1955), 166, 174.

Mansell, Jenny Solidago, "Chickweed, Yellow Dock, & Lambsquarters," in *Herbal*

Allies & Plant Profiles: *A Practitioner's Guide to Essential Medicinal Herbs,* vol. 2 of *Materia Medica,* ed. Jesse Wolf Hardin and Kiva Rose Hardin (*Plant Healer Magazine,* 2020), 104.

Sinadinos, *The Essential Guide to Western Botanical Medicine,* 130–32.

Skenderi, *Herbal Vade Mecum,* 97.

Tilford and Wulff, *Herbs for Pets,* 81–82.

Wood, *The Earthwise Herbal,* vol. 1, 472–74.

Cleavers

Garran, *Western Herbs according to Traditional Chinese Medicine,* 111–12.

Levy, Juliette de Bairacli, *The Complete Herbal Handbook for the Dog and Cat* (Faber and Faber, 1955), 162, 207.

Popham, Sajah, "Cleavers Monograph," Materia Medica Monthly course materials (volume 49), from the School of Evolutionary Herbalism, 2021.

Sinadinos, *The Essential Guide to Western Botanical Medicine,* 137–39.

Skenderi, *Herbal Vade Mecum,* 38.

Tilford and Wulff, *Herbs for Pets,* 82–84.

Wood, *The Earthwise Herbal,* vol. 1, 267–71.

Couch Grass

Holmes, *The Energetics of Western Herbs,* 172.

Skenderi, *Herbal Vade Mecum,* 115.

Tilford and Wulff, *Herbs for Pets,* 91–94.

Wood, *The Earthwise Herbal,* vol. 1, 60–63.

Dandelion

Holmes, *The Energetics of Western Herbs,* 172.

Levy, Juliette de Bairacli, *The Complete Herbal Handbook for the Dog and Cat* (Faber and Faber, 1955), 150, 154, 181.

Popham, Sajah, "Dandelion Monograph," Materia Medica Monthly course materials (volume 31), from the School of Evolutionary Herbalism, 2019.

Skenderi, *Herbal Vade Mecum,* 128.

Sinadinos, *The Essential Guide to Western Botanical Medicine,* 175–79.

Tilford and Wulff, *Herbs for Pets,* 94–97, 286.

Wood, *The Earthwise Herbal,* vol. 1, 478–83.

Echinacea

Garran, *Western Herbs according to Traditional Chinese Medicine,* 95–98.

Holmes, *The Energetics of Western Herbs,* 606.

Popham, Sajah, "Echinacea Monograph," Materia Medica Monthly course materials (volume 16), from the School of Evolutionary Herbalism, 2018.

Sinadinos, *The Essential Guide to Western Botanical Medicine*, 185–89.

Skenderi, *Herbal Vade Mecum*, 139.

Tilford and Wulff, *Herbs for Pets*, 99–104, 219, 267, 290.

Wood, *The Earthwise Herbal*, vol. 2, 135–39.

Elecampane

Garran, *Western Herbs according to Traditional Chinese Medicine*, 171–72.

Holmes, *The Energetics of Western Herbs*, 289.

Sinadinos, *The Essential Guide to Western Botanical Medicine*, 195–98.

Skenderi, *Herbal Vade Mecum*, 142.

Tilford and Wulff, *Herbs for Pets*, 104–5.

Wood, *The Earthwise Herbal*, vol. 1, 301–7.

Fennel

Holmes, *The Energetics of Western Herbs*, 146.

Levy, Juliette de Bairacli, *The Complete Herbal Handbook for the Dog and Cat* (Faber and Faber, 1955), 120–21.

Sinadinos, *The Essential Guide to Western Botanical Medicine*, 211–14.

Skenderi, *Herbal Vade Mecum*, 151.

Tilford and Wulff, *Herbs for Pets*, 106–7.

Wood, *The Earthwise Herbal*, vol. 1, 257–59.

Ginger

Cuthbert, Emily, "Herb Monograph: Ginger," Ayurvedic Health Center website, March 2, 2022.

Sinadinos, *The Essential Guide to Western Botanical Medicine*, 211–14.

Skenderi, *Herbal Vade Mecum*, 169.

White, B., "Ginger: An Overview," *American Family Physician* 75, no. 11 (2007): 1689–91.

Wood, *The Earthwise Herbal*, vol. 1, 533–37.

Goldenrod

Holmes, *The Energetics of Western Herbs*, 176.

Popham, Sajah, "Allergies and Asthma," the School of Evolutionary Herbalism website, April 14, 2021.

Sinadinos, *The Essential Guide to Western Botanical Medicine*, 246–48.

Skenderi, *Herbal Vade Mecum*, 175.

Tilford and Wulff, *Herbs for Pets*, 120–22.

Wood, *The Earthwise Herbal*, vol. 1, 468–70.

Goldenseal

Garran, *Western Herbs according to Traditional Chinese Medicine*, 72–75.

Holmes, *The Energetics of Western Herbs*, 629.

Skenderi, *Herbal Vade Mecum*, 175.

Tilford and Wulff, *Herbs for Pets*, 232–33.

Wood, *The Earthwise Herbal*, vol. 2, 193–98.

Gotu Kola

Bradwejn, J., Y. Zhou, D. Koszycki, and J. Shlik, "A Double-Blind, Placebo-Controlled Study on the Effects of Gotu Kola (*Centella asiatica*) on Acoustic Startle Response in Healthy Subjects," *Journal of Clinical Psychopharmacology* 20, no. 6 (2000): 680–84.

Holmes, *The Energetics of Western Herbs*, 726.

Sinadinos, *The Essential Guide to Western Botanical Medicine*, 249–51.

Skenderi, *Herbal Vade Mecum*, 176.

Tilford and Wulff, *Herbs for Pets*, 125–27.

Wood, *The Earthwise Herbal*, vol. 1, 174–76.

Gravel Root

Holmes, *The Energetics of Western Herbs*, 317.

Sinadinos, *The Essential Guide to Western Botanical Medicine*, 249–51.

Skenderi, *Herbal Vade Mecum*, 210.

Wood, *The Earthwise Herbal*, vol. 2, 153–57.

Hawthorn

Garran, *Western Herbs according to Traditional Chinese Medicine*, 173–75.

Holmes, *The Energetics of Western Herbs*, 297.

Masé, Guido, "Hawthorn," in *Herbal Allies & Plant Profiles: A Practitioner's Guide to Essential Medicinal Herbs*, vol. 2 of *Materia Medica*, ed. Jesse Wolf Hardin and Kiva Rose Hardin (*Plant Healer Magazine*, 2020), 150.

Popham, Sajah, "Hawthorn Materia Medica," Materia Medica Monthly course materials (volume 28), from the School of Evolutionary Herbalism, 2018.

Sinadinos, *The Essential Guide to Western Botanical Medicine*, 261–65.

Skenderi, *Herbal Vade Mecum*, 184.

Tilford and Wulff, *Herbs for Pets*, 130–33.

Wood, *The Earthwise Herbal*, vol. 1, 211–17.

Juniper Berry

Holmes, *The Energetics of Western Herbs*, 360.

Skenderi, *Herbal Vade Mecum*, 184.

Tilford and Wulff, *Herbs for Pets*, 138–40.

Wood, *The Earthwise Herbal*, vol. 2, 211–15.

Lemon Balm

Garcia, Charles, "Lemon Balm," in *Herbal Allies & Plant Profiles: A Practitioner's Guide to Essential Medicinal Herbs*, vol. 2 of *Materia Medica*, ed. Jesse Wolf Hardin and Kiva Rose Hardin (Plant Healer Magazine, 2020), 159.

Holmes, *The Energetics of Western Herbs*, 514.

Sinadinos, *The Essential Guide to Western Botanical Medicine*, 301–4.

Skenderi, *Herbal Vade Mecum*, 31.

Wood, *The Earthwise Herbal*, vol. 1, 342–44.

Licorice

Bergner, Paul, "Vitalist Teachings & Radical Thinking, More on the Dark Side of Adaptogens," in *Herbal Clinician IV: Herbal Treatments for Lungs, Liver, Kidneys, Bladder & Heart*, ed. Jesse Wolf Hardin and Kiva Rose Hardin (independently published, 2020), 47.

Holmes, *The Energetics of Western Herbs*, 292.

Sinadinos, *The Essential Guide to Western Botanical Medicine*, 305–11.

Skenderi, *Herbal Vade Mecum*, 225.

Tilford and Wulff, *Herbs for Pets*, 142–45.

Wood, *The Earthwise Herbal*, vol. 1, 283–84.

Marshmallow

Garran, *Western Herbs according to Traditional Chinese Medicine*, 179–80.

Holmes, *The Energetics of Western Herbs*, 468

Popham, Sajah, "Marshmallow Materia Medica," Materia Medica Monthly course materials (volume 29), from the School of Evolutionary Herbalism, 2019.

Sinadinos, *The Essential Guide to Western Botanical Medicine*, 324–27.

Skenderi, *Herbal Vade Mecum*, 242.

Tilford and Wulff, *Herbs for Pets*, 145–48.

Wood, *The Earthwise Herbal*, vol. 1, 79–80.

Meadowsweet

Garran, *Western Herbs according to Traditional Chinese Medicine*, 63–64.

Holmes, *The Energetics of Western Herbs*, 375.

Sinadinos, *The Essential Guide to Western Botanical Medicine*, 328–30.

Skenderi, *Herbal Vade Mecum*, 245.

Tilford and Wulff, *Herbs for Pets*, 207.

Wood, *The Earthwise Herbal*, vol. 1, 255–57.

Milk Thistle

Garran, *Western Herbs according to Traditional Chinese Medicine*, 177–78.

Holmes, *The Energetics of Western Herbs*, 415.

Levy, Juliette de Bairacli, *The Complete Herbal Handbook for the Dog and Cat* (Faber and Faber, 1955), 182.

Popham, Sajah, "Milk Thistle Materia Medica," Materia Medica Monthly course materials (volume 27), from the School of Evolutionary Herbalism, 2017.

Sinadinos, *The Essential Guide to Western Botanical Medicine*, 331–34.

Skenderi, *Herbal Vade Mecum*, 248.

Tilford and Wulff, *Herbs for Pets*, 148–50.

Wood, *The Earthwise Herbal*, vol. 1, 465–68.

Milky Oats

Bennett, Robin Rose, "Oats," in *Herbal Allies & Plant Profiles: A Practitioner's Guide to Essential Medicinal Herbs*, vol. 2 of *Materia Medica*, ed. Jesse Wolf Hardin and Kiva Rose Hardin (*Plant Healer Magazine*, 2020), 177.

Garran, *Western Herbs according to Traditional Chinese Medicine*, 181–82.

Popham, Sajah, "Milky Oats Monograph," Materia Medica Monthly course materials (volume 13), from the School of Evolutionary Herbalism, 2017.

Sinadinos, *The Essential Guide to Western Botanical Medicine*, 361–64.

Skenderi, *Herbal Vade Mecum*, 272.

Tilford and Wulff, *Herbs for Pets*, 155–57.

Wood, *The Earthwise Herbal*, vol. 1, 124–25.

Mullein

Holmes, *The Energetics of Western Herbs*, 474.

Sajah Popham, "Mullein Materia Medica," Materia Medica Monthly course materials (volume 21), from the School of Evolutionary Herbalism, 2018.

Sinadinos, *The Essential Guide to Western Botanical Medicine*, 345–49.

Skenderi, *Herbal Vade Mecum*, 248.

Tilford and Wulff, *Herbs for Pets*, 150–52, 271.

Wood, *The Earthwise Herbal*, vol. 1, 507–10.

Nettle

Garcia, Charles, "Stinging Nettle," in *Herbal Allies & Plant Profiles: A Practitioner's Guide to Essential Medicinal Herbs,* vol. 2 of *Materia Medica,* ed. Jesse Wolf Hardin and Kiva Rose Hardin (*Plant Healer Magazine,* 2020), 245.

Garran, *Western Herbs according to Traditional Chinese Medicine,* 116–18.

Holmes, *The Energetics of Western Herbs,* 443.

Levy, Juliette de Bairacli, *The Complete Herbal Handbook for the Dog and Cat* (Faber and Faber, 1955), 182.

Popham, Sajah, "Stinging Nettle," Materia Medica Monthly course materials (volume 21), from the School of Evolutionary Herbalism, 2018.

Sinadinos, *The Essential Guide to Western Botanical Medicine,* 354–60.

Skenderi, *Herbal Vade Mecum,* 265.

Tilford and Wulff, *Herbs for Pets,* 150–52, 271.

Wood, *The Earthwise Herbal,* vol. 1, 496–500.

Olive

Skenderi, *Herbal Vade Mecum,* 273.

Wood, *The Earthwise Herbal,* vol. 1, 364–66.

Oregon Grape Root

Garran, *Western Herbs according to Traditional Chinese Medicine,* 75–79.

Holmes, *The Energetics of Western Herbs,* 690.

Popham, Sajah, "Oregon Grape," Materia Medica Monthly course materials (volume 7), from the School of Evolutionary Herbalism, 2017.

Skenderi, *Herbal Vade Mecum,* 277.

Tilford and Wulff, *Herbs for Pets,* 157–60.

Wood, *The Earthwise Herbal,* vol. 2, 85–89.

Parsley

Farzaei, M. H., Z. Abbasabadi, M. R. Ardekani, R. Rahimi, and F. Farzaei, "Parsley: A Review of Ethnopharmacology, Phytochemistry and Biological Activities," *Journal of Traditional Chinese Medicine* 33, no. 6 (2013): 815–26.

Levy, Juliette de Bairacli, *The Complete Herbal Handbook for the Dog and Cat* (Faber and Faber, 1955), 184–89.

Sinadinos, *The Essential Guide to Western Botanical Medicine,* 381–85.

Skenderi, *Herbal Vade Mecum,* 280.

Tilford and Wulff, *Herbs for Pets,* 162–64.

Wood, *The Earthwise Herbal,* vol. 1, 378–81.

Passionflower

Akhondzadeh, S., H. R. Naghavi, M. Vazirian, A. Shayeganpour, H. Rashidi, and M. Khani, "Passionflower in the Treatment of Generalized Anxiety: A Pilot Double-Blind Randomized Controlled Trial with Oxazepam," *Journal of Clinical Pharmacy and Therapeutics* 26, no. 5 (2001): 363–67.

Garran, *Western Herbs according to Traditional Chinese Medicine*, 195–96.

Holmes, *The Energetics of Western Herbs*, 690.

Sinadinos, *The Essential Guide to Western Botanical Medicine*, 389–92.

Skenderi, *Herbal Vade Mecum*, 280.

Wood, *The Earthwise Herbal*, vol. 2, 262–65.

Pau d'Arco

Holmes, *The Energetics of Western Herbs*, 635.

Skenderi, *Herbal Vade Mecum*, 280.

Plantain

Garran, *Western Herbs according to Traditional Chinese Medicine*, 195–96.

Holmes, *The Energetics of Western Herbs*, 614.

Popham, Sajah, "Plantain," Materia Medica Monthly course materials (volume 6), from the School of Evolutionary Herbalism, 2017.

Sinadinos, *The Essential Guide to Western Botanical Medicine*, 408–10.

Skenderi, *Herbal Vade Mecum*, 310.

Tilford and Wulff, *Herbs for Pets*, 164–66.

Wood, *The Earthwise Herbal*, vol. 1, 385–89.

Red Clover

Garran, *Western Herbs according to Traditional Chinese Medicine*, 104–5.

Holmes, *The Energetics of Western Herbs*, 665.

Sinadinos, *The Essential Guide to Western Botanical Medicine*, 421–24.

Skenderi, *Herbal Vade Mecum*, 316.

Tilford and Wulff, *Herbs for Pets*, 168–70.

Wood, *The Earthwise Herbal*, vol. 1, 489–91.

Rose

Clarke, Natasha, "Rose," in *Herbal Allies & Plant Profiles: A Practitioner's Guide to Essential Medicinal Herbs*, vol. 2 of *Materia Medica*, ed. Jesse Wolf Hardin and Kiva Rose Hardin (*Plant Healer Magazine*, 2020), 228.

Holmes, *The Energetics of Western Herbs*, 334.

Sinadinos, *The Essential Guide to Western Botanical Medicine*, 435–40.

Skenderi, *Herbal Vade Mecum,* 321.

Tilford and Wulff, *Herbs for Pets,* 170–72.

Wood, *The Earthwise Herbal,* vol. 2, 262–65.

Rosemary

Holmes, *The Energetics of Western Herbs,* 350.

Popham, Sajah, "Rosemary Monograph," Materia Medica Monthly course materials (volume 6), from the School of Evolutionary Herbalism, 2017.

Sinadinos, *The Essential Guide to Western Botanical Medicine,* 441–45.

Skenderi, *Herbal Vade Mecum,* 322.

Tilford and Wulff, *Herbs for Pets,* 173–74.

Wood, *The Earthwise Herbal,* vol. 1, 427–33.

Skullcap

Holmes, *The Energetics of Western Herbs,* 507.

Sinadinos, *The Essential Guide to Western Botanical Medicine,* 471–74.

Skenderi, *Herbal Vade Mecum,* 346.

Tilford and Wulff, *Herbs for Pets,* 182–84.

Wood, *The Earthwise Herbal,* vol. 2, 323–26.

Slippery Elm

Tilford and Wulff, *Herbs for Pets,* 184–96.

Wood, *The Earthwise Herbal,* vol. 2, 342–47.

Solomon's Seal

Grieve, Maud, "Solomon's Seal," in *A Modern Herbal* (1931), posted in a hypertext edition on the Botanical.com website.

Larde, Ray, "Solomon's Seal Monograph," Sovereign Birch Herbal website, August 29, 2019.

O'Bryant, Colleen, "Solomon's Seal: The Musculoskeletal Healing Wizard," blog post, Wild Roots Apothecary, May 7, 2021.

Wood, *The Earthwise Herbal,* vol. 2, 274–78.

St. John's Wort

Garran, *Western Herbs according to Traditional Chinese Medicine,* 200–202.

Holmes, *The Energetics of Western Herbs,* 504.

Popham, Sajah, "St. John's Wort," Materia Medica Monthly course materials (volume 4), from the School of Evolutionary Herbalism, 2017.

Sinadinos, *The Essential Guide to Western Botanical Medicine,* 479–81.

Skenderi, *Herbal Vade Mecum,* 359.

Tilford and Wulff, *Herbs for Pets,* 171–80.

Wood, *The Earthwise Herbal,* vol. 1, 228–30.

Turmeric

Adi, Virginia, "Turmeric," in *Herbal Allies & Plant Profiles: A Practitioner's Guide to Essential Medicinal Herbs,* vol. 2 of *Materia Medica,* ed. Jesse Wolf Hardin and Kiva Rose Hardin (*Plant Healer Magazine,* 2020), 259.

Holmes, *The Energetics of Western Herbs,* 404.

Sinadinos, *The Essential Guide to Western Botanical Medicine,* 495–500.

Skenderi, *Herbal Vade Mecum,* 380.

Wood, *The Earthwise Herbal,* vol. 1, 228–30.

Usnea

Garran, *Western Herbs according to Traditional Chinese Medicine,* 99–100.

Popham, Sajah, "Usnea," Materia Medica Monthly course materials (volume 40), from the School of Evolutionary Herbalism, 2019.

Sinadinos, *The Essential Guide to Western Botanical Medicine,* 501–3

Skenderi, *Herbal Vade Mecum,* 382.

Uva-Ursi

Sinadinos, *The Essential Guide to Western Botanical Medicine,* 504–7.

Skenderi, *Herbal Vade Mecum,* 383.

Tilford and Wulff, *Herbs for Pets,* 188–90.

Wood, *The Earthwise Herbal,* vol. 2, 74–76.

Violet

Maier, Kat, *Energetic Herbalism* (Chelsea Green, 2021), 304–7.

Popham, Sajah, "Violet," Materia Medica Monthly course materials (volume 23), from the School of Evolutionary Herbalism, 2021.

Wood, *The Earthwise Herbal,* vol.1, 515–18.

Wood Betony

Easley, Thomas, and Steven Horne, *The Modern Herbal Dispensatory: A Medicine Making Guide* (North Atlantic, 2016), 324.

Popham, Sajah, "Wood Betony," Materia Medica Monthly course materials (volume 8), from the School of Evolutionary Herbalism, 2017.

Wood, *The Earthwise Herbal,* vol.1, 136–38.

Yarrow

Garran, *Western Herbs according to Traditional Chinese Medicine*, 37–41.

Holmes, *The Energetics of Western Herbs*, 736.

Popham, Sajah, "Yarrow," Materia Medica Monthly course materials (volume 25), from the School of Evolutionary Herbalism, 2018.

Sinadinos, *The Essential Guide to Western Botanical Medicine*, 532–36.

Skenderi, *Herbal Vade Mecum*, 398.

Tilford and Wulff, *Herbs for Pets*, 194–96.

Wood, *The Earthwise Herbal*, vol. 2, 51–57.

Yellow Dock

Garran, *Western Herbs according to Traditional Chinese Medicine*, 86–88.

Holmes, *The Energetics of Western Herbs*, 675.

Sinadinos, *The Essential Guide to Western Botanical Medicine*, 537–41.

Skenderi, *Herbal Vade Mecum*, 133.

Wood, *The Earthwise Herbal*, vol. 1, 428–43.

Medicinal Mushrooms

Carroll, Lee, Mastering Medicinal Mushrooms Beta Course, Herba Meditari, November 1, 15, 29 and December 13, 2022.

Hobbs, Christopher, *Christopher Hobbs's Medicinal Mushrooms: The Essential Guide* (Storey Books, 2020).

Poltavets, Eugene, and Svetlana Poltavets, *A Guide to the Medicinal Mushrooms of the Pacific Northwest: Health Benefits and Other Therapeutic Uses* (Hancock House, 2020).

Rogers, Robert, *The Fungal Pharmacy: The Complete Guide to Medicinal Mushrooms & Lichens of North America* (North Atlantic Books, 2011).

Semwal, Kamal Ch., Steven L. Stephenson, and Azamal Husen, eds., *Wild Mushrooms and Health: Diversity, Phytochemistry, Medicinal Benefits, and Cultivation* (CRC Press, 2023).

Silver, Rob, DVM, expert mushroom practitioner, personal communication with the author, March 9, 2024.

Wood, *The Earthwise Herbal*, vol. 1 (for details on reishi mushroom).

Phytoembryonics

Blake, Stephen, *Gemmotherapy for Our Animal Friends* (independently published, 2011).

Greaves, Marcus, *Gemmotherapy and Oligotherapy Regenerators of Dying Intoxicated Cells: Tridosha of Cellular Regeneration* (independently published, 2002).

Halfon, Roger, *Gemmotherapy: The Science of Healing with Plant Stem Cells* (Healing Arts Press, 2005).

Nicoletti, Marcello, and Fernando Piterà di Clima, *Gemmotherapy, and the Scientific Foundations of a Modern Meristemotherapy* (Cambridge Scholars Publishing, 2020).

Rozencwajg, Joe, *Dynamic Gemmotherapy. Beyond Gemmotherapy,* vol. 1 (independently published, 2016).

Speroni, Anthony, *Gemmotherapy and Oligotherapy for Natural Health Practitioners* (College of International Holistic Studies, 2009).

Tetau, Max, *Gemmotherapy: A Clinical Guide* (Editions Similla, 2010).

Flower Essences

Bach, Edward, M.D., and F. J. Wheeler, M.D. *The Bach Flower Remedies* (Keats, 1997).

Graham, Helen, and Gregory Vlamis, *Bach Flower Remedies for Animals* (Findhorn Press, 1999).

Kaminski, Patricia, and Richard Katz, *Flower Essence Repertory: A Comprehensive Guide to North American and English Flower Essence for Emotional and Spiritual Well-Being* (Flower Essence Society, 1994).

Wood, Matthew, *Seven Herbs: Plants as Teachers* (North Atlantic Books, 1987).

Appendix 1. Herbal Actions

1. Paul Bergner, "Vitalist Teachings & Radical Thinking, More on the Dark Side of Adaptogens," in *Herbal Clinician IV: Herbal Treatments for Lungs, Liver, Kidneys, Bladder & Heart,* ed. Jesse Wolf Hardin and Kiva Rose Hardin (independently published, 2020), 47.

Index

About the Author

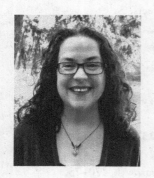

Rita Hogan is a clinical canine herbalist with more than two decades of experience specializing in holistic canine herbalism. She is an educator, speaker, writer, formulator, and herbal medicine maker.

Rita uses a combination of diet, flower essences, herbs, mushrooms, and phytoembryonic therapies, addressing dogs' mind, body, and spirit. Her work involves helping dog owners, natural practitioners, and veterinarians understand how to use herbs according to plant language. She believes in integrative, holistic care where traditional herbalism complements and supports integrative veterinary medicine.

Rita's full-time practice is based in Olympia, Washington, where she lives with her partner, five dogs, and two cats.

Visit her online at **TheHerbalDog.com**